Health Informatics

(formerly Computers in Health Care)

Kathryn J. Hannah   Marion J. Ball
Series Editors

Health Informatics Series
(formerly Computers in Health Care)

Series Editors
Kathryn J. Hannah   Marion J. Ball

Rajeev K. Bali   Ashish N. Dwivedi
Editors

Healthcare
Knowledge
Management

Issues, Advances, and Successes

Foreword by Philip C. Candy, PhD

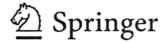 Springer

Rajeev K. Bali, PhD
Knowledge Management for Healthcare
  (KMH) subgroup,
Biomedical Computing and Engineering
  Technologies Applied Research
  Group (BIOCORE)
Coventry University
Coventry
West Midlands CV1 5FB
United Kingdom
r.bali@ieee.org

Ashish N. Dwivedi, PhD
The University of Hull Business School
Hull, HU6 7RX
United Kingdom
a.dwivedi@hull.ac.uk

Series Editors:
Kathryn J. Hannah, PhD, RN
Adjunct Professor, Department of
  Community Health Science
Faculty of Medicine
The University of Calgary
Calgary, Alberta T2N 4N1, Canada

Marion J. Ball, EdD
Vice President, Clinical Solutions
2 Hamill Road
Quadrangle 359 West
Healthlink, Inc.
Baltimore, MD 21210
and
Adjunct Professor
The Johns Hopkins University
  School of Nursing
Baltimore, MD 21205, USA

Library of Congress Control Number: 2006923639

ISBN-10: 0-387-33540-4
ISBN-13: 978-0-387-33540-7

Printed on acid-free paper.

9 8 7 6 5 4 3 2 1

springer.com

For our families

We're drowning in information and starving for knowledge.
—RUTHERFORD D. ROGERS

Foreword

Knowledge Management: Stand Here to View the Landscape

In 1818, the then Surgeon-General of the US Army, Joseph Lovell, directed each army surgeon attached to a military fort, camp, or detachment throughout the country to "...keep a diary of the weather..." and to note "...everything of importance relating to the medical topography of his station, the climate [and] diseases prevalent in the vicinity..." [1, p. 209].[1] All over the US, including the most remote frontier territories, Army medical personnel were engaged in a huge, distributed project to obtain information about local weather conditions, and to pool this information in order, as a latter-day commentator has said, "to learn about climate effects on disease" [2][2].

This might well be thought of as an early example of knowledge management in health, but it is far from the first. Indeed, although the term "knowledge management" may be relatively new and unfamiliar in the field of health, as the chapters in this book so clearly show, the basic practices to which it refers are as old as healthcare itself. Since time immemorial, doctors and other practitioners have collected and shared information about their healing practices, about specific illnesses and medicines, and about their patients, both as individuals and as groups or communities.

However, while it may be inappropriate to assume that knowledge management in health care has no precedent (because, clearly, it has important historical antecedents), it would be equally incorrect to see the current wave of technologically supported knowledge management as nothing more than an extension of past practices. In reality, modern technologies are providing clinicians, administrators, leaders, and patients with unimaginable amounts of information of unprecedented

---

[1] Smart, C. (1893). The Connection of the Army Medical Department with the Development of Meteorology in the United States, *U.S. Weather Bureau Bulletin* 11, pp. 207–16.

[2] Conner, G. (1995). Kentucky Climate Center Fact Sheet: Newport Barracks. Available online at http://kyclim.wku.edu/factsheets/newport_barr/ [accessed 28 May 2002].

complexity. So, this book performs the unusual but much needed role of reminding us that knowledge management has a long history in health, while arguing that recent developments and advances are truly novel and ground breaking.

As with any anthology or edited collection of essays, there are differences here in the focus, style, and tone of the individual chapters. Nevertheless, collectively they provide a distinctive (even unique) window onto a significant and emerging field of practice and research, and bring together in one place a diverse range of perspectives.

While there are several different *conceptual models and definitions* of knowledge management offered by the various authors, they all share the view that it is a more or less formal process of gathering, analyzing, and sharing information and insights based on health data that have been collected in various ways for various purposes. Because of its elegance, simplicity and prima facie plausibility, a particularly useful typology is that proposed by Frize, Walker, and Catley, who argue that knowledge management comprises four major elements: access to quality clinical data; knowledge discovery; knowledge translation; and, finally, knowledge integration and sharing. To a greater or lesser extent, something like this seems to underpin virtually all the chapters, although many of them are concerned with how this process has been affected by the development and widespread adoption of advanced information and communication technologies.

The first striking feature of this collection is the realization that knowledge management has a *long and noble history in healthcare*, albeit less formalized and less systematic in bygone years. As these chapters so ably demonstrate, knowledge management in the sense of sharing information and stories has been a fundamental part of medical practice since the very beginning. While one might tend to think of knowledge management as largely or even exclusively a product of the widespread use of technologies, doctors and clinicians have always made notes for their own purposes, as well as sharing information with each other, with administrators, and even with their patients.

While some of the chapters emphasize these softer (even poetic and narrative) aspects of healthcare and healing, and in particular the sharing of stories which are the prototype of knowledge management, others take a more overtly technical point of view, emphasizing the way in which technologies are simultaneously increasing the complexity of information collected, and at the same time enhancing people's capacity to utilize the dramatically greater amounts of information available. One theme in several chapters is *how patients and clinicians make sense* of the information that is collected, and harmonize it with their existing or emerging understandings and views.

Linked with this, at least one of the chapters deals with the intriguing question of whether, or *how well, technologies map onto the basic dynamics* of both the clinical interaction and the diagnostic thought processes of clinicians. Not unexpectedly, the more naturalistic and less intrusive approaches are preferred.

Related to this is the *complex reciprocal relationship developing between healthcare and technology*, where advances in one are calling forth developments in the other in a constantly repeated cycle of action and reaction. With the rapidly expanding amount and complexity of information, combined with the national and even international mobility of people along with their health conditions, technology is evolving in tandem with the problems it is seeking to manage.

A distinctive feature of much healthcare as it has evolved over the centuries has been the specialization of clinical practice and the consequent fragmentation of the care pathway from the patient's point of view. At its most basic, there are already two sets of data and two sets of perceptions: those of the clinician and the patient. But even relatively straightforward healthcare often involves information being distributed between patients, clinicians, local surgeries, and pharmacies; and as the case complexity increases, it is not long before specialists, hospitals, testing services, insurers, and others all have information and knowledge about individual cases. One of the challenges for knowledge management, and accordingly one of the themes in this book, is how to deal with the *separation of aspects of healthcare and the distributed nature of knowledge about individual patients.*

Clearly, this poses significant logistical problems (having all the information needed in the same place at the right time), but it also raises important questions about making sense of information collected in different ways and presented in diverse formats using a variety of professional protocols. Accordingly, some chapters are concerned with the harmonization and standardizations of information, including *technical interoperability and establishment of standards* between local, regional, national, and international systems.

The very fact that so much information is so readily available in so many different forms inevitably raises concerns that some of this information could fall into the wrong hands or be used for inappropriate purposes. Accordingly, an important theme within the book is the interweaving of ethical, legal, and technological strands to ensure that *the privacy of individual patients, families, or communities* is not compromised, and that the confidentiality of their data is respected. It is instructive and reassuring that those interested in promoting knowledge management are concerned with the welfare of patients, protecting and respecting their rights to confidentiality, while ensuring that information is available to improve clinical practice and, where appropriate, organizational and systemic efficacy.

One of the benefits of knowledge management, in particular the recent advances in the application of technologies, is the way in which they *amplify the capacity of people to deal with huge amounts of information*, and to interpret or discern trends that might otherwise be invisible. These trends can be at the micro level—looking for the relationship between various symptoms in a single patient—right through to the macro or epidemiological level, where trends in an entire community or population can be spotted more easily than hitherto.

Linked to this is the *empowerment of individual clinical practitioners*, who can often operate in silos with consequent feelings of isolation or even alienation. The disciplines of knowledge management, combined with the increasingly available technologies to support them, can have a transformative effect on how information, experience, and insights are combined, compared, and shared in ways not previously encountered. This, in turn, can enhance individual as well as organizational effectiveness, and allow individual practitioners to feel part of a distributed community of practice. It can also act as a powerful incentive to continuing learning, as well as providing access to information and resources using essentially the same infrastructure used to capture and store information.

At first sight, knowledge management might seem to be a rather dry, technical aspect of healthcare, with little to offer in the way of fresh insights into clinical practice. However, as this remarkable book demonstrates, it is in fact *a prism through which other aspects of medicine and healthcare can be viewed.* Ranging as it does from traditional healing to the most advanced and sophisticated uses of knowledge, technology, and therapies, it also touches on those most basic and primal of shared values: the sanctity of life, the preservation of health, and the importance of communication with others. It provides a fascinating insight into how clinicians conduct their work, how they relate to patients, and how they improve their practice.

If knowledge management is simultaneously a time-honored practice and an emerging field of study, it is likely that this book will come to be seen as a *landmark in the complex topographies of knowledge management on the one hand and of healthcare on the other hand.* The fact that the authors come from so many different countries underscores the international nature of the phenomenon; the fact that they approach the topic from such different perspectives emphasizes its breadth. Those who are concerned that the management of knowledge in healthcare settings is being dominated by experts (clinicians, administrators, health economists, and policy makers) will be heartened to find in the collection thoughtful essays about the need for a balanced approach, including sharing information with those about whom the records are being kept and shared. And those who are worried about what they see as the excessive technologization of health, should be encouraged to read about human aspects of knowledge management: how doctors, patients, and administrators make sense of the complex array of information they both produce and acquire from others.

The practice of medicine, and more generally the provision of healthcare, touches on everyone and is a near-universal practice shared by humanity the world over. This book makes a timely, significant, and valuable contribution to ensuring that the quality of that healthcare continues to improve for everyone.

Philip C. Candy, PhD
Director of Education, Training and Development
National Health Service "Connecting for Health," UK

References

1. Smart C. The connection of the Army Medical Department with the development of meteorology in the United States, *U.S. Weather Bur Bull* 1893;11: 207–216.
2. Conner G. *Kentucky Climate Center Fact Sheet: Newport Barracks*; 1995 Available from: http://kyclim.wku.edu/factsheets/newport_barr/ [28 May 2002].

Preface

Information is not knowledge.
—ALBERT EINSTEIN

Advances in information technology (IT), particularly in (a) database technologies and (b) Internet technologies and telecommunications, have brought about fundamental changes throughout the healthcare process [1,2] and, consequently, are transforming the healthcare industry [3–6]. These modern developments in IT have enabled a number of countries to implement a national electronic patient record (EPR) system by linking their existing healthcare information systems [7–12]. For example, in the UK, the main current objective of the National Health Service (NHS) is to ensure that the medical records of all its residents are available electronically [8,11,13,14]. The NHS aims to provide relevant healthcare stakeholders access to EPR data in order to improve clinical efficiency. Moreover, the NHS aims to empower patients by giving them access to their own EPR. This emphasis put on the EPR system can be gauged by the fact that the NHS has invested about US$ 10.80 billion in EPR and other related technologies [15].

The change process undergone is not limited to Europe alone, as confirmed by research which stated that, in the period 1997–2000, 85% of healthcare organizations have undergone some sort of transformation [16]. It would be fair to state that a significant focus of the transformation of the healthcare sector from a technological perspective has been on the manner in which patient records are accessed during the process of medical diagnosis and treatment.

However, in the last two decades, the synergistic interaction between the biomedical knowledge and genetic engineering revolutions is further transforming the healthcare sector and is simultaneously also creating an information explosion in healthcare. Advances in modern-day genetic sciences have increased the number of potential drug compositions from a mere 400 to over 4000 [17]. This has happened despite the fact that the rate of adoption of computer applications in healthcare is slower in comparison with other industries [18].

Perhaps the biggest tragedy in the history of modern science was the fact that the announcement regarding the completion of the Human Genome project (mapping the entire human genetic code) did not create any significant ripples in the minds of healthcare decision makers and academics, nor did it propel a new wave of healthcare discoveries [19]. We hypothesize that this situation is not likely to prevail for very long. The impact of the completion of the Human Genome project will profoundly change the concept of healthcare itself within the next 25 years [19], as physicians move away from the germ theory of disease to genetics.

An indicator of the impact of the biomedical knowledge and genetic engineering revolutions on healthcare is the exponential increase in biomedical knowledge in the National Library of Medicine's Medline database (4500 journals in 30 languages, dating from 1996) of published literature in health-related sciences. In 2002, Medline contained 11.7 million citations and, on average, about 400,000 new entries were being added per year [20]. If a typical modern-day healthcare stakeholder, who wanted to get updated with the current literature, was to read one article a day, it would take him or her 1100 years to get updated with the new literature added every year.

The calculations above ignore the existing literature level of 11.7 million items and also ignore the projected increase in the growth of new research. It is judicious to assume that not all of the literature would be of relevance to a particular healthcare stakeholder. If we assume that about 1% of the new literature added every year is of relevance to a healthcare stakeholder, then it would still take a stakeholder 10 years (reading an average of one article a day) to be updated with the healthcare advances of 1 year. This information explosion is further compounded by the fact that biomedical literature is doubling every 19 years.

We contend that if the impact of the above is seen together, then the conclusion from a healthcare informatics perspective is clear. Twenty-first century clinical practitioners have to acquire proficiency in understanding and interpreting clinical information so as to attain knowledge and wisdom whilst dealing with large amounts of clinical data—clinical data that will be dynamic in nature and would call for the ability to interpret context-based healthcare information. This challenge cannot be met by an IT-led solution. The solution has to come from a domain that supports all three integral healthcare system components (i.e. people, processes, and technology) of the future. There is only one such domain: the knowledge management paradigm.

The purpose of this book is to contribute to the building of a healthcare knowledge management paradigm and facilitate critical thinking in healthcare knowledge management. This book does this by bringing together healthcare knowledge management theorists and practitioners so as to allow them not only to identify and discuss key issues for research in healthcare knowledge management, but also to allow others interested in healthcare knowledge management to acquire information and knowledge from the experiences and thinking documented in this book.

Organization of the Book

Section I (*Healthcare Knowledge Management: Innovations and New Understanding*) has five chapters which present the case for incorporating knowledge management concepts in healthcare. This section also looks at how knowledge management concepts can be applied to the healthcare sector. Chapter 1 (*Building New Healthcare Management Paradigms: A Case for Healthcare Knowledge Management*) by Dwivedi, Bali, and Naguib begins this section of five chapters and investigates why the coming of age of healthcare knowledge management is essential if the healthcare sector is to overcome its challenges. This chapter discusses in detail the information management challenges facing the healthcare industry and argues that the inability of existing healthcare management paradigms to tackle the information explosion in healthcare (in conjunction with the coming of age of knowledge management) is an ideal opportunity for healthcare knowledge management to present its case for alleviating the information challenges facing the healthcare industry.

Chapter 2 (*Clinical Knowledge Management: A Model For Primary Care*) by de Lusignan and Robinson argues that opportunities for the application of knowledge management to primary care have grown in the last two decades due to the widespread implementation of information and communication technologies (ICT). They argue that, owing to the extensive implementation of ICT, the healthcare process (particularly relating to medical record-keeping and requirements to audit quality standards) has undergone drastic changes. The authors further argue that future healthcare knowledge management models need to take into account the unique nature of the primary care speciality and propose a novel knowledge management model for primary care.

Chapter 3 (*Role of Information Professionals as Intermediaries for Knowledge Management in Evidence-Based Healthcare*) by Fennessy and Burstein describes the challenges associated with the implementation of knowledge management for evidence-based healthcare and, in particular, reflects on the role of intermediaries in meeting the information needs of healthcare professionals. They describe a study which investigated how the objectives of evidence-based medicine could be enhanced by healthcare knowledge management concepts.

Chapter 4 (*Healthcare Knowledge Management and Information Technology: A Systems Understanding*) by Chowdhury examines why healthcare knowledge management has developed into a topical field of investigation. The chapter argues that although it is easy to become mesmerized by IT in knowledge management, it is the consideration of the wider organizational, political, and socio-cultural dimensions that can enable any information system and any knowledge management strategy to work effectively. The author discusses why concentrating solely on IT will mean adopting a one-sided view of healthcare knowledge management and presents an argument in favor of a systems understanding of the role of IT in healthcare knowledge management.

Finally in this section, Chapter 5 (*Medical Technology Management in Hospital Certification in Mexico*) by Posadas looks at how certification of standards can be applied in the healthcare sector. The author describes several projects developed in different hospitals (public and private) with different health levels in Mexico City, with each of them contributing to the certification of different clinical processes. The evolution of the NMX-CC standards family, the Mexican equivalent of the ISO 9000 standards family, is explained, together with the need for knowledge sharing.

Section II (*Approaches, Frameworks, and Techniques for Healthcare Knowledge Management***)** consists of seven chapters which present novel approaches, frameworks, and techniques for healthcare knowledge management. Chapter 6 (*Healthcare Knowledge Sharing: Purpose, Practices, and Prospects*) by Abidi envisages an ideal healthcare knowledge management environment and how this could be created using a novel healthcare knowledge-sharing framework.

Chapter 7 (*Healthcare Knowledge Management: Incorporating the Tools, Technologies, Strategies, and Process of Knowledge Management to Effect Superior Healthcare Delivery*) by Wickramasinghe and von Lubitz emphasizes the need to take a knowledge management perspective for improving efficiency in healthcare delivery. The author argues that, given the voluminous nature of healthcare databases and repositories, IT-led systems are essential to ensure that there is access to relevant information when required. It is elaborated that it is possible to create such an environment by integrating healthcare knowledge management intelligence continuum concepts. The work is supported by a case study example.

Chapter 8 (*The Hidden Power of Social Networks and Knowledge Sharing in Healthcare*) by Liebowitz highlights that the healthcare industry is a knowledge-based service. As such, specialized knowledge resides in healthcare providers, professionals, and staff in many areas. It is explained that, owing to the impact of a "graying" workforce within the healthcare sector, workforce development and succession planning issues will be increasingly important to healthcare organizations. It is argued that, in the future, the ability to integrate, share, and disseminate knowledge across functional silos in healthcare organizations will continue to remain a challenge. It is submitted that social network analysis and knowledge audits can be combined to provide a solution to this problem by providing mechanisms for locating knowledge flows and gaps in organizations in the healthcare field.

Chapter 9 (*Constructing Healthcare Knowledge*) by Zhu continues the sociological stream of thought on healthcare knowledge management. It is postulated that healthcare knowledge is socially constructed and the management of it is essentially context specific. There are constructive processes via which concerned actors interact with each other so as to accomplish socio-cognitive changes.

Chapter 10 (*Narratives in Healthcare*) by Lee and Foo discusses how hospitals can effectively deal with many of the problems associated with scheduling and overcrowding, and improve the quality of care through the use of automated patient management systems. In this chapter, narrative is defined and three lenses (organizational narratives, illness narratives, and practice of narrative medicine) through which the role of narratives in healthcare can be elucidated are discussed.

Chapter 11 (*Application Service Provider Technology in the Healthcare Environment*) brings about a shift (from sociological influences to technological influences) in the stream of healthcare knowledge management thought. Cruz, Rodríguez, Barr, and Sanchez note that the widespread use of software tools in a healthcare setting has the requirement (both from productivity and efficiency legislative points of view) of standardizing requirements of information management software tools and looks at how application service provider technology can assist healthcare stakeholders in this context.

Chapter 12 (*Secured Electronic Patient Records Content Exploitation*) by Puentes, Coatrieux, and Lecornu emphasizes the need for providing secure information security to multimedia electronic patient records. The authors describe the structure and protection strategy of a novel secured specialized electronic patient record which allows fir the exchange of multimedia medical data.

Section III (*Healthcare Knowledge Management Implementations: Evidence from Practice*) consists of five chapters and builds upon the preceding sections and presents lessons from current and previous healthcare knowledge management implementations. Chapter 13 (*Knowledge Management and the National Health Service in England*) by De Brún starts the section with a chapter on the application of healthcare knowledge management, with a particular focus on the NHS in England. A number of examples where knowledge management initiatives have been successfully applied to support clinical decision making and improve patient safety are discussed.

Chapter 14 (*Knowledge Management and the National Health Service in Scotland*) by Harding and Wales provides a discussion on the advances made in terms of developing the NHS in Scotland (NHSiS) as a knowledge-based organization and presents a brief case study of one such NHSiS healthcare knowledge management project: the National Pathways Project.

Chapter 15 (*Knowledge Management for Primary Healthcare Services*) by Eardley and Czerwinski examines the characteristics of UK-based healthcare organizations. The chapter argues that the concept of healthcare knowledge management is a viable concept and, in support of this hypothesis, presents an analysis of a number of knowledge management initiatives (i.e. the National Electronic Library for Health and the Map of Medicine™).

Chapter 16 (*We Haven't Got a Plan, so What Can Go Wrong? Where is the NHS Coming from?*) by Copper takes into account organizational issues surrounding the NHS in the UK and its implication for the service in terms of its development as a knowledge-based organization.

Chapter 17 (*Healthcare Knowledge Management: Knowledge Management in the Perinatal Care Environment*) by Frize, Walker, and Catley concludes this section and the book. The authors describe how knowledge management can be applied in the perinatal care environment to facilitate clinical decision support.

We have managed to solicit chapters from countries as diverse as France, Japan, Cuba, Mexico, Australia, Scotland, Singapore, the USA, and the UK, which we hope validates the coming of age of healthcare knowledge management. We trust that academics, clinical and nonclinical practitioners, managers, and students will find issues of interest and value in the ensuing pages.

Rajeev K. Bali, PhD
Coventry University, UK

Ashish N. Dwivedi, PhD
Hull University, UK
January 2006

References

1. Krause M, Brown L. Information security in the healthcare industry. *Inf Syst Secur* 1996;5: 32–40.
2. Raghupathi W, Tan J. Strategic IT applications in health care. *Commun ACM* 2002;45:56–61.
3. Applebaum SH, Wohl L. Transformation or change: some prescriptions for health care organizations. *Managing Serv Qual* 2000;10:279–298.
4. Baker GR. Healthcare managers in the complex world of healthcare. *Front Health Serv Manage* 2001;18:23–32.
5. Nash MG, Gremillion C. Globalization impacts the healthcare organization of the 21st century demanding new ways to market product lines successfully. *Nurs Admin Q* 2004;28:86–91.
6. Smith C. New technology continues to invade healthcare. What are the strategic implications/outcomes? *Nurs Admin Q* 2004;28:92–98.
7. Bos JJ. Digital signatures and the electronic health records: providing legal and security guarantees. *Int J Bio-Med Comput* 1996;42:157–163.
8. Brindle D. Electronic NHS in seven years. *The Guardian*, 1998; p. 006.
9. Immonen S. Developments in health care, the increasing role of information technology: security issues. *Int J Bio-Med Comput* 1996;43:9–15.
10. Janczewski L, Shi FX. Development of information security baselines for healthcare information systems in New Zealand. *Comput Secur* 2002;21:172–192.
11. McClelland R, Thomas V. Confidentiality and security of clinical information in mental health practice. *Adv Psychiatr Treat* 2002;8:291–296.
12. Takeda H, Matsumura Y, Kuwata S, Nakano H, Sakamoto N, Yamamoto R. Architecture for networked electronic patient record systems. *Int J Med Inform* 2000;60:161–167.
13. Department of Health. *Information for health: an information strategy for the modern NHS 1998–2001*. London: HMSO; 1998.
14. Lewis A, Health informatics: information and communication. *Adv Psychiatr Treat* 2002;8:165–171.
15. May C, Finch T, Mair F, Mort M. Towards a wireless patient: chronic illness, scarce care and technological innovation in the United Kingdom. *Social Sci Med* 2005;61:1485–1494.
16. Sherer J. The human side of change. *Healthcare Exec* 1995;12:8–14.
17. Pavia L. The era of knowledge in health care. *Health Care Strat Manage* 2001;19:12–13.
18. Johns PM. Integrating information systems and health care. *Logist Inf Manage* 1997;10:140–145.
19. Jones WJ. Genetics: year zero. *Health Forum J* 2001;44:14–18.
20. Masys DR. Effects of current and future information technologies on the health care workforce. *Health Aff* 2002;21:33–41.

Acknowledgments

This book would not have been possible without the cooperation and assistance of many people: the authors, reviewers, our colleagues, and the staff at Springer. In particular, we would like to thank Michelle Schmitt-DeBonis (for green-lighting the project) and for keeping us sane by way of her good-humored communications during the pre-publication process. We thank Robert Albano and Kathy Cacace for taking up the reigns and for answering our many questions, as well as enabling us to keep this project on schedule.

Sincere thanks to Dr Philip Candy (Director of Education, Training and Development, NHS Connecting for Health, UK) for providing us with such a fine Foreword and for his much-valued support. We further thank the authors of chapters in this book and the reviewers for their support and cooperation.

We appreciate the expressions of interest and stimulating discussions with numerous people we encountered in conferences, workshops, and symposia during our travels.

Finally, we would like to acknowledge our respective families for their support throughout this project.

Rajeev K Bali, PhD
Coventry University, UK

Ashish N Dwivedi, PhD
Hull University, UK
January 2006

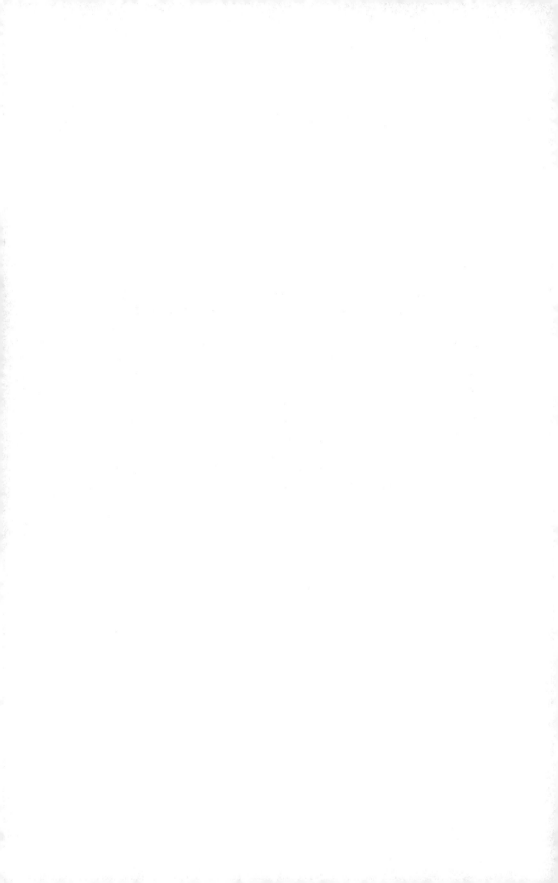

Contents

Contributors

Abidi, Syed Sibte Raza, PhD, Associate Professor and Director of Health Informatics, Faculty of Computer Science, Dalhousie University, CANADA

Bali, Rajeev K., PhD, Reader, Head of the Knowledge Management for Healthcare (KMH) research subgroup. Biomedical Computing and Engineering Technologies (BIOCORE) Applied Research Group. Coventry University, UK

Burstein, Frada, PhD, Associate Professor, Monash University, AUSTRALIA

Cameron, Barr, B.Eng, Higher Technical University, CUBA.

Catley, Christina, PhD Candidate, Carleton University, CANADA

Chowdhury, Rajneesh, PhD Candidate, University of Hull, UK

Coatrieux, Gouenou, PhD, Assistant Professor, GET École Nationale Supérieure des Télécommunications de Bretagne, FRANCE

Copper, Annette, MSc, Knowledge Management Consultant, UK

Cruz, A. Miguel, PhD, Higher Technical University, CUBA

Czerwinski, Alex, BSc, Programme Manager, Shropshire and Staffordshire Strategic Health Authority, UK

De Brún, Caroline, MA, Information Scientist, NHS National Library for Health Specialist Library for Knowledge Management, Milton Keynes Primary Care Trust, UK

de Lusignan, Simon, MBBS, MRCGP, St George's University of London, UK

Dwivedi, Ashish N., PhD, Lecturer, University of Hull, UK

Eardley, Alan, PhD, Head of Postgraduate Research Studies, Faculty of Computing, Engineering and Technology, Staffordshire University, UK

Fennessy, Gabby, PhD, Royal Australian and New Zealand College of Obstetricians and Gynaecologists, AUSTRALIA

Foo, Schubert, Professor and Vice Dean, School of Communication & Information, Nanyang Technological University, SINGAPORE

Frize, Monique, PhD, Professor, Carleton University, and University of Ottawa, CANADA

Harding, Oliver, MBchB, MSc, MFPHM, Information Services (ISD), SCOTLAND

Lecornu, Laurent, PhD, Assistant Professor, INSERM–U650, Brest, FRANCE

Lee, Chu Keong, MSc, Lecturer, Division of Information Studies, School of Communication and Information, Nanyang Technological University, SINGAPORE

Liebowitz, Jay, D.Sc., Professor, Graduate Division of Business and Management, Johns Hopkins University, USA

Naguib, Raouf, PhD, Head of the Biomedical Computing and Engineering Technologies (BIOCORE) Applied Research Group, Coventry University, UK

Ortiz Posadas, Martha R., PhD, Professor at Electrical Engineering Department, Universidad Autónoma Metropolitana-Iztapalapa, MEXICO

Puentes, John, PhD, Assistant Professor, GET-ENST Bretagne, France and Associate Researcher, French Institute of Health and Medical Research, FRANCE

Robinson, Judas, PhD Candidate, St George's University of London, UK

Rodríguez, Denis E., PhD, Higher Technical University, CUBA

Sanchez, M.C., MSc, Higher Technical University, CUBA

Wales, Ann, NHS Education for Scotland, SCOTLAND

Walker, Robin C., MB, ChB in medicine, FRCPC, FAAP, Professor of Paediatrics at the University of Ottawa, and Medical Director of Critical Care at the Children's Hospital of Eastern Ontario, CANADA

Wickramasinghe, Nilmini, PhD, Associate director, Center Management Medical Technologies (CMMT), Associate Professor, Stuart Graduate School of Business, Illinois Institute of Technology, USA

Zhu, Zhichang, PhD, Senior Lecturer, University of Hull, UK, Visiting Research Professor, Advanced Institute of Science and Technology, JAPAN, South China Normal University, CHINA

About the Editors

Rajeev K. Bali. Dr. Bali is currently a Reader at Coventry University, UK. He is the leader of the Knowledge Management for Healthcare research subgroup, which works under the Biomedical Computing Research group (BIOCORE). He is an invited reviewer for several journals, conferences, and organizations. His primary research interests are in healthcare knowledge management, clinical governance, engineering management, organizational behavior, and medical informatics. He has recently published a text on Clinical Knowledge Management. Dr. Bali has served as an invited reviewer and associate editor for several journals, including the *Transactions on Information Technology in Biomedicine*, and was the Publications Chair for the IEEE–EMBS Information Technology Applications in Biomedicine (ITAB) conference 2003, held in Birmingham, UK.

Ashish N. Dwivedi. Dr. Dwivedi is currently a lecturer at the Business School, University of Hull. Dr. Dwivedi is also associated with the management of the high-tech Management Learning Laboratory and is the program leader for a newly created Masters in Knowledge Management (MSc in KM). His primary research interests are in knowledge management (in which he obtained his PhD), organizational behavior, healthcare management, and information and communication technologies. Dr. Dwivedi has served as an invited reviewer and associate editor for several journals, including the *Transactions on Information Technology in Biomedicine*.

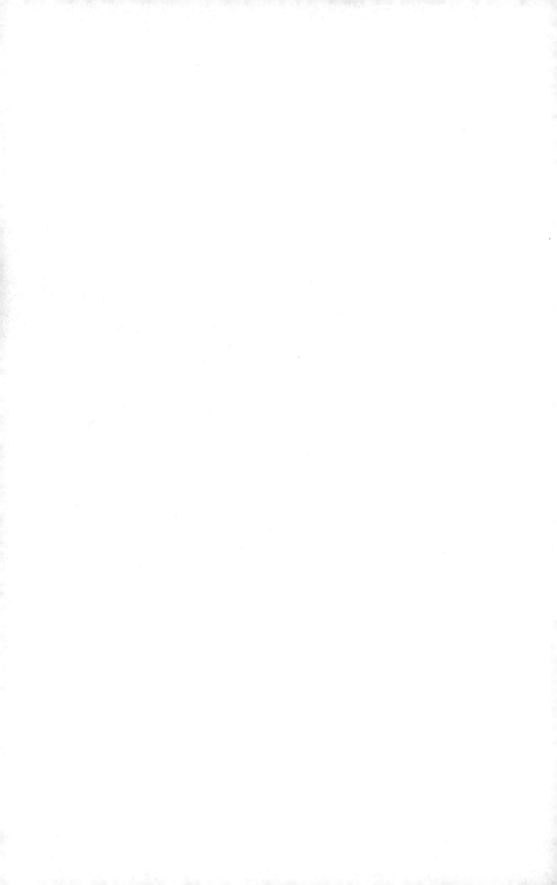

Section I
Healthcare Knowledge Management: Innovations and New Understanding

1
Building New Healthcare Management Paradigms: A Case for Healthcare Knowledge Management

A.N. DWIVEDI, R.K. BALI AND R.N.G. NAGUIB

Abstract

Advances in information technology have made it possible for medical stakeholders to have access to almost all existing health information available. However, as a result of these advances, physicians, and other medical stakeholders are facing an information overload and, in some cases, paradoxical information. This chapter presents evidence that (a) highlights the extent of the information explosion in healthcare and (b) elucidates the extent to which the information explosion in healthcare is adversely affecting the ability of medical stakeholders in the process of medical diagnosis and treatment. This chapter then discusses the concept of knowledge management (KM) as applicable to the healthcare sector (i.e. healthcare KM and clinical KM). Finally, this chapter presents a case for the incorporation of the KM paradigm as the driving force in the healthcare sector.

1.1   The Role of Information Technology in Health

Technology strongly influences the way we work and is creating opportunities and new demands for a range of different approaches to health [1]. Telecommunications have evolved and have been accompanied by an evolution in attitudes to information and communications technologies [2]. Technology-led change opens up opportunities for new working methods in three main ways, namely by allowing existing activities to be carried out more rapidly, with more consistency, and at a lower cost than could previously be achieved.

Today, the explosive growth of the Internet has promoted the trend for investment in information and communication devices, and the healthcare industry is an active participant in this trend [3]. Advances in information technology (IT), particularly in (a) database technologies and (b) Internet technologies and telecommunications, are transforming the healthcare industry [4–6]. Advances in portal devices such as smart mobile phones and PDAs [7,8], as well as in communications technologies

3

such as the Universal Mobile Telecommunications System (UMTS) and Digital Video Broadcasting (DVB-T), are promoting the Internet as the standard communication medium between medical practitioners and patients.

These modern developments in IT have enabled a number of countries to implement a national Electronic Health Record (EHR) by linking their existing Healthcare Information Systems [9–17]. It would be fair to state that advances in communications technology are dramatically changing the delivery of healthcare services [18].

1.2   Impact of Information Technology on Healthcare, Particularly in the Process of Medical Diagnosis and Treatment

Exchanging medical information between different medical information systems is an accepted norm for hospitals and medical practitioners all over the world. As mentioned in the preceding section, advances in IT have made it easier for medical stakeholders to share information. However, despite creating a technological infrastructure for sharing medical information, most medical stakeholders are facing an information explosion.

Medical stakeholders have to deal with over "10,000 known diseases, 3,000 drugs, 1,100 lab tests, 300 radiology procedures, 1,000 new drugs and biotechnology medicines in development and 2,000 individual risk factors" [19]. This situation is further aggravated by advances in hardware technologies which are further accentuating this information overload in healthcare. For example, "Organ and tissue scanning speed is doubling every 26 months, making tests both faster and cheaper.... Image resolution is doubling every 12 months" [19].

Advances in modern-day genetic sciences are acting as a key driving force behind the development of pharmaceutical drugs and have augmented the number of potential drug compositions from a meager 400 to over 4,000 in a very short time span [19]. This is validated by another study (by Egger) in which it has been estimated that, in the near future, new pharmaceutical compounds could replace 50% of today's in-patient services [20].

Medical stakeholders, apart from dealing with the impact of advances in hardware technologies and genetic sciences, also have to deal with information overload caused by advances in biomedical knowledge.

A marker of the impact of the biomedical knowledge and genetic engineering revolutions on healthcare is the exponential increase in biomedical knowledge in the National Library of Medicine's Medline database (4500 journals in 30 languages, dating from 1996) of published literature in health-related sciences. In 2002, Medline contained 11.7 million citations and, on average, about 400,000 new entries were being added per year [20]. If a typical modern-day healthcare stakeholder who wanted to get updated with this amount of current literature was to read one article a day, then it would take 1100 years to get updated with the new literature added every year.

The calculations above ignore the existing literature level of 11.7 million and also ignore the projected increase in the growth of new research. It is prudent to assume that not all the literature would be of relevance to a particular healthcare stakeholder. If we assume that about 1% of the new literature added every year is of relevance to a healthcare stakeholder, then it would still take a stakeholder 10 years (reading an average of one article a day) to be updated with the healthcare advances of 1 year. The above statistics validate the contention put forth by this chapter, that the healthcare industry is information intensive and immediately requires a resolution to the problem of information overload, a point supported by other studies [21–25].

It is argued that it is no longer possible for medical stakeholders to possess all the pertinent knowledge in their domain of specialty [19,26]. This notion is confirmed by Masys [20], who notes that

against a background of an explosively growing body of knowledge in the health sciences current models of clinical decision making by autonomous practitioners, relying upon their memory and personal experience, will be inadequate for effective twenty-first-century health care delivery.

1.3   Healthcare Knowledge Management: Solution to Medical Stakeholders' Informatics Woes

The healthcare sector has witnessed the incorporation of many management paradigms that were supposed to alleviate the information explosion in healthcare; in practice, though, none of them has been successful [27]. The failure of existing healthcare management concepts to tackle the information overload in healthcare has strengthened the case for incorporating the knowledge management (KM) paradigm in healthcare [28–31].

KM is often regarded as an interdisciplinary management paradigm which looks at the entire spectrum of knowledge activities (knowledge creation, identification, codification, and dissemination) [32]. Owing to this wide-ranging remit, there is no universally accepted definition of KM [33]. Almost all the definitions of KM state that it is a multidisciplinary paradigm [34] and that the main aim behind any strategy of KM is to ensure that knowledge workers have access to the right knowledge, to the right place, at the right time [35].

Though many definitions of KM have been proposed, we would like to adopt the definition of healthcare KM (i.e. KM defined in a healthcare context) proposed by Wickramasinghe [36]:

KM is a discipline that promotes an integrated approach to identifying, managing, and sharing all of an enterprise's information assets, including database, documents, policies and procedures, as well as unarticulated expertise and experience resident in individual workers.

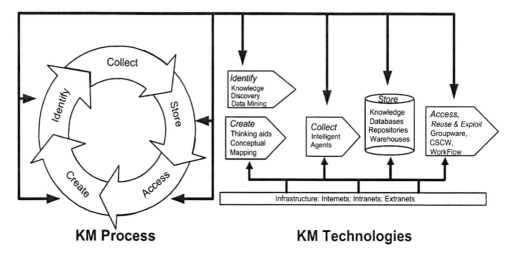

KM Process   **KM Technologies**

FIGURE 1.1. The KM cycle (modified from Skyrme [37]).

The entire spectrum of KM activities has been documented by Skyrme [37]; see Figure 1.1.

1.4   Healthcare Knowledge Management and Clinical Knowledge Management: An Overview

We would like to make the distinction between clinical KM and healthcare KM by arguing that the prime objective of clinical KM systems is to enable medical stakeholders to define, select, and implement treatment(s) within the process of medical diagnosis and treatment, whereas the objective of healthcare KM systems is to change the way that medical stakeholders think about patients and their needs and treatments.

Healthcare KM systems is a much broader concept and is primarily concerned with how medical stakeholders perceive, process, and communicate information flowing from activities relating to medical practice, medical education, medical research, and medical information dissemination

In order to assist healthcare KM in overcoming the information challenges facing the healthcare sector, it is important to look at why previous healthcare management paradigms have not succeeded. We would argue that the main reason for the failure of previous healthcare management paradigms can be traced to the inability to combine healthcare organizational processes with technology.

An ideal starting point in support of our argument is to obtain a better understanding of the theoretical propositions underpinning the nature of knowledge. There are currently two main schools of thought, which hold contrasting views on the nature of knowledge [38]. The first school of thought, known as the *cognitivist perspective*, contends that knowledge is universal for all and that any two systems (biological or machine) should be able to achieve and hold the same representation of the world. This implies that knowledge is explicit, capable of being encoded, stored, and disseminated. The cognitivist perspective has influenced the development of artificial intelligence.

The second school of thought, known as the *constructionist perspective*, states that "knowledge resides within our bodies and is closely tied to our previous experiences"; consequently, knowledge is tacit, highly personal, not easily expressed and, therefore, cannot be easily shared [38].

A number of leading management researchers have further elaborated that the Hungarian chemist, economist, and philosopher Michael Polanyi was among the earliest theorists who popularized the concept of characterizing knowledge as "tacit or explicit" which is now recognized as the de facto knowledge categorization approach [34,39,40].

Explicit knowledge typically takes the form of company documents and is easily available, whilst tacit knowledge is subjective and cognitive. One of the characteristics of explicit knowledge is that it can be easily documented and is generally located in the form of written manuals, books, procedures, reports and/or found in electronic databases [41]. As such, it is easily accessible and in many cases available on an organization's intranet.

As briefly mentioned, researchers who focus on the cognitivist perspective, believe that knowledge is explicit and capable of being encoded and stored and disseminated. The focus is on identification of knowledge and its subsequent codification, refinement, and storage for effective dissemination.

Researchers in the cognitivist perspective have created medical informatics applications that are IT led and based upon technologies like Knowledge Discovery In Databases (KDD), data warehousing, artificial intelligence, and expert systems. All of these technologies tend to focus on IT to model organizational processes. This is often carried out at the expense of the human aspect of the healthcare processes. A number of studies [42–45] have further noted that overdependence on IT results in the healthcare initiatives, and we argue the same is happening to healthcare KM.

It has been argued that future healthcare stakeholders would need to combine management skills with clinical knowledge [46]. The way forward for healthcare institutions is to "integrate clinical knowledge bases at the point of care . . . thereby rendering it more accessible," which would call for streamlining clinical knowledge into the workflow of healthcare processes [47]. This argument has also found support in other study by Jurisica et al. [48], who note that systematic KM (i.e. support for acquisition, representation, organization, usage and evolution of knowledge in its many forms) can alleviate problems caused due to the information explosion in the biomedical domain.

We further argue that the high failure rate of healthcare initiatives based upon the cognitivist perspective has further strengthened the need of incorporating the constructionist perspective in creating healthcare KM applications. This implies that healthcare KM as a discipline has to combine both the cognitivist perspective and the constructionist perspective, a combination that is lacking in previous healthcare management paradigms.

1.5   Conclusions

The information explosion in healthcare has adversely affected the ability of healthcare professionals, particularly physicians, in providing accurate and timely medical diagnosis and treatment. The information explosion in healthcare is likely to be further accentuated by advances in biomedical knowledge and genetic engineering.

It is argued that if the impact of all these factors is seen together, then the conclusion from a healthcare informatics perspective is clear: 21st century clinical practitioners have to acquire proficiency in understanding and interpreting clinical information so as to attain knowledge and wisdom whilst dealing with large amounts of clinical data. These data will be dynamic in nature and would call for the ability to interpret context-based healthcare information [49].

Previous healthcare management paradigms, despite their initial promise, were unable to offer solutions to the information management crisis in healthcare. This chapter has discussed the concept of KM as applicable to the healthcare sector and has argued that organizational aspects of healthcare management need to be incorporated within the healthcare system, alongside technological implementations in a manner where people, processes, and technology are in harmony. We believe this can be achieved by effective design of healthcare KM systems that combine both cognitivist and constructionist perspectives on knowledge creation and transfer.

References

1. Feldman D, Gainey T. Patterns of telecommuting and their consequences: framing the research agenda. *Hum Resource Manage Rev* 1997;7(4):369–388.
2. Stanworth C. Telework and the information age. *New Technol Work Employ* 1998;13(1):51–62.
3. Kazman W, Westerheim AA. Telemedicine leverages power of clinical information. *Health Manage Technol* 1999;20(9):8–10.
4. Krause M, Brown L. Information security in the healthcare industry. *Inf Syst Secur* 1996;5(3):32–40.
5. Liu D-R, Wu I-C, Hsieh S-T. Integrating SET and EDI for secure healthcare commerce. *Comput Stand Interfaces* 2001;23(5):367–381.
6. Raghupathi W, Tan J. Strategic IT applications in health care. *Commun ACM* 2002;45(12):56–61.
7. Olla P, Patel NV. A framework for delivering secure mobile location information. *Int J Mobile Commun* 2003;1(3):289–300.
8. Olla P, Atkinson C. Developing a wireless reference model for interpreting complexity in wireless projects. *Ind Manage Data Syst* 2004;104(3):262–272.
9. Takeda H, Matsumura Y, Kuwata S, Nakano H, Sakamoto N, Yamamoto R. Architecture for networked electronic patient record systems. *Int J Med Inform* 2000;60(2):161–167.
10. McClelland R, Thomas V. Confidentiality and security of clinical information in mental health practice. *Adv Psychiatr Treat* 2002;8(4):291–296.
11. Janczewski L, Shi FX. Development of information security baselines for healthcare information systems in New Zealand, *Comput Secur* 2002;21(2):172–192.

12. Bos JJ. Digital signatures and the electronic health records: providing legal and security guarantees. *Int J Bio-Med Comput* 1996;42(1–2):157–163.
13. Gritzalis D, Tomaras A, Katsikas S, Keklikoglou J. Data security in medical information systems: the Greek case. *Comput Secur* 1991;10(2):141–159.
14. Immonen S. Developments in health care, the increasing role of information technology: security issues. *Int J Bio-Med Comput* 1996;43(1–2):9–15.
15. TradePartners UK. Health and medical market in Finland. Available from: http://www.tradepartners.gov.uk/,1997/healthcare/finland/profile/overview.shtml [accessed 18 Nov 2002].
16. Dwivedi A, Bali RK, Meletis BA, Naguib RNG, Every P, Nassar NS. Towards a holistic healthcare information security model for healthcare. In: *Proceedings of 4th Annual IEEE EMBS Special Topic Conference on Information Technology Applications in Biomedicine*, Birmingham, UK, 2003; pp. 114–117.
17. Cross M. Europe's wrestling with electronic patient record. *Doc World* 2000;5(1):30–33.
18. Schooley AK. Allowing FDA regulation of communications software used in telemedicine: a potentially fatal misdiagnosis. *Fed Commun Law J* 1998;50(3):731–751.
19. Pavia L. The era of knowledge in health care. *Health Care Strategic Manage* 2001;19(2):12–13.
20. Masys DR. Effects of current and future information technologies on the health care workforce. *Health Affairs* 2002;21:33–41.
21. Dawes M, Sampson U. Knowledge management in clinical practice: a systematic review of information seeking behavior in physicians. *Int J Med Inform* 2003;71(1):9–15.
22. De Lusignan S, Pritchard K, Chan T. A knowledge-management model for clinical practice. *J Postgrad Med* 2002;48(4):297–303.
23. Hall A, Walton G. Information overload within the health care system: a literature review. *Health Inf Libr J* 2004;21(2):102–108.
24. Gray JAM. Where's the chief knowledge officer? *Br Med J* 1998;317(7162):832–840.
25. Dwivedi AN, Bali RK, Naguib RNG. Knowledge management in healthcare: overview of empirical evidence. *J Inf Technol Healthcare* 2005;3(3):141–148.
26. Rockefeller R. Informed shared decision making: is this the future of health care? *Health Forum J* 1999;42(3):54–56.
27. Melvin K, Wright J, Harrison SR, Robinson M, Connelly J, Williams DRR. Effective practice in the NHS and the contribution from public health: a qualitative study. *Br J Clin Govern* 1999;4(3):88–97.
28. Mercer K. Examining the impact of health information networks on health system integration in Canada. *Leadership Health Serv* 2001;14(3):1–30.
29. Health Canada. Vision and strategy for knowledge management and IM/IT for Health Canada. 1998. Available from: http://www.hc-sc.gc.ca/iacb-dgiac/km-gs/english/vsmenu_e.htm [accessed 20 Mar 2001].
30. Sharma SK, Wickramasinghe N, Gupta JND. Knowledge management in healthcare. In: Wickramasinghe N, Gupta JND, Sharma SK, editors, *Creating knowledge-based healthcare organizations*. Hershey, PA, USA: Idea Group Publishing; 2004, pp. 1–13.
31. Desouza KC. Knowledge management in hospitals. In: Wickramasinghe N, Gupta JND, Sharma SK, editors, *Creating knowledge-based healthcare organizations*. Hershey, PA, USA: Idea Group Publishing; 2004, pp. 14–28.

32. Choo CW. *The knowing organization: how organizations use information to construct meaning, create knowledge, and make decisions.* New York: Oxford University Press; 1998.
33. Beckman TJ. The current state of knowledge management. In: Liebowitz J, editor, *Knowledge management handbook.* New York: CRC Press; 1999.
34. Gupta B, Iyer LS, Aronson JE. Knowledge management: practices and challenges. *Ind Manage Data Syst* 2000;100(1):17–21.
35. Dove R. Knowledge management response ability and the agile enterprise. *J Knowl Manage* 1999;3(1):18–35.
36. Wickramasinghe N. Practising what we preach: are knowledge management systems in practice really knowledge management systems? *Bus Process Manage J* 2003;9(3):295–316.
37. Skyrme D. *Knowledge networking, creating the collaborative enterprise.* Butterworth-Heinemann; 1999.
38. Stefanelli M. Knowledge and process management in health care organizations. *Methods Inf Med* 2004;43(5):525–535.
39. Hansen MT, Nohria N, Tierney T. What's your strategy for managing knowledge? *Harvard Bus Rev* 1999;77(2):106–116.
40. Zack MH. Managing codified knowledge. *Sloan Manage Rev* 1999;40(4):45–58.
41. Dwivedi A, Bali RK, James AE. OCKD: a conceptual KM framework for gaining competitive advantage in the knowledge-based economy of the future. In: *Proceedings of 7th Annual Conference of the UK Academy for Information Systems*, Leeds, UK, 2002; pp. 216–225.
42. Cole-Gomolski B. Users loathe to share their know-how. *Computerworld* 1997;31(46):6.
43. Robertson M, Sørensen C, Swan J. Survival of the leanest: intensive knowledge work and groupware adaptation. *Inf Technol People* 2001;14(4):334–352.
44. Holsapple C, Joshi K. An investigation of factors that influence the management of knowledge in organizations. *J Strategic Inf Syst* 2000;9(2–3):235–261.
45. Silver CA. Where technology and knowledge meet. *J Bus Strat* 2000;21(6):28–33.
46. Stefl ME. The commentaries: a summary. *Front Health Serv Manage* 1997;13:26–27.
47. Blumenfeld B. Integrating knowledge bases at the point of care. *Health Manage Technol* 1997;18:44–46.
48. Jurisica I, Wolfley JR, Rogers P, Bianca MA, Glasgow JI, Weeks DR, et al. Intelligent decision support for protein crystal growth. *IBM Systs J* 2001;40(2):394–409.
49. Dwivedi A, Bali RK, James AE, Naguib RNG, Johnston D. Merger of knowledge management and information technology in healthcare: opportunities and challenges, In: *Proceedings of IEEE Canadian Conference on Electrical and Computer Engineering (CCECE)*, Winnipeg, Canada, 2002; pp. 1194–1199.

2
Clinical Knowledge Management: A Model for Primary Care

SIMON de LUSIGNAN AND JUDAS ROBINSON

Abstract

Opportunities for the application of knowledge management to primary care have grown in the last two decades with the implementation of information communication technology, resultant changes in medical record keeping, and requirements to audit quality standards. Knowledge management models for primary care need to take into account the unique nature of this speciality with emphasis on first-contact care, longitudinality, comprehensive services, and coordination. This chapter proposes a knowledge management model for primary care based on the division of the area into four prototypical subject areas: tacit versus explicit knowledge, and learner-centered versus information-centered knowledge management. In summary, we feel that the complexity of primary care does not lend itself to a single knowledge management solution, especially one that is entirely technology based or sees evidence-based medicine (EBM) as the only important paradigm. Instead, primary care requires a portfolio of solutions. We suggest that these should include one element from the following four areas: EBM, community of practice, clinical audit, and mentorship.

2.1   Introduction

Knowledge management (KM) has the potential to improve the working lives of primary care professionals at a time of changing roles and expectations. In previous decades, primary care physicians were the repository of clinical knowledge concerning their area of practice, they worked far more as individuals with their own list of patients, and they used information and communications technology (ICT) relatively little. Their medical records were hand written on individual medical record cards, which were stored together in that patient's medical record envelope. Their readily available knowledge sources generally consisted of a limited number of text books and a pharmacopoeia, as well as contact with colleagues. However, over the last two decades things have changed dramatically with contractual changes within primary care and the introduction of ICT. Data from computerized medical

records are almost instantaneously searchable in contrast to their paper prede-
cessors; and bibliographic databases and other on-line resources provide ready
access to up-to-date evidence [1]. The latter also help provide selective access to
the exponential growth in the volume of medical information. Consequently, this
role of the primary care professional has changed. Clinicians no longer know all
of the pertinent information, but instead need to know where to find the required
information. At the level of the individual patient, mastery of a generic problem-
solving process is more critical than factual knowledge. At the practice population
level, primary care professionals have the ability to audit quality standards in their
practices in a way that has not been previously possible. Health services can ensure that practices are implementing quality standards and have systems in place
to learn from critical incidents. Table 2.1 illustrates how many of the changes in
primary care over the last two decades have created an environment within which
cultural and organizational change, including the deployment of ICT, have created
an environment within which KM programs have a greater potential for success.

The increasing volume of medical knowledge and the constant search for an improved managerial effectiveness within health services also create an environment
within which KM has the potential for an increased role. The volume of medical
information is increasing, and, as a generalist, the primary care professional needs
to stay abreast of a broad corpus of information. It has been estimated that the
number of medical journals doubles on a 19-year basis and that there are over
40,000 biomedical journals in circulation [2,3].

A sample of 22 practices in 1998 revealed over 28 kg of guidelines [4]. Faced
with this ever-mounting growth in knowledge, primary care practitioners are almost
obliged to rely on ICT and KM to overcome information overload. Simultaneous
with the increase in medical knowledge, healthcare costs are rising. Healthcare
managers face the unenviable task of discovering approaches that are better, faster,
and cheaper. With this task in mind, the new concepts and paradigms that have
come to their attention in recent years are [5]:

- evidence-based medicine (EBM) [6];
- model of integrated patient pathways (MIPP/IPP) [7];
- clinical governance (CG) [8];
- in the UK, a financially incentivized Quality and Outcomes Framework (QOF)
  that has defined 20 clinical targets that GPs should achieve [9];
- KM [10].

KM is a broad, multidisciplinary field encompassing some of the other approaches, such as EBM. Broadly speaking, KM can be defined as capturing, organizing, and storing knowledge and experiences of individual workers and groups
within an organization and making this information available to others in the organization [11]. The concept of KM should also include accelerating learning;
a strategy that captures and codifies knowledge [12]. EBM is a highly structured
formed of explicit knowledge, which can be readily codified. Whilst much has been
written about EBM and its implementation in primary care [13] much less is know
about how to utilise this knowledge as part of a KM strategy for primary care.

TABLE 2.1. Evolution of primary care and scope to deploy clinical KM programmes

	Primary care in 1985	Primary care in 2005
Professional attitude	Reluctance to question clinical judgment—largely held by individuals	Clinical governance is expected Review and question processes and errors Systemic responsibility
Responsibility	Personal lists with 24-h responsibility for patient care	Practice-based registration, with most practices opting out of 24-h care provision
Knowledge	Held by physician	Clinician is problem solver with access to large amount of knowledge—online and sometimes integrated with computer record
Knowledge sources	Texts, sometimes quite old Pharmacopoeia—commercially produced MIMS is the most popular Postgraduate centre contact with colleagues and library access	Texts Paper BNF still remains popular despite online drug information Email access to information Digital libraries, e.g. Primary Care Electronic Library (PCEL) Postgraduate centers and library as before
Clinical records	Individual records on paper Narrative data Maybe a summary card and repeat prescription card Separate notes held by general practitioners (GPs), district nurses, health visitors, etc.	Computerized records consisting of structured data and associated narrative free text Whilst coding of diagnosis in some areas is incomplete, prescribing data is complete and reliable Single computerized record system used across primary care, linked to laboratories, and moves to integrate across the health service
Clinical audit	Nothing compulsory, some primary care professionals undertook: random case discussions; audit of a sample of cases Manual age–sex register provides a mechanism for searching records	Computerized records make searches of all records nearly instantaneous Computerized records mean that disease registers can be instantly created Comparative audit of standards between practices is possible
Quality standards	No formal mechanism other than new entrants must be vocationally trained	Annual appraisal, an intermediate step towards revalidation Appraisal includes review of critical incidents and participation in audit 2005 contract includes financially incentivized quality points for achieving specific targets for chronic disease management (CDM)
Training	Focus on narrative, learning from a trainer Formative assessment Very few practices had computers or Internet linkage	Much more structured: MCQ knowledge test Summative assessment of consulting ability Basic life support formally tested On going need to maintain standards All primary care clinical professionals have a desktop computer, specialist computerized medical records, email and the Internet (via NHSnet, the National Health Service's (NHS's) own fire-walled intranet), and an increasing number of electronic links to laboratories, pharmacy, and telelmonitoring devices
Scope to deploy KM	Low	High

This chapter sets out what is unique in primary care, a speciality where continuity and long-term relationships are critical. Next, we discuss the evolution of the primary care records and the potential to use knowledge derived from them to improve clinical practice. Many of the current strategies for quality improvement, listed above, are easy to use in areas where there is a large body of EBM that can be readily applied. They are much more difficult to apply in primary care, where the longitudinal relationship and social and psychosocial factors may outweigh those of evidence-based practice. Freeman and Sweeney [14] discussed reasons why GPs did not implement evidence. Practitioners' consideration of psychosocial factors and knowledge of a patient's personal situation may influence implementation of evidence. Also, personal experience is very powerful and may override the evidence base. For example, one doctor reported he was reluctant to anticoagulate elderly people after one 88-year-old woman kept falling and frequently ended up in casualty being stitched and bandaged up. Local circumstances can also affect decision making. When discussing the potential side effects of Warfarin, one participant said, "It's not a minor bleed if your patient is 30 miles from the nearest transfusion service." One doctor said

"The problem is starting him on ACE (the correct evidence-based therapy) is because he is very anxious about any medication change, and every time you change the medication it entails another four or five visits to go and see him and to try and reassure him that he is on the right medication".

These examples illustrate the logistical problems faced by practitioners, i.e. logistical problems that may conflict with the implementation of evidence-based practice. Taking the unique attributes of this speciality into account, this chapter explains how a balanced approach to KM is needed in primary care.

2.2   The Unique Nature of Primary Care

Primary care is generally recognized to be a unique speciality with its own distinct knowledge needs. Numerous definitions of primary care emphasize this; see Figure 2.1 [15–18]. KM, as applied to primary care, will have specific models and requirements. Indicative of this unique role is the emergence of a sub-speciality of medical informatics, i.e. primary care informatics [19], which has much to contribute to KM in primary care.

Current definitions of primary care emphasize first-contact care, longitudinality, comprehensive services, and coordination. Despite the fact that the inability to quantify these phenomena reduces their usefulness to planners and evaluators [20], they adequately describe the unique nature of primary care. Additional aspects of primary care which distinguish it from other areas of practice are its ready acceptance of psychosocial considerations as addenda to the biomedical model, and decision making based on heuristic rules of thumb, rather than deductive reasoning, which is used to advantage in situations when patients often present with nondescript symptoms or problems unrelated to illness. Primary care also has

Primary health care is essential health care based on practical, scientifically sound and socially acceptable methods and technology made universally accessible to individuals and families in the community through their full participation and at a cost that the community and country can afford to maintain at every stage of their development in the spirit of self-reliance and self-determination. It forms an integral part both of the country's health system, of which it is the central function and main focus, and of the overall social and economic development of the community. It is the first level of contact of individuals, the family and community with the national health system bringing health care as close as possible to where people live and work, and constitutes the first element of a continuing health care process [15].

Primary care is first-contact, continuous, comprehensive, and coordinated care provided to populations undifferentiated by gender, disease, or organ system [16].

Primary care is the provision of integrated, accessible health care services by clinicians who are accountable for addressing a large majority of personal health care needs, developing a sustained partnership with patients, and practicing in the context of family and community [17].

General practice / family medicine is an academic and scientific discipline, with its own educational content, research, evidence base and clinical activity, and a clinical specialty orientated to primary care [18].

FIGURE 2.1. Definitions of primary care.

its own clinical coding systems and unique clinical computer systems designed to provide access to the longitudinal medical records of primary care. Many of these have links to applications that belong to KM, decision-support and information systems which improve the quality of care.

Therapeutic decisions in primary care are frequently made on a heuristic basis (intelligent rules of thumb) [21]. The "rules" reflect the health beliefs and experience of that practitioner: the nature of a problem may be elucidated over several consultations. The contrast of the nature of family practitioner and hospital decision making is illustrated in Table 2.2. Although an oversimplification, it serves to illustrate the fundamentally different environment within which the primary care professional is required to operate. Inevitably there will be many circumstances in which the hospital doctor will practice in a way that is similar to the family practitioner, and vice versa. The nature of this decision-making process, in which a definite diagnosis is not always made, has implications for the certainty with which diagnostic labels can be applied, and what meaning can be attached to codes applied. For example, at what point should chest pain on exercise be labeled angina? The implication of using the angina label is that patients with this label may be called in for all sorts of preventive procedures that may or may not be appropriate.

The conventional approach to medical problem solving is to use deductive reasoning. The theoretical approach to developing computerized decision-support tools to assist is described by Musen [22] as having two components, which need definition:

The domain ontology: defining the concepts and their interrelation within the area under study.

The problem solving method: this has to be defined in general terms. This might be an algorithm, a statistical approach, or one of many other methods, alone or in combination.

TABLE 2.2. Polar views of the decision-making environment in general practice and hospital (adapted from Essex [21]).

Issue	General/Family practice	Hospital
Problem type	Unselected	Selected
Who makes decisions	Alone, in isolation	Often made with other doctors and colleagues
Influence of knowledge of the family	Decisions affected	Decisions often made with no knowledge of the family
Time available	Short consultations, little time	More time to take history and examine fully
Seriousness and urgency of problem	Decision made by GP outside hospital	Decided on before admission or referral
Type of problem	Worried about something, minor illness, chronic disease	Mainly major illness, chronic disease
Stage in natural history the disease is seen	Often early	Usually late
Type and range of decisions	Very broad, with several problems presented at once	More focused, often on an organ or system, depending on specialty
Review of decisions	Easily reviewed	Hard to review after discharge

Success with this analytical approach has been found using software that detects drug interactions [23], and its utility has been demonstrated in primary care [24,25]. Clearly, in the area of drug interaction detection, structured recording of medication has advantages for medical care. However, there are doubts expressed as to whether technology that is clearly useful in detecting drug interactions can be extrapolated more broadly across primary care.

Fugelli [26] questions whether limitation to a single domain is possible in primary care:

Doctors in other parts of medicine are devoted to a particular organ or a technology. They practice according to what the Germans call "Das Schemata. . . .

"Das Schemata" is not workable within general practice.

Over 15 years ago, Suchman provided insight into why this view may be correct [27]. She concluded that human–computer interfaces that propose set cognitive models (*das Schemata*) are likely to fail for three reasons:

1. *Context predominates.* The immediate context may predominate: if it is important to a patient with heart failure to tell a clinician about their grandchildren and their worries, then this agenda will fill the consultation, not the decision-support tool for heart failure.
2. *Rules are only a guide.* Guidelines and rules are only a tool around which individuals organize their own conduct, e.g. patients may not take their medicine as prescribed.
3. *Experience and commonsense modulate decision making.* Professional judgment drawn from experience modulates what happens: a child may have

symptoms suggestive of illness, but the physician's experience suggests that this person is well.

Studies showing how little decision-support tools were used in the management of chronic disease [28–30] lend support to Suchman's views.

Whilst it might be expected that simple heuristic "rules" might be modeled easily, in reality they are complex, depending on a unique set of factors that come together within that particular consultation. Things are further complicated by the recognition that the doctor–patient relationship is in itself therapeutic [31].

Primary care informatics should, therefore, examine complexity [32] and complex adaptive systems [33] as potential sources of insight into how to model the consultation. Chapman [34] describes the divide that needs to be bridged:

"IT experts are extremely good at linear, reductionist positivist thinking, and not so good at constructing social solutions and appreciating other perspectives. So there is an inherent mismatch between the mode of thinking required to develop robust social solutions and the thinking required to develop robust technical solutions."

To summarize, the following are some of the features that make primary care unique:

• continuity of care;
• comprehensive nature of care;
• first point of contact;
• longitudinal records;
• primary care specific computer systems and clinical coding;
• psychosocial factors taken into consideration;
• short consultations;
• patients seen early in the history of the disease;
• heuristic rules applied rather than deductive reasoning.

Any KM model needs to take account of these features. The experiential learning of the authors is that, because of time pressures, primary care clinicians tend to need to retrieve information in consultation (e.g. look up drug doses, the correct therapy, the level of cholesterol to intervene at, etc.); more reflective learning takes place at the end of the surgery session, when there is more time and space to formulate and answer questions. The use of the Doctor's Desk and PCEL reflect this pattern of use, i.e. peaks of use at the end of morning and evening surgery [35,36].

2.3   The Evolution of the Primary Care Medical Record

The evolution of the primary care record from paper to computer is a key enabler of KM in primary care. Themes can be identified in the evolution of the medical record in primary care [37]. Records started in an unstructured format, with the data they contained being of little value other than to the person who wrote it. The next step in development was the introduction of the use of coded data that

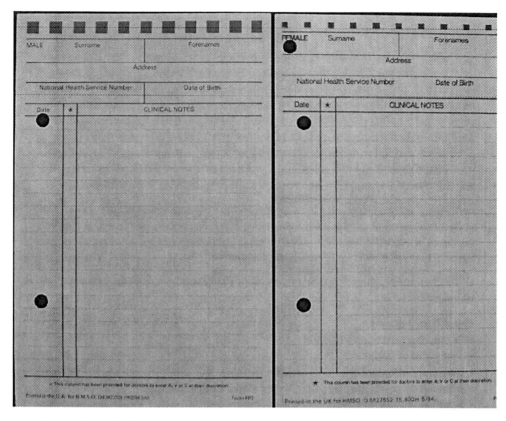

FIGURE 2.2. Continuation cards from UK general practice medical records, used 1911 onwards.

allows others to assimilate key information quickly. This process started long before computerization. There has been progressive change, from the Victorian doctor who might make notes in his journal or diary about the patients seen that day, to individual patient records; then to data recorded in a way that allow it to be aggregated from many records, so that the health status of whole populations can be assessed. The recognition of the need for structured data preceded computerization.

The written records system, which is only finally disappearing from use in the first decade of the 21st century has its roots in the UK's 1911 National Insurance Act. These records are often referred to after the originator of that act, as the "Lloyd George" records. The continuation cards on which the record was written are shown in Figure 2.2. They encouraged brevity, and had the advantage of being easy to scan visually. When medical records were reviewed in 1920 it was decided to keep the same format so that the same filing cabinets that kept the old records could be used. There was one record envelope per patient. There was space for information on the outside of the envelope, and a continuous chronological list of consultations would be created inside on continuation cards. There was no

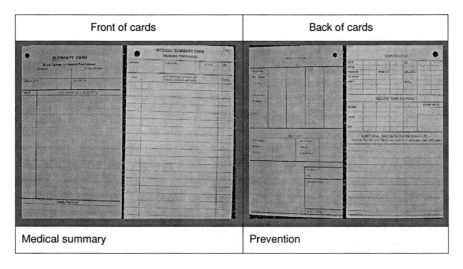

Front of cards	Back of cards
Medical summary	Prevention

FIGURE 2.3. Front and back of medical summary cards from GP records.

structured data in these records, only narrative. It was to be a permanent transferable record, kept by the doctor on whose list the patient resided at that time. This format remained unchanged until the 1950s, when it was suggested that a distinctive colored summary card be introduced.

These records became progressively more structured through the addition of extra cards to the record. However, progress was piecemeal, rather than as a result of health service planning. Most of the structuring of the record was directed at improved chronic illness management, and prevention. The first extra cards added to the record were summary cards added in the 1950s, followed by repeat prescription cards [37]. Later, additional cards relating to specific illnesses and conditions were added, e.g. asthma, hormone replacement therapy, diabetes, hypertension, pregnancy, and so on. Through this process, general practice started to define its own ontology (concepts and their interrelationships) which defines it as a specialty. It is the beginning of an evolutionary process of structuring the data in the record, and towards the creation of a coding system. Examples of these cards are provided in Figure 2.3.

More recently there have been attempts to transform the record to one which is problem orientated [38]. "Weed's SOAP" was a common format used: S was for subjective (or what the patient complained of); O was for objective (any objective findings, e.g. blood pressure measurement); A was for analysis (the doctor's judgment as to diagnosis); and, P was for plan, as to what action to take or prescription given. Although adding structure to the record, information could be recorded in any handwritten format. However, with the exception of stickers (sometimes used on the outside of records), data like blood pressure (which was always recorded in one format) and some practices' use of age–sex cards, the recording of data that these cards structured was where the narrative was recorded rather than coding of the data. The creation of records with properly structured data did not happen until computerization.

Computer systems allow data to be recorded in a structured format. Good quality computerized medical records contain ever-increasing amounts of structured data; recorded at every patient encounter. In the written record, additional cards (e.g. the bright yellow Royal College of General Practitioners asthma card) enabled the doctor or nurse to ascertain quickly that the patient had asthma, rather than scan up and down pages of consultations. The equivalent way of making the diagnosis visible in a computer record is to "code" it. Good computer records, therefore, rely on the clinician coding all the relevant information. There are no national standards about what should be coded, or how many items in a consultation. However, good records should have a coded problem title (diagnosis or symptom code), and other key data (relevant co-morbidities, family history, symptoms and signs) coded as well. There should be sufficient information for another clinician to be able to pick up the care of that patient, and for patients to benefit from computer searches to find patients who may be suboptimally managed, or who need an additional intervention (e.g. calling in for a flu immunization). Since April 2004, computerized records in the UK have been used to monitor progress towards delivering financially incentivized quality-based targets for CDM.

Routinely collected computer data are readily available for clinical audit, quality improvement, and research. The creation of the readily searchable computerized medical record has greatly improved the potential for KM activity within primary care [39]. Much of what is currently done is retrospective, involving relatively straightforward data processing [40]; however, health service managers cited their inability to access routinely collected data as one of their principal barriers to managing effectively [41]. Once mastered, though, it is inevitable that more advanced data-mining techniques will be used to generate better information in the future.

2.4   Knowledge Needs of Primary Care Professionals

Primary care professionals have a broad range of knowledge needs. Biomedical knowledge is essential to primary care professionals, and included in this is EBM, covering many aspects of diagnosis, treatment, and prescribing. Emphasis in the UK has recently been put on the management of chronic conditions, across the NHS as well as in primary care, with the introduction of National Service Frameworks and the activity of the NHS Modernisation Agency [42]. The role of primary care professionals is changing to one focused on CDM, with less out-of-hours activity. In addition to caring for patients, UK primary care professionals are also asked to take on a managerial role within the health system. There have been a series of initiatives with in the UK health service which have given primary care a powerful role in commissioning care. The objective of these reforms could be interpreted as incentivizing practitioners to reform the way they deliver care and manage demand. These reforms have included:

- fundholding,
- primary-care-led NHS,
- personal medical services, and most recently
- practice-based commissioning.

Emphasis on CDM and commissioning care have prioritized knowledge needs associated with the biomedical approach to disease, which are potentially different to the knowledge needs when caring for people without a definite diagnostic category.

It has been demonstrated that all professional groups in primary care welcome and support evidence-based practice. In support of the view that primary care professionals are suffering from information overload, the most important facilitator for the use of EBM was found to be protected time [43]. As well as welcoming and supporting EBM, information supporting evidence-based practice has been shown to be used and valued by the majority of doctors in an Australian study [44]. But as discussed in Section 2.1, primary care has its own barriers to the implementation of evidence-based medicine.

2.5   Knowledge Management Model for Primary Care

A comparison of the decision-making environment in general practice and hospital serves to illustrate some of the speciality specific needs of primary care. As noted by Balint [31], the primary care consultation is a complicated phenomenon. Doctors themselves are a "drug" with effects and side effects which perhaps deserve their own pharmacology. ICT solutions offered by KM tend to overlook aspects of the consultation such as this and are in danger of supplying unwanted solutions. We have already discussed how decisions in primary care are often made on a heuristic basis (intelligent rules of thumb) rather that using deductive reasoning; this, in turn, leads us to the view that human–computer interfaces that set cognitive models (except in a small number of well-defined disease areas) are likely to fail [27].

Knowledge can be either tacit or explicit (explicit knowledge can be found in the form of guidelines and is easily available, whereas tacit knowledge is subjective and cognitive). As tacit knowledge is often stored in the minds of healthcare professionals, one of the objectives of KM is to transform tacit knowledge into explicit knowledge to allow effective dissemination. This transfer of tacit knowledge to explicit knowledge is exemplified by databases such as Medline [45] and the Turning Research into Practice (TRIP) [46], and online collections of guidelines such as Prescribing Rationally in General Practice (PRODIGY) [47] and the National Institute of Clinical Excellence (NICE) [48]. Resources such as these enable clinicians to cope with the ever-expanding body of medical knowledge, and information retrieval systems have been shown to improve the quality of answers provided by clinicians to typical clinical problems [49].

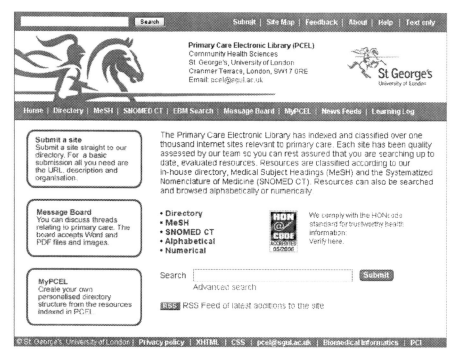

FIGURE 2.4. Primary Care Electronic Library (PCEL).

As well as the tacit/explicit knowledge dichotomy, KM projects can be divided into information- and learner-centered activities. Information-centered KM disseminates existing knowledge, whereas learner-centered KM aims to create opportunities to accelerate learning. It has been suggested that KM activities fall into four groups on the basis of the tacit/explicit nature of knowledge and information/learner-centered activities [50]. EBM is perhaps the most well known instance of KM, falling in the information-centered and explicit knowledge area.

Our own project in KM is the PCEL. This is a KM application that fits into the explicit knowledge and information-centered model area. We have worked in this area for some time, initially through the Doctor's Desk [35], then developing the primary care virtual branch library of the National Electronic Library for Health [51]. PCEL is our most recent development [52]. It is a case study of information-centered KM designed to disseminate specialist information (Figure 2.4). PCEL fits with one of the key aims of KM: the transformation of tacit knowledge into explicit knowledge, in order that it can be shared amongst colleagues. This objective is achieved by PCEL, in that the resources which are presented online are quality assured and assessed for their relevance to primary care. Every resource in the library has an electronic index card which presents metadata concerning each entry. The electronic indexing is designed to allow rapid searching of over 1000 resources stored within a database. These index cards can be searched via free text

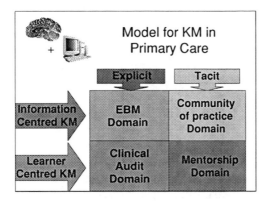

FIGURE 2.5. A KM model for primary care.

or an advanced search and can also be browsed alphabetically or numerically. The index cards are also cross-referenced by MeSH (Medical Subject Headings) terms [53], allowing browsing or retrieval of resources indexed with the same term.

Our proposed KM model seeks to balance, if not reconcile, the need for both explicit and tacit knowledge; as well as both the information- and learner-centered styles. It has been suggested that a combined approach to KM is inappropriate [54]; we do not agree with this, believing that this is needed to cope with the complexities of primary care. Primary care has to deal with individuals with their unique health beliefs, ideas, concerns, and expectations, whilst having to achieve evidence-based health gains for populations.

The model (Figure 2.5), in it simplest form, is a two-by-two matrix of explicit and tacit knowledge on its x-axis and information- and learner-centered activities on its y-axis. The model aims to encourage primary care professionals to have a portfolio of information management tools, as well as to be participating in learning activities. The model also encourages connecting with and learning about tacit information, as well as explicit information. Four prototypical activities or learning types for the model are proposed; however, this is not to say that, prescriptively, they have to be part of each primary care professional's KM portfolio. They should be regarded as exemplars, of how the set of knowledge activities might be made up, and what the place of information technology might be within the model.

2.6   Summary

In summary, we feel that primary care needs a broad approach to KM. Its complexity does not lend itself to a single approach. The complexities of primary care reflect that people have multiple complex problems contextualized by their own health beliefs and life experiences. Primary care practitioners need to form relationships over a long time period with their patients and know how to consult effectively, dispensing what Balint described as "drug doctor." Alongside this they need to implement nationally and locally agreed evidence-based targets for disease management, but they need to do so in an environment that manages demand and controls costs. The proposed model takes cognizance of needs for tacit and explicit knowledge and of learner- and information-centered KM. Our assertion is that the unique speciality of primary care needs a portfolio of KM, rather than any single tool.

References

1. de Lusignan S, Lakhani M, Chan T. The role of informatics in continuing professional development and quality improvement in primary care. *J Postgrad Med* 2003;49(2):163–165. URL: http://www.jpgmonline.com/article.asp?issn=0022-3859;year=2003;volume=49;issue=2;spage=163;epage=5;aulast=de.
2. Wyatt CJ. Reading journals and monitoring the published work. *J R Soc Med* 2000;93:423–427 Available from: http://www.jrsm.org/cgi/reprint/93/8/423?ijkey=fca389c6a4b4ec26eea825e25d81a1c9e33e0d46&keytype2=tf_ipsecsha [accessed October 2005].
3. Wyatt J. Use and sources of medical knowledge. *Lancet* 1991;338:1368–1373. Available from: http://www.ncbi.nlm.nih.gov/entrez/query.fcgi?cmd=retrieve&db=pubmed&list_uids=1682745&dopt=Abstract [accessed October 2005].
4. Hibble A, Kanka D, Pencheon D, Pooles F. Guidelines in general practice: the new Tower of Babel? *Br Med J* 1998;317:862–863 Available from: http://bmj.bmjjournals.com/cgi/content/full/317/7162/862 [accessed November 2005].
5. Bali RK (editor). Issues in clinical knowledge management: revisiting healthcare management. In: *Clinical knowledge management: opportunities and challenges.* Idea Group Publishing; 2005, chapter 1. Available from: http://www.idea-group.com/downloads/excerpts/Bali01.pdf [accessed September 2005].
6. Sackett DL, Rosenberg WMC, Muir Gray JA, Haynes RB, WSRichardson. Evidence based medicine: what it is and what it isn't. *Br Med J* 1996;312:71–72. Available from: http://bmj.bmjjournals.com/cgi/content/full/312/7023/71 [accessed September 2005].
7. Schmid K, Conen D. Integrated patient pathways: "MIPP"—a tool for quality improvement and cost management in health care. Pilot study on the pathway "Acute Myocardial Infarction." *Int J Health Care Qual Assur* 13(2):87–92 [Online] Available from: http://www.emeraldinsight.com/Insight/html/Output/Published/EmeraldFullTextArticle/Articles/0620130205.html [accessed September 2005].
8. Halligan A, Donaldson L. Implementing clinical governance: turning vision into reality. *Br Med J* 2001;322:1413–1417 Available from: http://bmj.bmjjournals.com/cgi/content/full/322/7299/1413 [accessed September 2005].
9. Roland M. Linking physicians' pay to the quality of care—a major experiment in the United Kingdom *New Engl J Med* 2004;351:1448–1454.
10. Bali R. Preface. In: *Issues in clinical knowledge management—opportunities and challenges.* Idea Group Publishing; 2005. Available from: http://www.idea-group.com/books/additional.asp?id=4892&title=Preface&col=preface [accessed September 2005].
11. American Health Informatics Management Association. Available from: http://library.ahima.org/xpedio/groups/public/documents/ahima/pub_bok1_025042.html [accessed September 2005].

12. Senge P. Reflection on "A leaders new work: building learning organisations." In Moorey D, Maybury M, Thuraisingham B, editors, *Knowledge management: classic and contemporary works*. Cambridge, MA; MIT Press; 2000.

13. de Lusignan S, Wells S, Singleton A. Why general practitioners do not implement evidence. Learning environments must be created that capitalise on teams' wealth of knowledge. *Br Med J*. 2002;324(7338):674.

14. Freeman C, Sweeney K. Why general practitioners do not implement evidence: qualitative study. *Br Med J* 2001;323:1100. Available from: http://bmj.bmjjournals.com/cgi/content/full/323/7321/1100 [accessed November 2005].

15. WHO/Europe. Declaration of Alma-Ata; 1978. Available from: http://www.euro.who.int/AboutWHO/Policy/20010827_1 [accessed October 2005].

16. Starfield B. Is primary care essential? *Lancet* 1994;344(8930):1129–1133. Available from: http://www.sbmfc.org.br/site/bib/download/isprimarycare.pdf [accessed October 2005].

17. Institute of Medicine, Committee on the Future of Primary Care. *Primary care: America's health in a new era*. Washington, DC: National Academy Press; 1996.

18. WONCA Europe. The European definition of general practice/family medicine; 2002. Available from: http://www.woncaeurope.org/Web%20documents/European%20Definition%20of%20family%20medicine/The%20European%20Definition%20of%20General%20Practice%20and%20Family%20Medicine.pdf [accessed 2005 November].

19. de Lusignan S. What is primary care informatics? *J Am Med Inform Assoc* 2003;10(4):304–309. Available from: http://www.ncbi.nlm.nih.gov/entrez/query.fcgi?cmd=Retrieve&db=pubmed&dopt=Abstract&list_uids=12668690&query_hl=3 [accessed November 2005].

20. Starfield B. Measuring the attainment of primary care. *J Med Educ* 1979;54(5):361–369. Available from: http://www.ncbi.nlm.nih.gov/entrez/query.fcgi?cmd=Retrieve&db=PubMed&list_uids=374735&dopt=Abstract [accessed November 2005].

21. Essex B. *Doctors dilemmas and decisions*. London: BMJ Books; 1994.

22. Musen M.A. Medical Informatics: searching for underlying components. *Methods Inf Med* 2002;41:12-9.

23. Poirier TI, Giudici RA. Drug interaction microcomputer software evaluation: PDR's drug interactions and side effects diskettes. *Hosp Pharm* 1990;(9):839-42, 851

24. Lobato Madueno F, Portillo Strempel J, Perez Vicente A, Garcia Lopez A, Garcia Raso MA, Morilla Herrera JC. Detection by a computer program of drug interactions in chronic patients. Its practical usefulness in a health center *Aten Prim* 1997;19(3):138–141

25. Hunt DL, Haynes RB, Morgan D. Using old technology to implement modern computer-aided decision support for primary diabetes care. *Proc AMIA Symp* 2001;274–278.

26. Fugelli P. Trust—in general practice. *BJGP* 2001;51:575–579.

27. Suchman L. *Plans and situated actions*. Cambridge: Cambridge University Press; 1987

28. Eccles M, McColl E, Steen N, Rousseau N, Grimshaw J, Parkin D, et al. Effect of computerised evidence based guidelines on management of asthma and angina in adults in primary care: cluster randomised controlled trial. *Br Med J* 2002;325:941–944.

29. Rousseau N, McColl E, Newton J, Grimshaw J, Eccles M. Practice based, longitudinal, qualitative interview study of computerised evidence based guidelines in primary care. *Br Med J* 2003;326:314.

30. Maviglia SM, Zielsttorff RD, Paterno M, Teich JM, Bates DW, Kuperman GJ. Automating complex guidelines for chronic disease: lesson's learned. *J Am Med Inform Assoc* 2003;10(2):154–165.
31. Balint M. *The doctor, his patient, and the illness*. London: Tavistock Press; 1957.
32. Griffiths F, Byrne D. General practice and the new science emerging from the theories of "chaos" and complexity. *Br J Gen Pract* 1998;48(435):1697–1699.
33. Miller WL, Crabtree BF, McDaniel R, Stange KC. Understanding change in primary care practice using complexity theory. *J Fam Pract* 1998;46(5):369–376.
34. Chapman J. A systems perspective on computing in the NHS. *Inform Prim Care* 2002;10:197–199.
35. de Lusignan S. The Doctors Desk. One vision of how to deliver the future information and communication needs of general practice. *J Inform Prim Care* 1998;(May):19–22.
36. Robinson J, de Lusignan S, Kostkova P. The Primary Care Electronic Library (PCEL) five years on: open source evaluation of usage. *Inform Primy Care* 2005; 13(4):271–80.
37. Rithie LD. *Computers in primary care*. London: William Heinemann; 1984.
38. Weed LL. *Medical records, medical education and patient care*. Cleveland: Case Western Reserve Press; 1969.
39. de Lusignan S, van Weel C. The use of routinely collected computer data for research in primary care: opportunities and challenges. *Fam Pract* 2006 (Apr.); 23(2):253–63.
40. van Vlymen J, de Lusignan S, Hague N, Chan T, Dzregah B. Ensuring the quality of aggregated general practice data: lessons from the Primary Care Data Quality Programme (PCDQ). *Stud Health Technol Inform* 2005;116:1010–1015.
41. de Lusignan S, Wells S, Shaw A, Rowlands G, Crilly T. A knowledge audit of the managers of primary care organizations: top priority is how to use routinely collected clinical data for quality improvement. *Med Inform Internet Med* 2005;30(1):69–80.
42. Lewis R, Dixon J. Rethinking management of chronic diseases. *Br Med J* 2004;328:220–222. Available from: http://bmj.bmjjournals.com/cgi/content/full/328/7433/220 [accessed October 2005].
43. O'Donnell CA. Attitudes and knowledge of primary care professionals towards evidence-based practice: a postal survey. *J Eval Clin Pract* 2004;10(2):197–205. Available from: http://www.ncbi.nlm.nih.gov/entrez/query.fcgi?cmd=Retrieve&db=pubmed&dopt=Abstract&list_uids=15189386&query_hl=1 [accessed November 2005].
44. Westbrook JI, Gosling AS, Westbrook MT. Use of point-of-care online clinical evidence by junior and senior doctors in New South Wales public hospitals. *Intern Med J* 2005;35:399–404. Available from: http://www.ncbi.nlm.nih.gov/entrez/query.fcgi?cmd=Retrieve&db=pubmed&dopt=Abstract&list_uids=15958109&query_hl=3 [accessed November 2005].
45. PubMed. National Library of Medicine; 2005. Available from: http://www.ncbi.nlm.nih.gov/entrez/query.fcgi [accessed November 2005].
46. Turning Research into Practice (TRIP); 2005. Available from: http://www.tripdatabase.com/ [accessed November 2005].
47. PRODIGY; 2005. Available from: http://www.prodigy.nhs.uk/indexMain.asp [accessed November 2005].
48. National Institute for Clinical Excellence (NICE); 2005. Available from: http://www.nice.org.uk/ [accessed November 2005].
49. Westbrook JI, Coiera EW, Gosling AS. Do online information retrieval systems help experienced clinicians answer clinical questions? *J Am Med Inform Assoc* 2005;12(3):315–321. Available from: http://www.ncbi.nlm.nih.gov/entrez/query.

fcgi?cmd=Retrieve&db=pubmed&dopt=Abstract&list_uids=15684126&query_hl=11 [accessed November 2005].

50. de Lusignan S, Pritchard K, Chan T. A knowledge-management model for clinical practice. *J Postgrad Med* 2002;48(4);297–303. Available from: http://www.jpgmonline.com/article.asp?issn=0022-3859;year=2002;volume=48;issue=4;spage=297;epage=303;aulast=de [accessed September 2005].

51. Muir Gray JA, de Lusignan S. National Electronic Library for Health (NeLH). *Br Med J* 1999;319(7223):1476–1479.

52. Primary Care Electronic Library; 2005. Available from: http://www.pcel.info/ [accessed September 2005].

53. Medical Subject Headings—Home Page; 2005. Available from: http://www.nlm.nih.gov/mesh/meshhome.html [accessed September 2005].

54. Brown JS, Duiguid P. Balancing act—how to capture knowledge without killing it. *Harv Bus Rev* 2000;R00309:45–59.

3
Role of Information Professionals as Intermediaries for Knowledge Management in Evidence-Based Healthcare

GABBY FENNESSY AND FRADA BURSTEIN

Abstract

The common practice of evidence-based healthcare can also include information professionals as intermediaries in a socio-technical framework of knowledge management for supporting medical decision making. Intermediaries play a part in supporting task performance at the level of practical activity. This chapter describes challenges associated with implementation of knowledge management for evidence-based healthcare. In particular, we explore the role of intermediaries in meeting information needs of healthcare professionals. The chapter describes a field study that evaluated the impact of using intermediaries on indicators such as rigor, speed and completeness of information provision and appraisal and interpretation of knowledge selection.

3.1 Introduction

There is an anomaly between the amount of time, effort, and money that is invested in seeking and providing information to healthcare practitioners in order to help their decision making and the lack of what is generated from this process. This is a typical situation for somebody using evidence based healthcare to facilitate decision making. Knowledge management (KM) in the context of evidence-based healthcare creates a learning environment and ensures that "best practice" is captured and disseminated. KM in healthcare is a complex process involving many information processes that need special skills and support. A range of tools and techniques has been considered to improve the speed and quality of information provision. Some of those are technology based, others require people in roles specifically devoted to supporting the knowledge needs of healthcare practitioners. There is a challenge in establishing the right balance and combination of the technology and human skills so that decision-making needs are met in the most effective and efficient way.

   The common practice of evidence-based medicine in meeting information needs of medical practitioners may also include information professionals as intermediaries in a socio-technical framework of knowledge management. Intermediaries play a part in supporting information needs for task performance at the level of practical activity. Moreover, knowledge generated by these "intermediaries," at both an individual and a collective level, becomes a valuable resource that can be reused as a meta-knowledge of performing future requests for new evidence.

The role of information providers and the work they have to perform in an evidence-based practice context in turning information into meaningful knowledge has seldom been explored. Such a role is one of supporting decision making, by acting as an intermediary between the health practitioner and the large range of knowledge available. Up to now there has been some talk about a chief knowledge officer in evidence-based practice and the role of KM [1], but the extent of its application to this area of healthcare has not been elaborated. An extension of this concept to include information technology has also been hampered by a lack of support for such work close to where healthcare decisions are made about the patient [2].

This research builds on previous work [3, 4–5] which established that tacit knowledge and exploiting human understandings of the evidence was more important for KM than codified knowledge available through databases.

The use of intermediaries, information professionals, as part of the KM for decision support within the context of evidence-based practice has not been studied empirically [5]. Can information professionals enhance decision making as part of the KM process? Is this process improved compared with end users using technology for themselves? Current views are divergent on this issue [6–8]. These differ about whether practitioners are best placed to meet their own evidence-based information needs well, or whether intermediaries who have specific skills, time, and expertise could do this more effectively.

In this chapter we explore challenges associated with implementation of KM for evidence-based healthcare. In particular, we investigate the role of intermediaries in meeting information needs of healthcare professionals and compare this role with replacing it with technology solutions. The chapter reports on a field study that explored how intermediaries can be used to improve decision-making performance. We used indicators such as rigor, speed, and completeness of knowledge selection, appraisal, and interpretation as the basis for performance comparison.

3.2 Knowledge Management in Evidence-Based Healthcare

Defining knowledge is a core issue in the KM literature. In a healthcare context, the question of what makes up "knowledge" is also very complex. This type of knowledge has been mapped out by Eraut [9], and comprises tacit knowledge as its very important component. This practice knowledge, or set of working assumptions, is not brought to scrutiny on a routine basis. Such tacit knowledge can be broken down into:

- Empirical knowledge, i.e. the hard facts, which is usually owned by professionals, such as physiology.
- Process knowledge, which is about how to get things done and how the health process operates.
- Control knowledge, which is about dealing with feelings and emotions, designed to be used in ethical ways.
- Knowledge of people, which is concerned with anticipating how others will behave.

Using evidence to inform decision making will influence the first two types of tacit knowledge described here, i.e. informing both empirical and process knowledge. Within the hospital setting, health practitioners have questions about:

- What is best practice?
- Is it effective?
- How do interventions compare in terms of their relative effectiveness?

Such questions are raised in the day-to-day work of healthcare practitioners, but also as a means of problem solving at an organizational level. Providing information to support evidence-based decision making in healthcare is a complex and nonstructured component of KM, where information is acquired, retrieved, sifted, and appraised before being handed on to practitioners so that decisions can be informed [3]. The central role of information in evidence-based healthcare has always been widely recognized. Information provides a cornerstone for deciding what is the best available evidence and best practice [10,11].

Evidence-based practice has been defined as "the practice of . . . integrating individual clinical expertise with the best available external clinical evidence from systematic research" [10]. Using the best available evidence means identifying and integrating the most current research and practice results for effective care in order to support clinical decision making of the healthcare practitioners.

Evidence-based practice has evolved as a movement within healthcare systems to understand how health resources can be used most effectively to improve health outcomes and the quality of patient care. At an individual level it is a way of helping health practitioners who are overwhelmed with the information explosion, who have limited time and resources to pursue their questions. A range of people, tools, and techniques can be engaged to improve the speed and quality of decision making. From an organizational level, health services are under pressure to make use of finite resources; evidence-based practice may be one way of rationalizing expenditure.

From an early stage, information providers become knowledge workers within an evidence-based context [12]. They utilize their specialist skills to translate complex requests for evidence into a search for codified knowledge. Moreover, they use their knowledge to link the practitioner making the request to a range of tacit knowledge that exists within the organization.

The potential of knowledge creation within this context is a strong driver for introducing a system for managing such knowledge. The aim is to capture this knowledge at the point of when it is being created and make it available as part of decision support in similar contexts.

Up until now, decision support using evidence-based practice has been in the form of computer reminders, which integrate clinical guidelines and protocols [13,14]. These systems provide excellent summaries of good-quality evidence, making recommendations for practice, but they are usually limited in scope and topic coverage, due to the high cost and amount of time involved in developing them. At a pragmatic level, practitioners have a lack of skills, time, and understanding of what to look for [15]. Current decision-support systems, which can be viewed to overcome such problems, are not found in all areas of healthcare, and in many cases they may be based on "individual expert opinion" rather than the best available evidence [16]. The time required and the skills needed to use such systems are also issues, when practitioners view their time as best used in direct patient care, rather than involving information systems, which may slow down the healthcare process.

3.3 Exploratory Case Study

KM within a context of evidence-based healthcare gives the potential to improve quality of service. This section provides results from a project that explores a KM approach for knowledge workers from the Southern Health Care Network [17]. Participants were recruited when the researchers approached a specialist evidence center. This center was funded by the state government, to provide information about clinical effectiveness to all health practitioners within a network of four hospitals. The service has been running for over six years, and addressed enquiries from medics, professions allied to medicine, nurses, and midwives. The researchers observed that the range in difficulty and complexity of such enquiries, depended on the questions and especially on the types of evidence, which can be found and used to answer the question asked [4,18].

The major aim of this empirical study was to investigate how intermediaries can be used in to improve the performance in evidence-based healthcare decision making. Decision support within this context is based on communicating the right knowledge to the right user. In a general knowledge management context, the concept of "intermediaries" can be compared with that of a "chauffeur-decision-maker" [19], "a person who helps the users, perhaps merely as a clerical assistant, to push the buttons of the terminal, or perhaps as a more substantial staff assistant, to interact and make suggestions" [20]. It is acknowledged as a role, which is often needed to meet busy work requirements of the chief executive officers; however, advances in decision-support technologies are often driven by the aim of making decision-support systems more accessible and usable to the immediate decision makers. The example of evidence-based practice shows that the role of intermediaries may be needed regardless of the progress of technical systems, because of the sophistication of the questions and the complexity of knowledge available.

Intermediaries help decisions being made at all levels, knowing about healthcare and the politics that influence such decisions. They have access and contribute to information resources, and the skills to sift and find information. In particular, their role becomes critical when the decision maker does not know where to look for the evidence to support their judgment, not having the skills to work out what is high-quality information that can be used in the particular situation. The intermediaries are there to ask the right questions: searching for relevant information to supportg implementation of the decision, performing critical appraisal evaluation, and negotiation of the context-specific meaning of the information. All these activities of the intermediary are essential to overcoming the information barriers of the practitioner-decision-maker, as well as to generate potentially new knowledge for both participants.

By creating knowledge from information searching, acquisition, sifting, and interpretation, the intermediary brings knowledge to the decision-support process. In this respect, the role of intermediaries in decision support can be seen in supporting task performance, as well as in KM and learning within the organization [20]. Within a systems approach to decision support, intermediaries can be considered as part of a socio-technical decision-support system.

The research described in this section tests whether intermediaries can enhance a range of performance outcomes relating decision making based on the best available evidence. The performance measurement factors under investigation include:

- *Rigor*: how well evidence is appraised for its own internal rigor and validity, through critical appraisal; and its relevance to the question.
- *Completeness*: that a wider range of resources is searched, including databases, websites, and experts.
- *Timeliness*: that the two preceding indicators can be carried out within a reasonable amount of time between asking the question and finding evidence to support an answer

3.3.1   Empirical Study Design Model

The following model represents the basis for the empirical study described in this chapter (see Figure 3.1). It aims to test whether decision-making performance is improved when using intermediaries, and if they perform better in rigor, completeness, and timeliness of utilizing the evidence for decision making.

3.3.2   Field Study

A group of health practitioners and intermediaries within a large healthcare center in Melbourne, Australia [17], were used to test the contingency model. Participants for this research were approached after a search of the Internet was done, looking for organizations in Australia who work in the area of evidence-based practice information. The nature of their work follows the principles described in Section 3.3.

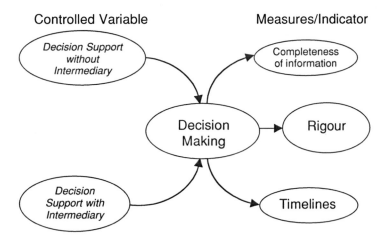

FIGURE 3.1. Evidence-based decision-support evaluation framework (adapted from [5], p. 69).

Health practitioners were recruited from the same organization. These were people who had knowledge of evidence-based practice and had also used the center. Choosing this subset of the practitioner population meant that participants could contrast their own experiences of searching and appraising the evidence with that of using the center as an intermediary.

3.3.3 Data Collection

To explore decision performance in evidence-based practice, ten healthcare practitioners and seven intermediaries were investigated using a range of data collection techniques. These included interviews, focus groups, and observation of practice.

Soft systems methodology (SSM) was used to map how key indicators were influenced and performed within the intermediary environment and within a health practitioner environment [4,21,22]. Rich pictures were used to illustrate the steps required in seeking the evidence; these were validated by both groups of participants, and as being the desired pathway that people should follow in order to get the best available evidence [22]. These steps in finding and appraising the evidence are reflected in the literature from a range of experts in the evidence-based practice community [23,24].

A range of interviews with intermediaries and a representative sample of health practitioners supplemented this, focusing on the relationship between intermediary and health practitioners. Other data analyzed were collected internally over a period of 18 months by the center in the form of user questionnaires, investigating why they used the center, and what they did with the evidence once they had it. Using a wide variety of data sources allowed many aspects of decision making, knowledge work, practice and interaction to be investigated within a short time frame so that data could be triangulated.

3.3.4 Analysis

Information seeking and knowledge flows were mapped out using rich pictures and conceptual modeling [4,22]. Participants also added their own perspectives about what was taking place, therefore validating the models and rich pictures. A group of international knowledge workers in the field of evidence-based practice also externally validated models. Interviews and qualitative comments from questionnaires were thematically analyzed using the qualitative software program NUDIST (nonnumerical unstructured data indexing, searching and theorizing) Nvivo™. Coding of the text was not simply a mechanical process of labeling, but itself formed part of the analysis process, with interpretation and formulation of theoretical perspectives as the analysis progressed.

3.3.5 Findings

3.3.5.1 Improvement of Indicators

Improvement in the information quality indicators, ie rigour, speed, completeness of selection, appraisal and interpretation is not clear cut. All measures identified for the purposes of this research are subjective and self-reported. To date, no objective measures of the completeness or rigor of searching and appraisal have been developed; there are only "rules of thumb" [23,25] or accepted standards set up by experts in the area. Further, in this chapter we present the results of the comparative analysis supported by the quotes taken from the interviews with practitioners (Pract) and information professionals used as intermediaries (Int) as part of knowledge management systems.

3.3.5.2 Intermediaries: Why Use Them?

Much of this research has explored issues of end users not solving evidence-based questions for themselves. This includes a lack of skills, time and understanding of what to look for [15]. Current knowledge management systems, which can be viewed to overcome such problems, are not found in all areas of healthcare, and in many cases may not be based on good-quality research [16]. The time and the skills required to use such systems are also an issue, when practitioners view their time as best used in direct patient care, rather than involving systems, which may slow down the healthcare process. One of the practitioners reflected:

"The only problem is that the area is so busy. It's actually making time when you're away from the phone and away from the work, to be able to take it on board. It is very, very hard to split yourself into two and say "ok 15 minutes to do this, I've got to listen to that phone or listen to that emergency bell", you just can't do it during work hours." (Pract)

Articulation of information needs relating to the problem at hand is the second problem. Until they talk to someone else about the issue, practitioners have a problem in expressing information needs and relating this to the problem at hand.

"Making sense" of complex problems as part of decision support may pose a challenge when practitioners have trouble trying to articulate the problem:

"I had no idea what I was looking for, I had hundreds of questions and no way of knowing how to ask them in a way that was focused". (Pract)

"... most of the questions we have to answer are not worded properly. They're not worded in an evidence-based way; in a way that they should be worded". (Int)

To resolve this, a conversation needs to take place between the practitioner and the intermediary. At this stage the practitioner can receive feedback about the viability of the question, whether a search for the best available evidence is appropriate, and whether there are a range of questions. Such a conversation becomes part of a transformation from question, to information sharing, to shared knowledge about the issue at hand. Another information professional reported:

"... it puts so much stress on you, you're trying to figure out what they're asking, you try and figure out the question, and try and find the answer to that question so that you interpret from the round about way they talk to you". (Int)

3.3.5.3   Rigor of Searching and Appraising the Evidence

Evidence-based practice, when described in the context of the Task-based Knowledge Management [25], presumes that past instances of task performance are stored in memory; the actor has an individual model of the task (implicit/explicit), as well as access to the shared knowledge and understanding of the task developed by other members of the team. To carry out the task at hand, the actor "makes real" the task model by filling it with current information relevant to the problem situation at hand. Making such a model a reality requires the actor's skills and tacit knowledge. Memory helps the actor to adapt task performance to meet the specifics of the current enquiry.

The individual memory helps the actor to provide the historical basis of developing, creating, and changing tasks to ensure that the information provider reaches his or her goals. However, often the medical practitioner get frustrated, because:

"Information gained was non-conclusive; the quality of the search is astounding. Lack of evidence inspires research". (Pract)

On the other hand, information professionals face different problems:

"I get many similar questions, so that I know where to search on the Web, and what sites are not useful, this makes the process relatively fast". (Int)

Uptake of the use of intermediaries also improved over time. Since the inception of the center, use has increased monthly, from just a few requests for the evidence, to an average of 40 questions, to the point of now rationing the service. This indicates that practitioners see the value, improved rigor, and speed at which intermediaries can add to decision making. One of them stated:

"If it's quiet, either management encourage you to go down to the library, that's the appropriate environment to be doing searches, or have a room that has a computer set up, away from the nurses' desk, away from the phones, where you can do your work without being interrupted. You get constantly interrupted if you are sitting at the desk. It's not the sort of environment where you want to be trying to look things up". (Pract)

This response is in contrast to that of the intermediary; by constantly carrying out the same tasks of retrieving and appraising the evidence. Here, they are consistently seeing a range of practitioners seeking the evidence, and thus building upon these experiences to provide faster, more sophisticated solutions to complex questions.

3.3.5.4 Appraisal

While there is some evidence that suggests that critical appraisal teaching has positive effects on attitudes, knowledge, and skills, there are gaps as to whether it impacts on decision making, or indeed whether any impact is large enough to be of practical significance [24]. The findings from this study show that health practitioners see intermediaries as "experts" who have the skills to do this more quickly and have a role to decide the value of the evidence on behalf of practitioners [4,5]. As one informant states:

"I was looking for comment on the worth of papers". (Pract)

On the other hand, information professionals confirm:

". . . look at the validity of the evidence we search, this is less bias because we are not based in clinical practice and concentrate on the methodology without worrying about the context around us". (Int)

These comments illustrate a wider view, that many practitioners do not have research methods training or the critical appraisal skills to do this type of work for themselves. It would, therefore, seem logical to utilize someone in a role removed from direct clinical practice that has experience of evaluating validity.

3.3.5.5 Completeness

The breadth of searching for the evidence has progressed beyond simple database searching. The evidence-based practice movement has moved towards more prescriptive and accepted pathways that should be searched in order to produce a complete result. This generally begins with the Cochrane library, and moves in conjunction with levels of evidence [26,30], i.e. from sources that look to reduce bias in reporting, such as systematic reviews of randomized controlled trials, to more biased sources of evidence of effectiveness, such as expert opinion. If questions are not fulfilled by level 1 and 2 sources, then levels 3 and 4 may need to be explored. Looking at levels of evidence beyond systematic reviews may require wider searches of the Internet, including the learned societies, and "gray" literature.

Such completeness in covering a range of sources was realized by practitioners who used intermediaries:

... very impressed by the range of databases able to search far more than I can access easily using university OVID databases, thanks. (Pract)

Information professional explains this:

... we have an agreed pathway to follow when we search for the evidence, the less level I and II evidence we find the wider we have to go, this means going to wider literature and appraising primary sources. (Int)

Confirmation that there was little or no evidence to support some decisions was deemed to be just as important, and was often much more difficult for both practitioners and intermediaries to conclude:

"... no information was available on the subject investigates. It's at least good to know that". (Pract)

"... the literature search done by the Centre was very thorough. However the studies to answer the question have not been done". (Pract)

This process of being inclusive in searching for the evidence contributes to the ongoing building of memory, which reflects experience and knowledge of the task. Such a complex task is influenced by past experience of the task of transforming questions for evidence into action. The intermediary takes the problem to develop their understanding not only relevant to this context, but also takes the "knowledge" that has been gained from this encounter to inform further encounters with other practitioners in a continuous KM.

3.3.5.6   Timeliness

The time that it takes to complete a rigorous search and appraisal of the evidence will vary according to the complexity of the question and the amount of evidence that can be found in searching. Measures of timeliness in delivering both of these tasks will, therefore, vary and be of a subjective nature. The speed with which intermediaries carried out both searching and appraisal of a wide range of evidence was illustrated through their own evaluation of work, the more evidence-based search they worked on, and the more efficient they became. Practitioners also reflected on whether they had the time to complete the task:

"... great service particularly for clinical staff who do not have the time during their working day to do this sort of thing". (Pract)

"... sometimes it takes us a few weeks to do the search for users, but even so, because there is so much rigour put into the process I doubt whether most medics would have the time or resources to do the same". (Int)

An evaluation of the intermediaries' performance was elicited by questions in interviews and questionnaires that asked about how the center had performed at carrying out requests:

"... this was a rush job that the Centre completed very quickly". (Pract)

"I was impressed by the timeliness and of contact and efforts made". (Pract)

Practitioners were at pains to point at that they had little time away from providing care to carry out searching for themselves. The alternative was to carry out the task in private time:

"Main barrier is time!! Even though I strongly believe evidence based practice is integral to my practice, I have little time to access and familiarise myself with the associated information". (Pract)

"Heavy workloads mean that all research or reading has to be done in my own time. Sometimes then too tired or fed up to put in extra time". (Pract)

3.4   Conclusion and Discussion

The findings from this study have implications for the provision of an evidence-based practice information service and the education of end users, i.e. health practitioners, in information seeking for clinical knowledge management. While it cannot be contended that excessive education in searching and appraising the evidence is a waste of time, it could be argued that investment in ad hoc training programs has little impact on health practitioner skills and effectiveness in retrieving and appraising the evidence. Monies invested by governments, professional organizations, and education providers in this area cannot currently be directly linked to improvements in decision making. Follow up, constant repetition of skills learned, and a conducive working environment must be in place before clinicians can hone their evidence-based skills to a level that makes it time and cost effective for them to take this role on themselves in continuous KM context. Perhaps resources could be better spent in investing in intermediaries who already possess the skills required to do the work on behalf of practitioners.

The move of health systems to using evidence-based practice has meant focusing on the need for clinicians to keep up to date and improve not only their own skills in seeking the evidence, but also to build on their own knowledge base of what effective practice is. Developing decision-support systems for health practitioners to answer questions about clinical effectiveness as part of systematic KM can be a way of improving decision making and improving on a range of performance indicators. However, as we have demonstrated in this study, there is a strong role for information management professionals to serve as an integral part of a socio-technical system of KM for decision support. If the performance measures outlined in this chapter are elected as being of importance to health practitioners, then using intermediaries gives a better overall result in decision making, compared with healthcare practitioners practicing an evidence-based approach and using the technology by themselves.

Acknowledgment. This research was partly funded by the Australian Research Council and a Monash University grant.

References

1. Muir Gray JA. Where's the chief knowledge officer? *Br Med J* 1998;317:832–840.
2. Smith I, Palmer J. Getting to the evidence. *Health Serv J* 1998;108(5606)(suppl):4–6.
3. Fennessy G. What's the evidence? Clinical effectiveness. *Nurs Stand* 1998;13(8):1–13.
4. Fennessy G. Knowledge management in evidence based practice: study of a community of practice. PhD thesis, Monash University; 2002.
5. Fennessy G, Burstein F. Empirical study of decision-making performance in evidence based health care. In: *6th International Conference of the International Society for Decision Support Systems*, Department of Information Systems and Computing, Brunel University, 2–4 July 2001, London, UK; pp. 66–73.
6. Urquhart C, Hepworth J. The value to clinical decision making of information supplied by NHS library and information services. R&D Report No. 6205. Boston Spa: British Library; 1995.
7. Walker C, McKibbon KA, Haynes R, Ramsden M. Problems encountered by clinical end users of MEDLINE and GRATEFUL MED. *Bull Med Libr Assoc* 1991;79(1):67–69.
8. Del Mar CB, Anderson JN. Epitaph for the EBM in action series. *Med J Aust* 2003;178(11):535–536
9. Eraut M. In: Black H, editor, *Knowledge and competencies: current issues in training and education*. Scottish Council for Research in Education in association with University of London, London; 1990.
10. Sackett D, Rosenberg W, Muir Gray J, Haynes R, Richardson W. Evidence based medicine: what it is and what it isn't. *Br Med J* 1996;312:71–72.
11. Sackett D. *Evidence-based medicine: how to practice and teach EBM*. New York: Churchill Livingstone; 1997.
12. Drucker PF. *Post-capitalist society*. Oxford: Butterworth-Heinmann; 1993.
13. Dickinson HD. Evidence-based decision-making: an argumentative approach. *Int J Med Inform* 1998;51(2–3):71–81.
14. Shiffman RN, Liaw Y, Brandt CA, Corb GJ. Computer-based guideline implementation systems: a systematic review of functionality and effectiveness. J Am Med Inform Assoc 1999;6(2):104–114.
15. Shaughnessy AF, Slawson DC. Are we providing doctors with the training and tools for lifelong learning? *Br Med J* 1999;319:1280.
16. Frank MS. Embodying medical expertise in decision support systems for health care management: techniques and benefits. *Top Health Inf Manage* 1998;19(2):44–54.
17. Anderson J. An evidence centre in a general hospital: finding and evaluating the best available evidence for clinicians. *Evidence Based Med* 1999;4(4):102–103.
18. Fennessy G, Burstein F. Developing a knowledge management system to support intermediaries in health care decision making. In: *IFIP WG 8.3 Conference "Decision support through knowledge management,"* 9–11 July 2000, Stockholm, Sweden; pp. 122–136.
19. Ahituv N, Getz I. A semiotics approach for evaluating DSS. In: Gray P, editor, *Decision support and executive information systems*. Prentice Hall; 1994, pp. 98–106.
20. Sprague R, Carlson E. *Building effective decision support systems*. Englewood Cliffs, NJ: Prentice Hall; 1982.
21. Fennessy G, Burstein F. Using soft systems as a methodology for researching knowledge management problems. In: *International Conference on Systems Thinking in Management Dynamics of Theory and Practice Incorporating the First Australasian Conference*

on System Dynamics and Sixth Australia and New Zealand Systems Conference, 8–10 November 2000, Melbourne, Australia; pp. 180–185.

22. Checkland P. *Systems thinking, systems practice*. Chichester: Wiley; 1981.
23. Booth A. Madge B. Finding the evidence. In: Bury T, Mead J, editors, *Evidence-based healthcare: a practical guide for therapists*. London: Butterworth-Heinemann; 1998.
24. Hunt DL, Jaeschke R, McKibbon KA. Users' guides to the medical literature: XXI. Using electronic health information resources in evidence-based practice. *J Am Med Assoc* 2000;283(14):1875–1879.
25. Burstein FV, Linger H. Supporting post-fordist work prectices: A knowledge management framework for supporting knowledge work: *Information Technology and people* 2003;16(3):289–305.
26. Oxford Centre for Evidence-Based Medicine. Levels of evidence and grades of recommendations; 2001. Available from: http://www.cebm.net/levels_of_evidence.asp [accessed December 2005].
27. Hyde C, Parkes J, Deeks J, Milne R. *Systematic review of effectiveness of teaching critical appraisal*. Oxford: ICRF/NHS Centre for Statistics in Medicine; 2000.
28. National Health and Medical Research Council (NHMRC). A guide to the development, implementation and evaluation of clinical practice guidelines. Commonwealth of Australia, Canberra; 1999.
29. NHS Centre for Reviews and Dissemination. *Undertaking systematic reviews of research on effectiveness: CRD's guidance for carrying out or commissioning reviews*, 2nd edition. York: NHS CRD; 2001.
30. Clarke M, Oxman A, editors. *Cochrane reviews' handbook 4.1*. Oxford: Cochrane Collaboration; 2000.

4
Healthcare Knowledge Management and Information Technology: A Systems Understanding

RAJNEESH CHOWDHURY

Abstract

Healthcare knowledge management (HKM) has developed into a topical field of investigation. Much of this stems from the current investments in information technology (IT) in health, the application of hi-tech information management systems for the capture, recording, and retrieval of health information, and the prevalent thinking that "the machine can do it all." The world of IT is a world of glitter and myth, which gives the impression that anything can be achieved at the click of a mouse. In contrast, the world of human activity is an extremely complex domain of thoughts and beliefs, culture and rituals, and individual comprehensions and apprehensions, none of which can be captured even by the most sophisticated IT system.

Although it is easy to become mesmerized by IT in knowledge management, it is the consideration of the wider organizational, political, and socio-cultural dimensions that can enable any information system and any knowledge management strategy to work with effectiveness. Concentrating solely on IT will mean adopting a one-sided view of HKM, ignoring the whole gamut of socio-cultural, political, and ethical dimensions of working in a healthcare organization.

What is required is an approach that recognizes the whole picture and embraces holism, rather than reductionism, in understanding the complexity of human cognition: in other words, a systems understanding of HKM.

Bearing from this understanding, the intention of this chapter is to present an argument in favor of a systems understanding of the role of IT in HKM, in the UK context, which can enable an effective comprehension of the opportunities and challenges associated with the same.

4.1   Introduction

Technology can be of tremendous aid in the capture, recording, and retrieval of information. This can lead to direct benefits for improvement in the quality of care, clinical audit, performance management, and, above all, knowledge management

(KM). A detailed analysis of IT systems implementation within a National Health Service (NHS) trust is presented. This exercise has been conducted using a viable systems model (VSM) exercise. The arguments and analyses presented in this chapter are akin to the opinion that, in any KM and information systems project, the human and the technical aspects should not be regarded as two disparate dimensions, but as interactive subsystems within one larger system.

The research leads to an argument in favor of a systems understanding of the role of information technology (IT) in healthcare KM (HKM), in the UK context, which can enable an effective comprehension of the opportunities and challenges associated within this domain. In the UK, the responsibility of the provision of health and social care welfare is under the UK Department of Health (DoH) and Social Security, which was formed in 1966 as a result of a merger between the Ministry of Health and the Ministry of Social Security [1]. The DoH is answerable to Parliament for the strategic control and direction of the NHS and social services [2]. This chapter will mainly draw insights from relevant contributions in the field of KM, from the policy context of the DoH, and from some of the findings from an investigation within a particular primary care trust (PCT) in the UK. A PCT is an NHS body to commission primary care services in a specific area.

These insights have been informed by systems thinking, which has also informed the methodologies employed to approach the situation.

4.2   Systems Thinking and Healthcare Knowledge Management

Systems thinking is a particular perspective in management thought, which seeks to approach a situation with a holistic view, rather than considering parts in themselves. It operates with the philosophy that *the whole is more than the sum of its parts*. Hence, rather than concentrating on parts per se, a systems approach would encourage one to observe the dynamics between the parts and how they interact and give character to the whole. It encourages the observer to be *systemic* rather than being *systematic*. A systems approach is an organization aspires to relate to all possible operative dimensions, viz. culture, people, technology, time, place, etc., within which organizations and their activities are positioned and within which they function.

As a fundamental critique to Descartes' [3] "reductionism," the systems approach is a revolutionary paradigm to approach, analyze, and comprehend organizations with holism, creativity, and criticality. Tracing back to established writers like Bernard, Wiener, and Von Bertalanffy in the 1940s and 1950s [4], systems thinking emerged as a challenging state of mind to visualize organizations as "goal directed," "purposive," "structurally interdependent" entities which exist in a "dimensional domain," yet changing its domain by its action. As Reed [5] remarks:

...the starting point for the systems framework is a conception of organisation as a goal-oriented, purposeful system constituted through a set of common underlying abstract variables or dimensions relating to structural properties which are geared to the functional needs of a more inclusive social system.

Descending from the Greek verb *sunistanai*, the word systems originally meant "to cause to stand together" [6]. Senge et al. [6] note that perception plays a crucial role here, as it fundamentally depends upon the observer who perceives what causes the system to stand together. Hence, the systems thinker is continually negotiating and renegotiating with a "boundary critique": a process where knowledge not only diverges from the observer, but also culminates into her/him from the environment. Sparrow [7] advocates that systems thinking is "about boundaries" and that our analysis is to be directed towards the generative mechanisms of systemic structures, yet which cannot be structurally reduced. The important message it carries is that the boundaries that healthcare organizations normally create between departments (IT, human resources, performance management, learning and development, commissioning, etc.) are not only based on insufficient and reductionist understanding, but also create artificial divisions between people. In this regard, Starbuck and Mezias [8] found in their research that organizations define their responsibilities and their environments "very narrowly," leading to a kind of a pathological compartmentalization; and this has to be overcome to achieve an intra-firm collaborative synergy.

Systems thinking can be of great benefit in approaching and designing an effective strategy for HKM. When there seems to be tremendous emphasis on IT to aid HKM, a systems perspective can help understand that providing an efficient IT infrastructure may serve as only one element, albeit important. IT can largely facilitate information management, which is the preceding stage to KM. The ability to capture relevant understanding pertaining to HKM demands transcendence from information management to KM. This is an interplay of both objective and subjective dimensions, which is beyond the provision of just an IT infrastructure. Objective dimensions would include consideration of the hardware and software elements for the recording, storage, and retrieval of information; and the subjective dimensions would include stakeholder participation, co-generative learning, and the ability to devise a strategy of how healthcare service providers can best make use of available information. KM is not just about the availability and accessibility of information through IT, but also how to harness the power of creative action that organizational members can engage in as a result of this availability and accessibility and its interpretation. Holistic approaches, facilitated by systems thinking, help link the human and technical aspects in HKM.

The analysis and understanding of the human element is of utmost importance in considering the successful introduction of new IT/communication systems. Whereas a reductionist approach may consider human and technical aspects in isolation, a systems approach will consider both the human and technical aspects as interconnected dimensions within one larger system. During (and before) the introduction of IT to facilitate KM, it has to be recognized that the technology is delivered to suit the users, and the users are adept in the usage of the technology. Rather than users existing for technology to work efficiently, technology ought to exist for users to work effectively. It will be relevant to note here that Mumford [9] developed a socio-technical methodology called ETHICS (Effective Technical and Human Implementation of Computer-based Systems). The key lies in getting the human and technical balance right. A failure to do so may result in the failure of entire projects, no matter however advanced the technology is. In this context, Clarke [10] notes that, although the development of information systems is functionally a technological and networking exercise, the system essentially has to work within a "social framework." The inability to recognize this has led to a large number of high-profile failures in IT systems implementation, including cases like the failures of the systems of the London Ambulance Service and the London Stock Exchange System [11]. Clarke [12] notes:

The London Ambulance Service (LAS) computer-aided dispatch system failed on 26 October 1992, its first day in operation. From its inception, the system has been treated as a technical problem, to which a viable solution could be found. But LAS exhibited social and political dimensions which the technology-based approach proved ill-equipped to address.

Understanding of the socio-political and cultural dimensions for the design of an information systems project may not be treated as an isolated one-off event, but as an iterative and ongoing process, so that the complexity in this context may be captured. As Davenport [13] comments: "One reason that Knowledge Management never ends is that the categories of required knowledge are always changing." The project may be designed to begin with stakeholder participation, leading on to co-generative learning from experiences. Please refer to further reading for a detailed discussion of co-generative learning. Only after the identification of these needs should investments be made to devise IT systems suited to the stakeholders' needs. Only this may lead to an effective strategy for HKM. However, once this stage is reached, the actions ought not to come to an end. As Davenport said, "one reason that KM never ends is that the categories of required knowledge are always changing." Thus, the route towards an effective HKM ought to be an iterative process. This idea has been conceptualized in steps in Figure 4.1.

The idea is not to present Figure 4.1 as a recipe for HKM, but rather as a conceptual model which appreciates the iterative criticality of HKM.

Systems approaches, in general, and critical systems thinking (CST) in particular, may greatly aid planners and designers to be critical of boundaries, and to be accommodative of stakeholder ideas whilst devising an information systems strategy for HKM. This may enable information systems design to be inclusive and more attuned to human requirement. According to Midgley [14], there are three fundamental commitments of CST:

• Critical awareness: examining and re-examining taken-for-granted assumptions, along with the conditions that give rise to them.

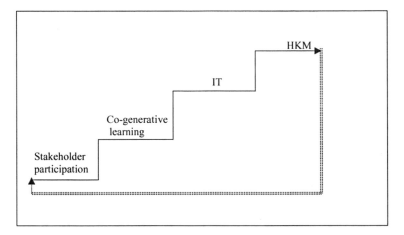

FIGURE 4.1. The route to an effective HKM.

- Emancipation: ensuring that research is focused on "improvement," defined temporarily and locally, taking issues of power (which may affect the definition) into account.
- Methodological pluralism: using a variety of research methods in a theoretically coherent manner, becoming aware of their strengths and weaknesses, to address a corresponding variety of issues.

A critical awareness is vital for HKM because, as has been addressed above, KM may be in danger of slipping into mere information management. Moreover, a boundary critique and re-examination of taken-for-granted assumptions will facilitate comprehending subsystems as part of a whole, rather than individual parts in themselves. This will help understanding the interlinkages between systems, and how the system evolves as a result of this interaction. Hence, CST can be a handy approach to devise an effective organizational development strategy, working particularly within rigid NHS boundaries and departments of the various strategic health authorities (SHAs), the PCTs, and the acute care trusts.

4.3   Healthcare Knowledge Management in the UK Department of Health

Concepts of HKM and learning are not entirely new to the NHS. Documents produced by the DoH, like *The new NHS—modern, dependable* [15], *Our information age* [16], *Information for health* [18], *An organisation with a memory* [18], amongst others, specifically strategize the management of knowledge in a learning environment. The NHS has also established the NKS, where the "K," which stands for knowledge, replaces the "H," which stands for health. The NKS seeks to "meet the needs of professionals, patients and the public for up-to-date, cross-referenced, evidence-based information by fully integrating the development of NHS knowledge systems" [19].

Presently, the NHS has invested over £6.2 billion (which independent observers claim will cost up to £30 billion) to put in place the National Programme for Information Technology (NPfIT), which is expected to deliver all management services electronically, like patient booking, service provider choice, prescription, and information sharing between the primary, secondary and tertiary sectors. The NPfIT is by far the most ambitious project of the NHS in the field of information systems and KM. The NPfIT is currently in its implementation stage, involving the following six stages according to the *National Programme Implementation Guide*, 2005 [20]:

0. *Preparation for implementation*. This must begin several months prior to the start of the implementation stage and consists of undertaking a series of activities that ensure that local health communities (LHCs) are ready at an organizational level. Activities in this stage should include an assessment of LHC maturity, gathering high-level planning information, benefits realization planning, and business justification.
1. *Initiate*. This includes sponsorship, resources, financial approvals, and other commitments ending in a signed-off project initiation document.
2. *Local design*. This has three elements: survey, local design (or tailoring of national/local service provider design), and procurement. This stage may be relatively short if a national application (e.g. "choose and book" or "electronic transcription of prescription") is being implemented.
3. *Prepare for go live*. This includes the undertaking of those activities required to prepare the process, people and IT environments for the deployment of the new solution, including hardware and network upgrades, clinical risk checks, data cleansing, testing, and training;
4. *Go live*. This includes the activities required to progress a new local service and the supporting systems, from test to live status are undertaken in a particular location; this is also commonly referred to as "cut over" or deployment. This stage may be relatively short.
5. *Support*. This includes the transition from users being directly supported by the local implementation teams, handover, deployment verification acceptance, and lessons learned.

The DoH has given considerable autonomy to local trusts to adopt and implement the above stages according to their local requirements and needs. Hence, the NHS appears to have made considerable strides in the area of KM and information systems with introducing some of the most impressive initiatives in the field of healthcare management.

However, setting aside the strategies and implementation documents, there seems to be a worrying degree of skepticism amongst the actual users regarding their involvement in the design and implementation of the systems, and an apprehension that, as a result of this, the new strategies are doomed to failure. For instance, when the Radio 4 *File On 4* survey was conducted, only 7% of the 500 general practitioners (GPs) and hospital doctors felt that they had been "adequately consulted," and a further three-quarters of doctors were not confident that the system will succeed [21]. The major danger of current HKM in the UK is that there is increasing attention being paid to the sole IT element, without realizing the importance of considering IT as an element of the wider system; and there is a lack of perception of a holistic picture of how and where different initiatives fit in, whereas the issue of HKM is endowed with extreme complexity and an effective and holistic healthcare service is a synthesis of a myriad of considerations. It is some of these apprehensions that Section 4.4 will turn to.

4.4   Analyzing Healthcare Knowledge Management: A Case Study

This section explores some of the insights and findings that have come to light as a result of a systems investigation on KM and information systems strategies of a particular PCT in Yorkshire. Let us call it PCT-1. Funded by the Economic and Social Research Council, this research project started as an initiative to inform a cardiac informatics protocol in line with the National Service Framework for Coronary Heart Disease [22], but it soon evolved to be a robust investigation into health informatics and KM strategies for the local area, with specific attention to NPfIT.

It was realized that, to approach the situation in a holistic manner, it is essential to understand where PCT-1 fits into the entire NHS system, and what kinds of constraints and opportunities it receives under the DoH. The method adopted to approach the situation was a VSM. Pioneered by Beer [23], and inspired by neurocybernetics, VSM is a structural analysis of any organization (in the state of a known-to-be viable system) to reveal its constituent parts and study how they interact with one another. The VSM was designed by Beer as a generic model which can be applied to any organization across time and space. He advocates that this model sets out to explain how systems are capable of independent existence due to the prevalence of fundamental laws of viability. The VSM is a structuralist endeavor to study not the system per se, but the relationship between the constituent systems.

VSM studies organizations in terms of five subsystems. "System 1" is the *implementation* system, where the actual operation of the organization takes place. Therefore, there may be several Systems 1. Each System 1 has its own localized management and deals with its own local environment. "System 2" is the *coordination* system, which is responsible for maintaining a harmonious balance of functions between each System 1. "System 3" is the *control* system, which ensures the optimal materialization of policies and goals in the subsystems of the larger organization. There is also a "System 3*," which gives System 3 direct access to the operational level through the "Audit channel." "System 4" is the *development* system, which Beer calls the "biggest 'switch'" in the organization [24]. This system is responsible for information passage between System 5 and the other subsystems, as well as for gathering information from the contingent environment. "System 5" is the *policy*-making and executive unit of the VSM, which Beer calls the "multimode," an elaborate and interactive integration for managers [25]. Based on the urgency and necessity, System 2 will filter information before passing it from System 3 to System 1. This link is called the "algedonic link." These five systems follow the law of "recursion" throughout the subsystems, which imply that all the five systems exist and operate within each system. As Beer advocates, VSM is a generic model, in the sense that a single person will play the role of all five systems if an organization is comprised of only one person.

A VSM for PCT-1 was conducted in September 2005, by the author with a performance analyst from PCT-1, with the objective to understand how the position of PCT-1 within the NHS structure facilitates or constrains its ability to take into consideration user opinion and perspective in implementing new IT strategies, which thereby impinges upon the effectiveness of the KM agenda. The VSM was applied as a guide in facilitating a better comprehension of the position of PCT-1 within the larger NHS.

According to the DoH strategy, the NPfIT was designed to be implemented in five waves, as below.

1	General Practice
2	PCT, Community, District Nursing, etc.
3 & 4	Acute/Maternity.
5	Ambulance.

The VSM referred to in this chapter was an initial attempt to understand the PCT-1, and considers the DoH as the system in focus. The recursion levels within the system have been studied in detail in subsequent VSMs. Considering PCT-1 as the primary implementation system for the DoH policies, the following systems were identified.

System 1: PCT-1 and other local PCTs.
System 2: does not exist; occasionally fulfilled by System 3.
System 3: SHA.
System 4: Accenture/NHS local IT service.
System 5: DoH.

A VSM placing PCT-1 as System 1 is given in Figure 4.2.

The four PCTs in the area were identified to be the Systems 1, the implementation system, named PCT-1, PCT-2, PCT-3, and PCT-4. It was found that responsibility for implementation of the NPfIT strategies lies in the PCT level, where the PCTs have considerable autonomy over how they choose to deliver the goals of the DoH.

The coordination system, System 2, seems to be a gray area, the reason being the absence of any formal body to coordinate between the four PCTs. Coordination

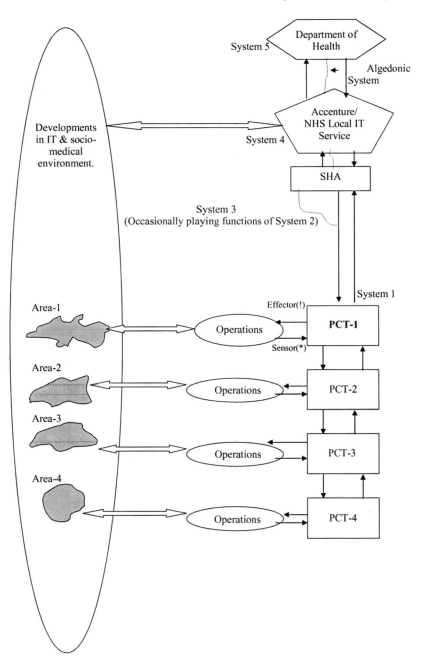

FIGURE 4.2. VSM for PCT-1.

occurs at an ad hoc level and there is no formal practice of inter-PCT linkage in this regard, apart from the fact that the Workforce Development team from the PCTs meet in the SHA once every 8 weeks. The PCTs report to the SHA, but there is no formalized body for coordination between them. They may share interests, but overall they are autonomous. Hence, we concluded that there is no formalized System 2, but the SHA occasionally plays this role.

System 3 is the control system. However, it was agreed that, in the present context, the control systems may not be considered as "control" per se, but more as a monitoring system. This function is fulfilled by the SHA, which oversees the work of the PCTs. However, the SHA does not hold any decision-making power over the PCTs. The SHA can only ask; it cannot demand.

System 4 is the "development" system, and this role is responsible for information passage between System 1 and the other subsystems, and gathers information from the environment. Dealing specifically with the implementation of IT systems within the NHS, it was agreed that the service provider for the region, Accenture, usually fulfills the functions related to this. Along with Accenture, the NHS local IT service also has a joint interest in the development function of the NPfIT, in terms of passage of information between System 5 and the Systems 1. Accenture and the NHS local IT service have direct communication with the PCTs.

System 5 is "policy," the highest level of decision making. This function is fulfilled at the ministerial level at the DoH. The DoH commissions the services and indicates the specifications, with some degree of flexibility, within which the services are to be delivered.

From the above model, it was identified that PCT-1 (System 1) operates as an autonomous entity, with its own independent decision-making body. It deals with its respective geographical area, i.e. Area-1. Each localized management has a set of instructions which it receives, based on which it will instruct its operational environment of actions. This is the "effector" function. From the operational environment, activities are monitored and transmitted back to the localized management. This is the "sensor" function.

The absence of a formalized coordination system means that there is no effective communication or linkage between the PCTs. Learning from any improvement in one PCT probably does not get transferred to another. The only systems which bind the PCTs are the payroll system, personnel records, and the informatics service, which is central to all the PCTs. Coordination at this level is entirely in terms of IT.

The SHA is the monitoring body, but it does not control the functioning of the PCT. The PCTs have been given autonomous roles on how NPfIT is to be implemented. There is no audit channel (3*), as the SHA oversees the PCTs directly anyway. Therefore, there is disparity in the progress different areas are making in this regard. Some PCTs are performance managing, some are in the initial stages of developing a performance management system, and, in some, performance management does not exist at all. PCT-1 claims high standards in performance management.

The PCTs have their own NPfIT targets, and delivery of these targets is PCT based, not SHA based. The DoH just issues the directives of what is to be delivered and the PCTs make their own decisions on how these will be delivered. For instance, the creation of a central electronic staff record was a DoH directive. To meet the demands of such directives and improve IT literacy, PCT-1 had recently invested in a hi-tech training center.

Hence, in a way, it can be advocated that PCT-1 is not controlled by any superior body for the implementation of the NPfIT. The higher bodies only issue directives and express a desire for what is to be implemented. Therefore, it is the responsibility of the PCT to design an effective strategy for involvement and stakeholder participation in the implementation of the new system. The PCT should interact with users, but there is no evidence that this is taking place.

The DoH had an anticipated time-frame for the desired implementation of NPfIT, within the constraints of time and resources. In this first wave/stage, user opinion was not given due attention, which bred skepticism of the new system and clinicians' possessiveness of their old systems. In this stage, the DoH seemed to perceive the new system totally in terms of IT, and overlooked the socio-political and human dimensions of change and work culture. Therefore, the second wave characterized "community focus groups," in which the individual local environments of the respective PCTs were taken into account, enabling Accenture to understand the complexity of the situation. A critical benefit from this was to illustrate and reinforce the very localized and specific ways healthcare is provided to a target population. Whilst services are similar in overview, their delivery differs markedly between PCTs and their recipient public. It is believed that the NPfIT solution will introduce uniformity without removing the flexibility with which services are tailored to their local communities. The community is itself a complex phenomenon, and it differs from PCT to PCT. The local factors and services of each PCT are different. Issues around social services and child welfare and their relation to civil society have not yet been addressed. This is a muddy area and full of complex issues that need clarification. It would be easier to indicate that many PCTs host services such as Sexual & Reproductive Health, Dentistry, and Prison Health, etc., some of which may be included in the initial NPfIT provision; however, there are areas where there are provisions which are out of the scope of the NPfIT program, e.g. the armed forces.

When the DoH issues its directives, it also allows a degree of flexibility, with the core element (e.g. the patient identifier) remaining intact. The flexibility may include the decision of the PCT of how to record patient information and make this available to other clinicians. Accenture and the NHS local IT service are responsible for consideration of the environmental factors and the hardware/software element of the new system. Accenture shares an interest with PCT-1 in the implementation of the NPfIT. Accenture and the NHS local health informatics service are answerable to the DoH for the delivery of services.

The "algedonic link," which transmits information directly from System 1 to System 5, based on urgency, may be activated in this situation if the IT security system in the PCT is threatened by hacking or other failure. Action to rectify any such fault may be directed directly to Accenture or the NHS local IT service.

The VSM analysis carries a mixed message about the level of consistency and standardization of the implementation of the NPfIT. The technical and human dimensions have been treated as entirely disparate concepts, with the assumption that, once a technology strategy is imposed, people will automatically adapt to it. Hence, although the DoH appears to grant flexibility to the PCTs to the manner in which they choose to implement the NPfIT in terms of local needs and user perspective, this is just pseudo-flexibility, as the DoH already has an established model of a high-tech information systems project, which it aspires to put in place. This has resulted in the end users in PCT-1 being left isolated and feeling imposed upon by the grand plans of the DoH.

The above opinion is reinforced by findings from questionnaire surveys that were being conducted amongst practice managers and GPs in the PCT-1 area. The objective of these surveys was to throw light on the level of awareness and involvement of clinicians and grass-roots-level management in the NPfIT.

Twenty-seven questionnaires were sent out to GPs and nine responses were received. All the GPs who responded indicated that they have not been involved in the planning and design of the NPfIT, and only one GP felt that the NPfIT will work as per the expectations of the DoH. There was one GP who was not even aware of the NPfIT until they received the questionnaire. In answers to the open-ended questions, whilst many GPs anticipated a good service support from the NPfIT, critical comments were also featured, and one GP commented that they are not confident that the system will work, and anticipates the system to be "beset with huge problems." Another GP commented that they did not know how the new system will impact on the quality of services. The main issue that was featured in most of the responses was that the system ought to be user friendly if it has to gain acceptance amongst clinicians, and patient confidentiality was noted as a priority. However, GPs do feel "pressurized" to shift to new systems all the time. Other interesting comments noted were that NHS IT strategies are a "waste of money" and are "laudable but impractical."

Similarly, 27 questionnaires were sent out to practice managers and 16 responses were received. Of these, only five felt that they have been involved in the design and implementation of the NPfIT, and 11 felt that they were not. In response to the open-ended questions, there was generally good anticipation from how the NPfIT will change the manner in which information is shared at present. Whilst practice managers did agree with the potential benefits that may be derived from the NPfIT, some answers did reveal issues of concerns as well. One of the interesting comments was skepticism with the change in the system, when GPs already feel committed to paper records. The issue that was mainly featured is the availability of adequate training to use the new system.

4.5   Afterword

The above investigation into the KM and information systems strategy of the NHS carries a mixed message for such strategies. The case study of PCT-1 depicts a road map towards an ambitious system which will be of tremendous assistance to addressing issues like maintaining information consistency, avoiding duplication, timely information sharing, and reduction of medical errors, carrying the message that a sound IT support strategy is not only desirable, but also necessary. And taking this into consideration, it is commendable that the NHS has a strategy which has the ability to address the issues mentioned above.

However, as this chapter demonstrates, the basis on which this strategy is founded creates a separation of the human and technological dimensions as two disparate aspects to be designed and delivered in isolation. This is a *systematic*, but not *systemic*, approach, with dangerous consequences. Whereas a systematic approach would break down the organization into departments and strategies into disparate chunks and approach them part by part, a systemic approach will look at the problem situation as a whole and attempt to understand not only how the different dimensions interact with each other, but also how the whole system evolves as a result of it.

The requirement is that of an effective "combination of human and computer-based resources that results in the collection, storage, retrieval, communication and use of data for the purpose of efficient management of operations . . . " [26]. In this quotation, it is crucial that we understand that what is important is both the human and the technical element, hence the "combination" of "human" and "computer-based" resources. The management of knowledge does not parallel the management of information. Whereas the latter may be *achieved* by adequately placed hardware and software, the former may be *attained* only by understanding how humans establish a working relationship with the organizational and IT provisions, within the climate of organizational activities.

Therefore, this chapter may be concluded with the opinion that there have been promising developments in the area of information-systems-enabled knowledge management in the UK healthcare sector, but there have been pitfalls as well. However, the recognition of such issues is the first step towards resolving them. And as it has been emphasized in this chapter that this should be regarded as an iterative process designed for continual learning. A systems perspective to approach and comprehend situations can enable a holistic understanding of integration of initiatives, inclusion in stakeholders, and an attempt towards greater effectiveness of organizational strategy making.

Acknowledgement. The author is grateful to Professor Steve Clarke, University of Hull Business School, for his valuable comments and advice.

References

1. Department of Health. (2005) History of the Department of Health. [Internet] London. Available from <http://www.DH.gov.uk>. [Accessed 01 October 2005].
2. Department of Health. (2005) History of the Department of Health. [Internet] London. Available from <http://www.DH.gov.uk>. [Accessed 01 October 2005].
3. Descartes R. *Discourse on method and the mediations*, Sutcliffe FE, translator. Harmondsworth: Penguin Classics; 1968.
4. Jackson MC. *Systems approaches to management.* Chichester: Wiley; 2000.

5. Reed MI. *The sociology of organisations: themes, perspectives and prospects.* Hertfordshire: Harvester Wheatsheaf; 1992, p. 7.

6. Senge, PM, Kleiner A, Roberts C, Ross R, Smith B. *The fifth discipline fieldbook: strategies and tools for building a learning organisation.* London: Nicholas Brealey Publishing; 1994, p. 90.

7. Sparrow J. *Knowledge in organisations: access to thinking at work.* London: Sage Publications; 1998.

8. Cited in: Starbuck WH, Hedberg B. How organisations learn from success and failure. In: Dierkes M, Berthoin Antal A, John Child J, Nonaka I, editors, *Handbook of organisational learning and knowledge.* Oxford: Oxford University Press; 2001.

9. Mumford E. *Effective systems design and requirements analysis.* Basingstoke: Macmillan; 1995.

10. Clarke S. *Information systems, strategic management: an integrated approach.* London: Routledge; 2001, p. 7.

11. Clarke S. *Information systems, strategic management: an integrated approach.* London: Routledge; 2001.

12. Clarke S. *Information systems, strategic management: an integrated approach.* London: Routledge; 2001, p. 10.

13. Davenport, TH (2005) Some principles of knowledge management [Internet]. The ITM Web network. Available from: <http://www.itmweb.com/essay538.htm>

14. Midgley G. What is this thing called CST? In: Flood RL, Romm NRA, editors. *Critical systems thinking: current research and practice.* New York: Plenum; 1996, pp. 11–24.

15. *The new NHS—modern, dependable.* London: Department of Health; 1997.

16. *Our information age.* London: Department of Health; 1998.

17. *Information for health.* London: Department of Health; 1998.

18. *An organisation with a memory.* London: Department of Health; 2000.

19. *Learning from Bristol.* London: Department of Health; 2002.

20. Connecting for Health (2005). National Programme Implementation Guide [Internet]. Available from: <www.connectingforhealth.co.uk>. Accessed on 15 October 2005.

21. BBC News. (2004) GPs doubtful about IT upgrade. [Internet] Available from: <http://news.bbc.co.uk/1/hi/health/3750474.stm>. Accessed on: 17 October 2004.

22. National Service Framework for Coronary Heart Disease. London: Department of Health; 2000.

23. Beer S. *Brain of the firm.* London: Allen Lane; 1972.

24. Jackson MC. *Systems approaches to management.* Chichester: Wiley; 2000, p. 162.

25. Jackson MC. *Systems approaches to management.* Chichester: Wiley, 2000, p. 161.

26. Lucey T. *Management information systems.* London: Letts Educational; 1997, p. 1.

Further Reading

For a detailed discussion on co-generative learning refer to:

1. Elden M, Levin M. *Cogenerative learning: bringing participation into action research.* Newbury Park, CA: Participatory Action Research, Sage; 1991, pp.127–142.

5
Medical Technology Management in Hospital Certification in Mexico

MARTHA R. ORTIZ POSADAS

5.1 Introduction

Mexican health policy is promoting the quality of health services by hospital certification meeting the NMX-CC standards family, which is the Mexican equivalent of the ISO 9000 standards family. These standards can help both product- and service-oriented organizations achieve standards of quality that are recognized and respected throughout the world in developing a quality management system (QMS).

In hospital certification, one important aspect to be evaluated is the availability of technical supplies. In this sense, the incorporation of technical support services into healthcare organizations has become very important. That is why many hospitals in Mexico, both public and private, have incorporated into their organization a Biomedical Engineering Department (BED) with the purpose of integrating all engineering and management processes for assurance of the optimal use of all technological supplies in the hospital, helping in the quality of health services provided to patients.

The purpose of this study is to show how the medical technology management done by the BED at the hospitals contributes both to health services quality and as an element required for certification. In general, it describes several projects developed in different hospitals (public and private) with different health levels in Mexico City. Each of them contributed to the certification of different clinical processes.

5.2 ISO 9000 Certification

ISO standards are voluntary. As a nongovernmental organization, ISO has no legal authority to enforce their implementation. Some ISO standards (mainly those concerned with health, safety, or the environment) have been adopted in some countries as part of their regulatory framework, or are referred to in legislation for which it serves as the technical basis. Such adoptions are sovereign decisions by the regulatory authorities or governments of the countries concerned; ISO itself does not regulate or legislate. However, although ISO standards are voluntary, they

55

may become a market requirement, as has happened in the case of the ISO 9000 QMSs. By QMS we understand a management strategy that is characterized by: a focus on process management; a focus on quality, based on the participation of all members in the organization; getting profit through client satisfaction and providing benefits to all members in the organization and in the society.

For governments, international standards provide the technological and scientific bases underpinning health, safety, and environmental legislation. For consumers, conformity of products and services to international standards provides assurance about their quality, safety, and reliability. For customers, the worldwide compatibility of technology that is achieved when products and services are based on international standards brings them an increasingly wide choice of offers, and they also benefit from the effects of competition among suppliers [1]. In this sense there are some important quality management principles: customer focus, leadership, involvement of people, process approach, system approach to management, continual improvement, factual approach to decision making, and mutually beneficial supplier relationships.

In particular, the process approach (from procedures to processes) is based on the following principles:

- identifying processes needful for the QMS;
- demonstrating the ability of processes to achieve planned results and monitor, measure, analyze, and improve them;
- developing information on characteristics and trends of processes;
- top management reviewing process performance and improving effectiveness;
- greater effectiveness when activities and resources are managed as a process;
- more customer focus;
- more cost effective;
- meeting business objectives.

5.3   ISO 9000 Family and its Mexican Equivalent NMX-CC

The term ISO 9000 refers to a set of quality management standards. ISO 9000 currently includes three quality standards: ISO 9000:2000, ISO 9001:2000, and ISO 9004:2000. The ISO 9000 2000 standards apply to all kinds of organizations in all kinds of areas and present the requirements, whereas ISO 9000:2000 and ISO 9004:2000 present the guidelines. All of these are process standards (not product standards).

This approach is based on the development of a QMS that meets the new quality standard, in order to control or improve the quality of your products and services, to reduce the costs associated with poor quality, or to become more competitive, or because your customers expect you to do so, or because a governmental body has made it mandatory. You then develop a quality management system that meets the requirements specified by ISO 9001:2000.

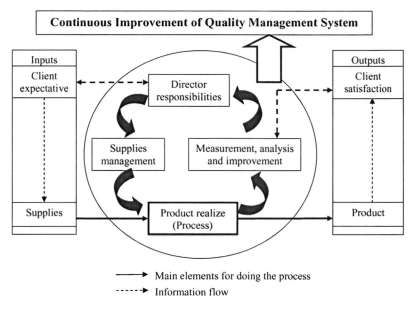

Continuous Improvement of Quality Management System

Inputs

Client expectative

Director responsibilities

Supplies management

Measurement, analysis and improvement

Supplies

Product realize (Process)

Outputs

Client satisfaction

Product

⟶ Main elements for doing the process
------▶ Information flow

FIGURE 5.1. The process-based approach for improving QMS.

In Mexico, the ISO 9000 2000 family have been translated by the "Spanish Translation Task Group," providing the Mexican standards NMX-CC, a set of standards to assist any organization with implementing a management quality system. In this study we just use the following Mexican standards:

- NMX-CC-9000-IMNC-2000. Quality Management System. Concepts and Vocabulary [2]. This describes the fundaments and specifies the terminology for the QMS.
- NMX-CC-9001-IMNC-2000. Quality Management System. Requirements [3]. This specifies the requirements for the QMS for any organization which needs to demonstrate its capability to provide products that comply with the legal and their clients' requirements, in order to improve their clients' satisfaction.

Figure 5.1 shows a process-based QMS approach using the Mexican set of standards NMX-CC. It shows the links between all parts involved with the inputs to the system and the main role the clients have in determining the input requirements.

5.4 Quality in Health Services: A National Policy

The National Crusade for Quality in Health Services is a government policy developed by the Health Ministry of Mexico. Its purpose is to lead to more effective medical services in all Mexican health institutions [4]. This policy proposes elevating quality in health services and standardizing it throughout the country. To achieve this purpose, the policy has been developed through 10 statements. One of these concerns the certification of organizations and individuals. This action helps public and private institutions improve the satisfaction of both the personnel and the customers (patients). It reduces heterogeneity in the quality level among different types of health service, whether public or private, throughout the country. In addition, the population will gain an improved perception about the quality of services with veridical information, which allows people's trust in the health system to be raised. Likewise, it will look to incorporating the population in supervision of quality health services.

5.5   Importance of Technology Management in Hospital Certification

Many hospitals in Mexico City have been working to comply with the requirements of the Mexican standards NMX-CC in order to become certificated. This procedure certificates each clinical service (in an individual way), which is considered as a *process* by the standard. In this sense, hospitals must develop the required documentation for all procedures related to each *process*, including clinical, technical, and administrative aspects.

With regard to technical aspects, the department generally in charge of the medical technology management at a hospital is the BED. Its main functions are medical equipment maintenance (preventive and corrective), medical equipment assessment, training, security, and risk management. However, the most important function that demands most of the technical personnel's time is medical equipment maintenance [5]. It is clear that all these activities have the objective of assuring optimal functionality of the available medical technology at the hospital. In this way, the technology management turns into a fundamental element in hospital certification, and thus all the services and procedures related to medical technology management provide by the BED must also comply with the Mexican standards family NMX-CC.

In what follows, we will describe some projects developed in different hospitals in Mexico City related to different clinical services (processes) where the BED developed several manuals about specific procedures for medical equipment management in order to contribute to the certification of these services.

5.5.1   Project 1: Guaranty Quality Program for a Radiology Service

Project 1 [6] was developed in a secondary care private hospital with 125 beds. This hospital had implemented a guaranty quality program, based on the NMX-CC-9001-IMNC-2000 standard. It was developed specifically for the management of radio-diagnostic equipment. This program includes procedures concerning physical inspection and equipment functionality according to the manufacturers' technical specifications, as well as quality control tests. Afterwards, the tests were applied according to the Mexican official norm NOM-158-SSA-1996 related to technical specifications for diagnostic medical equipment that uses X-rays. Preventive maintenance tests were developed. These included physical, mechanical, and electrical aspects for monitoring the most significant functionality parameters in the equipment, in order to assure their stability as a function of time. Quality tests were also developed. These evaluate functionality parameters with the objective to get a reference value (control value). These parameters were: focal point, exposure time, performance, field coincidence, center coincidence, fuzzy alignment, exposure rate for conventional fluoroscopy, and dose in breast tumor radiation. Both preventive maintenance and quality tests were applied to 12 items of radio-diagnostic equipment (which included X-ray, CAT, mastograph, and fluoroscopy equipment) at the hospital during three consecutive weeks. Failures were detected in some equipment, and the optimal functionality of other equipment was probed.

5.5.2   Project 2: Medical Equipment Maintenance Quality Plan for a Biomedical Engineering Department

Project 2 [7] was developed in a 125-bed private hospital that decided to implement a QMS based on the NMX-CC-9001-IMNC-2000 standard. The purpose was to assure the quality of the health services provided to their patients. The hospital developed a quality manual that provides information about the quality plans. These plans are documents that specify the facilities and activities necessary to realize the health processes in an effective way.

On the other hand, the hospital's BED has the function to maintain the medical equipment in optimal condition. That is why the objective of this study was to develop a quality plan (based on NMX-CC-9001-IMNC-2000) containing the process related to this activity, in order to support the implementation of a QMS and the certification of three specific health services at the hospital, namely pathology, clinical laboratory, and blood bank. Moreover, this quality plan also provides the necessary information to enable the technical personnel to carry out the maintenance process on the medical equipment.

First, we identified three processes related to maintenance. (1) Revision routines, which corresponds to visual and functionality inspection of hospital facilities and medical equipment done in a scheduled way. This requires diagnostic instrumentation, simulators, and noninvasive tests, such as fluids level analysis, temperature, and pressure tests. (2) Preventive maintenance, which is defined as a programmed serial inspection of functionality, security, and calibration realized in regular periods. The purpose is to avoid failures in medical equipment and enable hospital facilities to operate at optimal levels of efficiency. (3) Repair, which covers activities such as spark replacement, component adjustment, reconditioning, etc. whose purpose is to restore the normal function, performance, and security of the equipment in the least possible time. It is important to say that the equipment maintenance could be done by technical personnel from the hospital BED or by external technical personnel, depending on the technical complexity of the equipment.

The quality plan developed in this study contains the general procedure to realize each process with a flow diagram showing the graphics of the process. Likewise, it points out the register form (service order, revision process, etc.) required in each case.

5.5.3   Project 3: Procedures for the Right Use and Management of Medical Technology Utilized in Minimal Invasive Surgical Procedures

Project 3 [8] was developed in a private hospital with 100 beds. It has a surgical area consisting of 12 surgical rooms. Five of these have endosuites, surgical suites designed to create the optimal operating environment for the surgeon, staff, and, most importantly, the patient. Today it is the most versatile room design, and serves a large number of minimally invasive procedures (endoscopy, laparoscopy, and arthroscopy) [3]. The system's functions and images are displayed on multifunction flat-panel monitors, which are also capable of showing images.

The purpose of this study was to develop a procedures manual about the use and management of the medical technology utilized in minimally invasive surgeries at the hospital, in order to provide information about the adequate management of the equipment to the technical personnel from the DIB and adequate use of this equipment for the medical personnel, as well as to contribute to the certification of the surgical process.

The procedures were generated by clinical and technical information. The methodology for obtaining and organizing these procedures is described below.

1. Identification of the types of minimally invasive surgery done in the hospital. They were classified into five medical categories: gynecology, general surgery, thoracic, orthopedics, and otorhinolaryngology.
2. Identification of the medical technology used in each surgery. Six technology sets were defined, according to the medical categories identified. In the case of orthopedics, this requires two different technology sets, i.e. one for shoulder surgery and other for knee surgery.
3. We consulted 16 technical manuals with the purpose of obtaining the technical specifications of the equipment, as well as the manufacturers' recommendations for the use and management of the equipment.
4. Fourteen technical schedules were developed with the next information: (a) description of the equipment (including alarms); (b) physical inspection procedure; (c) management of the equipment (washing, sterilization (if necessary), warehoused, and care); and (d) warnings and precautions. This information was incorporated in the procedure in order to provide the technical elements about the functionality of the equipment to the technical personnel from the BED.

5. Six generic procedures about the use and management of electronic devices and medical equipment used in each minimally invasive surgery identified were elaborated. It is important to say that biomedical engineering helps the physician in all the procedures related to the minimally invasive surgeries done at the hospital. In this sense, the procedures included in the manual will be an instrument for technical and medical personnel for learning the adequate used of the medical technology, and so the optimization of the resources and the technical capability of the hospital.

The procedures developed here are actually incorporated into the documentation of the management quality system of the hospital. This system provides the regulation for optimal functionality of all services (medical and administrative) from the hospital.

5.5.4   Project 4: Procedures for Maintenance and Risk Management for Medical Equipment at a Research Center of Infectious Diseases

Project 4 [9] was developed at the National Health Institute in its Infectious Diseases Research Center (CIENI). The center works with the human immunodeficiency virus, *Mycobacterium tuberculosis*, influenza virus (H5N1) and the SARS corona virus. It has three laboratories designed with the necessary bio-safety standards, levels BSL2 and BSL3. The laboratory equipment has two kinds of contact with the infectious agents, namely *direct* and *indirect*. For example, pipettes have *direct* contact and CO_2 incubators have *indirect* contact because the virus is in Petri boxes. That is why the technology requires specific management and control.

The objective of this study was to develop preventive maintenance procedures for the laboratory equipment present in this center, involving aspects about risk management and quality control. The importance of these kinds of procedure is that activities related to the maintenance and the sanitation procedures attending bio-safety should decrease the biological risk for technical personnel. In this sense, the partial goals of this study were to provide to the technical personnel from the BED the bio-safety procedures necessary for minimizing biological risk during the execution of work:

- A complete preventive maintenance procedure for each specific piece of equipment.
- Technical and quality specifications required during the execution of the maintenance procedures and equipment calibration.
- Minimization of equipment failure, assuring continuous operation of the equipment and extending its useful time.

- Contribution to the certification process of several clinical and research laboratory processes at the center by complying with the Mexican standard MX-NMX-CC.

There were 13 pieces of equipment selected: (1) two doors sterilizer, (2) analytical digital balance, (3) extraction bench, (4) laminar flux bench, (5) centrifuge and micro-centrifuge, (6) refrigerated centrifuge and ultracentrifuge, (7) laser diffraction particle-size analyzer, (8) CO_2 incubator, (9) microscope, (10) pipettes, (11) digital potentiometer, (12) refrigerator, (13) ultra-freezer.

The procedures were structured as follows:

1. *Introduction.* This includes general information about the features of the different research laboratories at CIENI.
2. *General and security rules.* These provide the security procedures required for access to the center and for equipment maintenance.
3. *Procedure for preventive maintenance.* Each procedure contains the following information: maintenance periodicity, security procedures (the security equipment required for doing it), maintenance procedure (including general external cleaning, external inspection, internal cleaning, internal inspection, lubrication, spare parts replacement, calibration, revision of electrical security, and full functionality tests).
4. *Equipment, tools and spare parts.* This section provides information about the tools and spare parts necessary for carrying out preventive maintenance on the equipment, as well as consumables for the operation and calibration.
5. *Quality control.* Some actions recommended for quality control were included, such as: a daily register of parameters (temperature, pressure, humidity, etc.) in order to monitor their fluctuations; instrumentation necessary for maintenance, certified by the Mexican Entity of Accreditation [10].
6. *Registration form.* This form includes general data about the equipment (generic name, trademark, model, serial number, inventory number, and the clinic area where it is placed), periodicity of the maintenance, the report of the functionality tests, electrical security, and calibration.

Furthermore, there three appendices were incorporated: A_1. Cleaners and lubricators, A_2. Disinfectors' substances, and A_3. Procedures in accident cases [11].

5.6   Conclusion

This study had described four different projects related to medical technology management developed by BEDs in different hospitals in Mexico City. The primary objective of all these projects was to provide knowledge about the maintenance procedures and quality control tests to the technical personnel to carry out their jobs and to contribute to the certification process by the NMX standards for the clinical services at the particular hospital.

This study shows the importance of having documented procedures related to the management of medical technology in order to optimize the technical facilities available in the hospital, as well as for the certification.

In Mexico, hospital certification is a new process, and projects developed in this way will be very important in the hospital environment in order to guarantee the quality of the clinical services provide.

References

1. Overview of the ISO system. Available from: http://www.iso.org/iso/en/aboutiso/introduction/index.html [accessed October 2005].
2. Sistemas de gestión de la calidad—fundamentos y vocabulario. NMX-CC-9000-IMNC-2000.
3. Sistemas de gestión de la calidad—requisitos. NMX-CC-9001-IMNC-2000.
4. Cruzada Nacional por la Calidad de los Servicios de Salud. Available from: http://www.salud.gob.mx/unidades/dgcs/sala_noticias/campanas/2001-01-25/cruzada-nacional.htm [accessed September 2005] (in Spanish).
5. Ortiz-Posadas MR, Tafoya-Doñán F, Pimentel-Aguilar AB, Rodríguez-Vera R. Funciones de los Departamentos de Ingeniería Biomédica en Instituciones de Salud Pública y Privada en México. In: *IFMBE Proceedings 3rd Latin-American Congress on Biomedical Engineering "III CLAEB 2004,"* vol. 5, Joao Pessoa, Brazil, 2004; pp. 373–376.
6. Galán-Rodríguez SO. Programa de garantía de calidad para el servicio de radiología del Hospital Mocel. Proyecto terminal. Licenciatura en Ingeniería Biomédica, Universidad Autónoma Metropolitana-Iztapalapa, 2001.
7. Ortiz-Posadas MR, García Martínez AL, Arellano-Carbajal J. Plan de Calidad de Mantenimiento basado en ISO 9001-2000 para el Departamento de Ingeniería Biomédica del Hospital Ángeles Mocel. In: *Memorias XXVII Congreso Nacional de Ingeniería Biomédica*, Acapulco, México, 2004; pp. 28–31.
8. Ortiz-Posadas MR, González-Trejo R, García Martínez T. Procedimientos de Uso y Manejo de la Tecnología Médica relacionada con las Cirugías de Mínima Invasión en el Hospital Santa Fe. In *Memorias XXVIII Congreso Nacional de Ingeniería Biomédica*, Acapulco, México, 2005; pp. 5–8.
9. Jiménez-Quintana O, Ortiz-Posadas MR, Pimentel-Aguilar AB. Manual de Procedimientos de Mantenimiento y Prevención de Riesgos para Equipo del Centro de Investigación en Enfermedades Infecciosas del INER. In *Memorias XXVII Congreso Nacional de Ingeniería Biomédica*, Acapulco, México, 2005; pp 13–16.
10. Entidad Mexicana de Acreditación (EMA). Available from: http://www.ema.org.mx/index800.htm [accessed June 2004].
11. Emergency Care Research Institute (ECRI), Health Devices Inspection and Preventive Maintenance System, Third Edition, 1995.

Section II
Approaches, Frameworks, and Techniques for Healthcare Knowledge Management

6
Healthcare Knowledge Sharing: Purpose, Practices, and Prospects

SYED SIBTE RAZA ABIDI

6.1   Knowledge Sharing

In knowledge management parlance, knowledge sharing can be regarded as a systematically planned and managed activity involving a group of like-minded individuals engaged in sharing their knowledge resources, insights, and experiences for a defined objective. The objective of knowledge sharing may span from organizational learning, to collaborative problem solving, to peer support to capacity building. These objectives entail the explication of knowledge and facilitating its flow throughout a community of practice, i.e. a group of individuals who share a common interest, need, or enterprise towards the knowledge being shared. In a knowledge sharing set-up, the overall available knowledge is perceived as the collection of individual knowledge resources such that the entire knowledge resource is viewed as a community-owned commodity [1]. The dynamics of knowledge sharing are complex, involving an active interplay between an assortment of determinants, such as culture, community, incentives, medium, context, needs, motivation, facilitation, outreach, ubiquity, and, most importantly, trust [2].

Current knowledge management themes focus on the pragmatic effects of knowledge sharing resulting in the reuse of the knowledge by knowledge workers [3]. Advances in information and communication technology have led to the design of innovative knowledge-sharing environments and programs, whereby geographically dispersed individuals are virtually accessible to meet, collaborate, create, and share knowledge [4,5]: the Internet as a knowledge-sharing medium is a case in point [6]. Knowledge sharing, therefore, is not just an activity, but in itself is a knowledge resource.

Healthcare is knowledge rich, yet healthcare knowledge is largely underutilized due to various operational and functional barriers to knowledge flow and use, especially at the point of care [7]. Healthcare knowledge is generated at a significant rate and is represented in a variety of modalities, ranging from research-based publications, to problem-based discussions, to experience-based insights. More so, healthcare knowledge is created and consumed by a wide range of multidisciplinary healthcare stakeholders—including healthcare practitioners (specialists, physicians, nurses, therapists, etc.), administrators, policy makers, patients, care providers, support groups, and community-based healthcare workers—for a range of healthcare-related tasks.

Over the last few years there has been an increased interest in investigating the nature and utilization of healthcare knowledge through the lens of knowledge management theories, methodologies, and technical frameworks [8–10]. In essence, healthcare knowledge management is about the creation and utilization of healthcare knowledge to improve the quality of patient care. Yet, this rather simplistic objective is quite complex to achieve because healthcare knowledge management needs to support and coincide with the temporal evolution of the patient and the corresponding care processes. Healthcare knowledge management, therefore, needs to deal with: (i) heterogeneous healthcare knowledge modalities; (ii) a variety of knowledge resources; (iii) a range of knowledge-driven healthcare processes that need to modulate with the changing operational environments; (iv) a range of healthcare knowledge stakeholders with diverse capabilities, orientations, terminology, needs, and expectations; (v) dispersion of knowledge across different individuals, departments, and institutions; and finally (vi) clinical situations that are unique and hence demand specialized manipulation of the healthcare knowledge. This makes healthcare knowledge management both challenging and yet fulfilling, because there is the potential to design, develop, and deploy healthcare knowledge management solutions that can really impact patient care [11,12].

In the realm of healthcare knowledge management, the aim of healthcare knowledge sharing is to establish a *knowledge-centric* healthcare system, whereby healthcare stakeholders are able to seek and share both existing and new published and unpublished knowledge resources in a timely manner with respect to their immersed contexts. This presents an interesting set of challenges, because both the activity of knowledge sharing and the knowledge being shared need to respond systematically to the ever-changing knowledge needs of an evolving clinical situation whilst satisfying circumstantial constraints, such as: (i) operational workflows/protocols; (ii) proliferation of new knowledge at a rapid rate; (iii) abundance of knowledge resources; (iv) diversity of access mediums; (v) applicability of and trust in the shared knowledge, where both these elements largely depend on the knowledge consumer's capability and orientation; and finally (vi) the presence (or not) of a knowledge-sharing culture. Notwithstanding the complexity of healthcare knowledge sharing, the current state of knowledge management practice and technology is mature enough to be leveraged to formulate effective healthcare knowledge-sharing strategies and frameworks to bridge the perceived knowledge gaps within the healthcare system [13].

In the backdrop of the abovementioned healthcare knowledge management environment and knowledge-sharing considerations, in this chapter we define healthcare knowledge sharing and distinguish the different types of healthcare knowledge-sharing practices (Section 6.2), propose a novel healthcare knowledge-sharing framework to assist in specifying knowledge-sharing solutions (Section 6.3), highlight prevailing healthcare knowledge-sharing activities by characterizing them based on our unique extension to Nonaka's knowledge creation model

(Section 6.4), and finally conclude with a future outlook of healthcare knowledge sharing (Section 6.5).

6.2   Healthcare Knowledge Sharing

Healthcare knowledge sharing can be characterized as the explication and dissemination of context-sensitive healthcare knowledge by and for healthcare stakeholders through a collaborative communication medium in order to advance the knowledge quotient of the participating healthcare stakeholders. Healthcare knowledge sharing is practiced for a variety of reasons, including clinical decision making, patient education vis-à-vis patient empowerment programs, practitioner's education and experience enhancement, translation of knowledge to practices and vice versa, healthcare policy making, clinical protocol and guideline formulation, public health and community support for patients, capturing care-giver perspectives and feedback about practices and outcomes, and disseminating clinical research findings.

The aim of healthcare knowledge sharing can be characterized as:

1. To provide efficient and focused access to evidence-based knowledge resources, either by directly guiding the user to the knowledge artifacts or by providing peer recommendations to help find the relevant knowledge artifacts.
2. To explicate and share the "unpublished" intrinsic experiential know-how, insights, judgments, and problem-solving strategies of stakeholders to complement evidence-based knowledge.
3. To establish a culture for collaboration between like-minded stakeholders in order to stimulate collaborative learning, atypical problem-solving, practice evaluation, critical appraisal of evidence, practices and outcomes, leveraging peer experiences and knowledge, and feedback solicitation on practices and policies.

Healthcare knowledge sharing practices can be formally characterized as follows:

1. *Artifact-mediated knowledge sharing* involves the sharing of healthcare knowledge either *through an artifact* (such as a research article, clinical practice guideline, or a clinical document) or *around an artifact*. In the former case, the artifact serves as the knowledge object being that can be shared/retrieved through a knowledge repository (such as PubMed or Cochrane), or the artifact can be exchanged through a communication channel, e.g. e-mail, between stakeholders having a common interest. In the latter case, the artifact serves as the focal point for a critical discussion between interested stakeholders, and it is the canonical knowledge explicated through such discussions that serves as the knowledge object that is shared within a larger community of stakeholders. In both the abovementioned cases, the artifact serves as the stimulus for knowledge sharing.
2. *Experience-mediated knowledge sharing* involves the articulation and sharing of clinical, operational, and even psychosocial experiences, insights, and

know-how about a particular healthcare topic. Healthcare stakeholders, orig-
inating from different backgrounds and expertise levels, engage, collaborate,
and share their intrinsic knowledge and extrinsic work practices to address
a specific healthcare issue through a communication medium, e.g. an online
discussion forum or e-mail exchanges. To guide the knowledge-sharing
activity, the healthcare topic serves as the focal point for the exchange of
knowledge, whereas the explicated experiential knowledge (withholding a
diversity of opinions and perspectives from a variety of stakeholders) serves as
a tangible and sharable knowledge object that ultimately enriches the overall
knowledge quantum around the healthcare issue.
3. *Resource-mediated knowledge sharing* involves the identification of knowledge
resources as a by-product of actual knowledge-sharing activities between
healthcare stakeholders. In this case, actual sharing of knowledge objects
does not take place; rather, as context-sensitive knowledge is being shared,
the associated knowledge resources (e.g. domain experts, contact persons,
knowledge brokers, websites, discussion forums, knowledge artifacts, etc.)
are identified, registered, and shared as potential sources of knowledge for a
specific healthcare issue.

In healthcare, knowledge sharing is a necessity and a common practice, albeit it is
conducted in a rather ad hoc manner [7]. In routine practice, healthcare knowledge
sharing transpires during problems-solving conversations between healthcare colleagues about: a clinical case at hand; joint critical appraisals of a research article,
clinical situation, clinical guideline, or administrative policy; group-based formu-
lations of a clinical guideline or workflow; referrals to a subject specialist, published evidence, and reviews; and provision of therapeutic or health maintenance
information to patients (or their care givers). Typically, these knowledge-sharing
activities are orchestrated in an uncharted and informal manner and spanning a
limited period over which the healthcare issue is under consideration. Notwithstanding the success of such ad hoc healthcare knowledge-sharing activities, the
reality is that, most often: (a) the knowledge-sharing community (i.e. both donors
and seekers) is not sustained for future knowledge-sharing activities; (b) the knowledge created and shared during the process is not necessarily recorded for future
reference purposes; (c) the knowledge-sharing medium is not maintained for future knowledge-sharing exercises; and (d) the knowledge-sharing culture is not
promoted and consolidated. This brings to relief the need for technology-enriched
knowledge-sharing frameworks that can handle the sharing of different healthcare
knowledge modalities in a timely, ubiquitous, and sustained manner [11,14].

6.3   A Healthcare Knowledge-Sharing Model

To conceptualize healthcare knowledge-sharing frameworks we need a high-level
abstraction of the determinants of healthcare knowledge sharing (i.e. a generic
model that identifies and relates the determinants of healthcare knowledge sharing)

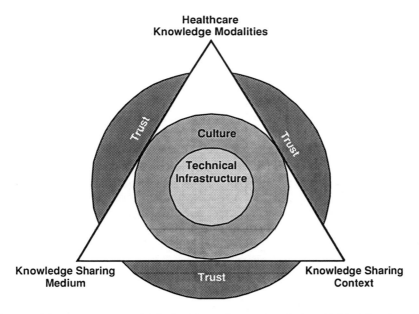

FIGURE 6.1. The LINKS model for healthcare knowledge sharing, highlighting the relationship between the conceptual, operational, and compliance levels.

in order to characterize and validate the functional and operational characteristics of a problem-specific knowledge-sharing solution.

We present a novel healthcare knowledge-sharing model named LINKS (Leveraging Internet-based Knowledge Sharing) illustrated in Figure 6.1. The LINKS model characterizes healthcare knowledge-sharing solutions at three interrelated levels, i.e. conceptual, operational, and compliance. The conceptual level predicates knowledge sharing as a function between three elements: *healthcare knowledge*, *knowledge-sharing context*, and a *knowledge-sharing medium*. The operational level addresses functional issues in terms of *technical infrastructure* design metrics, and occupational issues in terms of strategies to establish a *culture* of collaboration between stakeholders. The compliance level addresses the underlying issue of perceived *trust* in the validity of the knowledge being shared [15], which is the ultimate measure of the success of the knowledge-sharing activity and the operational efficacy of shared knowledge.

6.3.1 *Healthcare Knowledge Modalities*

To conceptualize healthcare knowledge sharing it is important to have a sense of the diversity of the healthcare knowledge modalities that exist and need to be shared between the stakeholders. We know that, typically, healthcare knowledge is broadly differentiated along the lines of *explicit* and *tacit knowledge* [16–18]. Explicit knowledge is codified knowledge represented by information in journals, clinical pathways, protocols, and procedures [19], and it describes *how things should work.* Tacit healthcare knowledge is the nonformalized innate knowledge of practitioners and embodies their experiential know-how, skills, and intuitive judgment about *what really works* and *how to make it work* [20,21].

Given the variety of objectives and practices for healthcare knowledge sharing, we have further characterized healthcare knowledge into more specialized knowledge modalities to pursue highly focused knowledge-sharing activities. For knowledge-sharing purposes, the characterization of healthcare knowledge spans from tacit knowledge, to experiential knowledge, to explicit knowledge, to data-induced knowledge. More specifically, the different healthcare knowledge modalities can be identified as: (a) the tacit knowledge of practitioners in terms of problem-solving skills, judgment, and intuition; (b) practitioners' clinical experiences (both recorded and observed) and lessons learnt through practice; (c) collaborative problem-solving discussions or consultations between practitioners; (d) published medical literature and clinical practice guidelines; (e) operational knowledge in terms of clinical protocols and pathways; (f) medical education content for practitioners; (g) patient-specific educational interventions; (h) psychosocial support and rehabilitation discussions between patient groups; (i) formal decision-support knowledge encapsulated as symbolic decision rules obtained from domain experts and/or decision models induced from data; (j) social networks involving members of a community of practice highlighting their communication patterns, interests, and maybe even expertise; and (k) data-mediated knowledge derived by mining healthcare data on clinical observations, diagnostic tests, and therapeutic treatments recorded in medical records and stored in a clinical data warehouse.

6.3.2   Healthcare Knowledge-Sharing Context

Healthcare knowledge sharing takes place within a context which epitomizes (a) the *topic* (or subject) of the shared knowledge, (b) the *motivation* for knowledge sharing, (c) the *temporal relevance* of the shared knowledge, and (d) the *orientation* of the multidisciplinary stakeholder(s) engaged in the knowledge-sharing exercise.

Let us establish the relevance of context in knowledge sharing. A rich knowledge-sharing activity realizes a compendium of wisdom via the gradual accumulation of validated healthcare knowledge contributed from a variety of sources. Despite the availability of this accumulated knowledge, during any knowledge-sharing exercise the stakeholders tend to carefully observe, align, and validate the available knowledge and then selectively uptake the most relevant knowledge based on their immersed context. In this case, the spectrum of knowledge-sharing context entails the stakeholder's needs (e.g. a current clinical case), interests, consumption capacity (e.g. degree of specialization), professional dispositions, personal preferences, operational applicability, and degree of trust towards the knowledge. What makes healthcare knowledge sharing so interesting is the diversity of contexts associated with a single knowledge-sharing exercise: i.e. different stakeholders may view both the available knowledge and the knowledge-sharing exercise from different perspectives; different stakeholders may pursue the same body of knowledge to satisfy their unique needs, motivations, outcomes, and experiences;

and the stakeholder's eventual uptake and operationalization of the knowledge may depend on their idiosyncratic professional and personal circumstances.

To understand healthcare knowledge sharing, especially for designing and implementing knowledge-sharing programs or technical frameworks, it is important (a) to specify the constituents of context vis-à-vis knowledge sharing and (b) to incorporate them as part of the functional specifications of the knowledge-sharing program or environment. We propose that context can be defined as a tuple {topic, motivation, temporal relevance, stakeholder}, where each element may have a domain of values and the combination of these values leads to the specification of different contexts. The elements of context are described in detail below.

6.3.2.1 Topic

Knowledge is classified in terms of real-world domains and within a domain it is identified by the domain-specific topic (or subject). For establishing the context of knowledge sharing, one needs to determine what the knowledge is about, i.e. the topic or subject of the shared knowledge within a certain knowledge-sharing program/environment. The determination of the knowledge-sharing topic may range from quite generic to extremely specific topics, depending on the objectives set by the stakeholder initiating the knowledge-sharing activity and the intended audience.

In designing a healthcare knowledge-sharing program/environment it is imperative to specify meaningful topics to streamline the knowledge-sharing exercise [22]. For a more flexible and all-encompassing knowledge-sharing exercise, a broad topic is better with an n-level hierarchy of subtopics to account for specializations within the topic, whereas a list of specific topics can be defined for focused knowledge sharing. It may be noted that it is unrealistic to expect the knowledge being shared to be strictly confined within the specified topics; rather, there will always be instances when a knowledge-sharing thread within a specific topic may not relate to the topic or may progressively (and maybe inadvertently) diverge from the specified topic. In such situations, the knowledge-sharing facilitator may create a new topic to accommodate the shift in the knowledge content (if no existing topic can be used), align to an existing and more relevant topic, or advise the stakeholders to revert to the predefined topic.

6.3.2.2 Motivation

Why does an individual/group want to share knowledge [23]? The motivations can be manifold, e.g.: (a) to instigate collaborative problem solving; (b) to inform and educate peers through personal/professional experiences, insights, and know how; (c) to be informed and educated; (d) to negotiate and validate one's thinking, practices, or even a "gray" knowledge artifact; (e) to exchange ideas in order to advance care planning, policies, and research; (f) to build capacity within a specific area of clinical practice, care, or research; (g) to serve as a knowledge broker by directing peers to healthcare knowledge resources; (h) to address knowledge gaps (in particular to address the rural–urban divide) beyond the traditional knowledge access methods; and (i) to form a viable community of practice around a certain topic. The aforementioned motivations may further be differentiated based on practitioner, patient, and community viewpoints (the viewpoints may be shaped by terms of engagement, perceived benefits, and expected outcomes) to share knowledge.

In designing healthcare knowledge-sharing programs/environments it is important to determine a priori the potential range of knowledge-sharing motivations for the participating stakeholders. In fact, it is even recommended to ask the participating stakeholders to state their motivation for participating in the knowledge-sharing exercise, as it would accordingly allow one to align the knowledge-sharing exercise and to measure the utility of the knowledge-sharing exercise objectively. In any knowledge-sharing practice it is important to attempt to satisfy the predetermined set of motivations, because it is practically infeasible to account for all possible motivations within a single knowledge-sharing program/environment. In fact, the predetermined motivations, typically derived from the knowledge-sharing objectives, serve as a design parameter to determine the nature, functional requirements, and implications of the knowledge-sharing program/environment.

6.3.2.3   Temporal Relevance

Patient care is a time-related activity that involves an active interplay between different healthcare knowledge modalities systematically applied in response to the evolving patient conditions. Knowledge-driven medical interventions need to be applied in a specific order and for a specific duration to achieve specific outcomes that are pertinent to the different temporal stages of patient care, i.e. diagnosis, prognosis, and therapy [24,25].

Healthcare knowledge sharing, from a patient care perspective, therefore, needs to be congruent to the knowledge needs at a specific stage of patient care. For instance, the type, scope, and functionality of knowledge is quite different to comprehend and respond to (i) the manifested symptoms, (ii) the interventions applied, (iii) the outcomes measured, and (iv) the effects of the interventions. We argue that, in principle, knowledge-sharing programs/frameworks should model the temporal progression of a clinical case in order to facilitate the sharing of temporally salient knowledge artifacts, support, judgments, and actions [26]. The rationale for this is that the application and implication of any healthcare knowledge is not uniform across all stages of patient care: knowledge pertinent to the etiology of the disease may not have much relevance at the treatment stage. However, in the current state of practice, the temporal relevance of knowledge is ignored whilst sharing it and, if noted, the stakeholder subjectively determines it.

The LINKS models, therefore, demand the temporal characterization of the knowledge-sharing context in designing knowledge-sharing programs/environments. In this regard, the context should inform the temporal relevance of the knowledge in order to improve the effectiveness of the sharing exercise and enhance the uptake of temporally relevant knowledge-driven interventions. Furthermore, for design purposes, the temporal reality of the clinical case and the knowledge demands for its administration help to determine the potential usability and impact of the candidate knowledge modalities and the sharing mediums.

6.3.2.4 Stakeholders

In determining the knowledge-sharing context, a characterization of the stakeholders is required to determine *how* and *what* knowledge is created and shared. The stakeholder's orientation influences the knowledge-sharing exercise; for instance, practitioners are largely interested in sharing problem-solving knowledge, patients are interested in sharing illness-specific experiences, whereas community care givers are interested in formulating support groups. Hence, knowledge sharing at different stakeholder levels is potentially different, whereby variations may exist in terms of (i) the terminology being used, (ii) the specificity of the concepts, (iii) the brevity and formality of the knowledge, (iv) the language constructs, (v) the nature and degree of the relationships (either actual or virtual) between participating stakeholders, (vi) the anticipated application and expected outcomes, (vii) the trust in the source and the content, and (viii) the success measuring criterion. The aforementioned discussion not only suggests the intrinsic make-up of the knowledge created and shared by different stakeholders, but, more crucially, it highlights a set of stakeholder-specific constraints that need to be satisfied to achieve effective stakeholder-centric knowledge-sharing programs/environments.

The LINKS model suggests the creation of a profile for each stakeholder (or each stakeholder group) in order to orchestrate the act of knowledge sharing and to modulate the knowledge being shared. Knowledge sharing guided by the stakeholder's profile will allow means to satisfy the aforementioned constraints and, in turn, will make the knowledge and the knowledge-sharing experience more relevant to the stakeholder. To create the stakeholder's profile, one may either: (a) explicitly seek their motivation/objective, intellectual level, operational workplace, knowledge expectations, levels of involvement in the knowledge sharing exercise, and topics of interest; or (b) infer through observations and analysis of the stakeholder's past knowledge-sharing activities. However, for the sake of operational convenience, it is recommended to determine the stakeholder's profile explicitly.

6.3.3   Healthcare Knowledge-Sharing Medium

Knowledge sharing is practiced via a medium. The sophistication of the medium may range from traditional face-to-face environments, such as person–person conversations and speaker(s)—audience interactions, to virtual meeting environments leveraging the Internet to enable stakeholders to meet and share knowledge virtually.

The LINKS model supports electronic knowledge sharing, grounded in knowledge management practices, and leverages the Internet as the knowledge-sharing medium. There are a range of Internet-based mediums that can be used for healthcare knowledge sharing, e.g.: (a) point-to-point or multipoint (i.e. broadcast) e-mails; (b) recommender system-to-patient e-mails comprising personalized knowledge content, recommendations, and even alerts; (c) Web-based portal to disseminate static healthcare knowledge; here, extensions are possible to personalize the knowledge towards a stakeholder's profile; (d) online discussion forum allowing stakeholders to engage in a virtual meeting place and, through discussions, collaboratively address problems/issues and educate participating stakeholders; (e) online training environments, such as WebCT; (f) peer-to-peer (P2P) networks for sharing knowledge between a dedicated community of practice; and (g) online healthcare knowledge repositories, such as PubMed, Cochrane, etc. A hybrid knowledge-sharing medium comprising more than one of the aforementioned mediums is also technically feasible. The aforementioned knowledge-sharing mediums differentiate the knowledge-sharing experience along the lines of the following modalities: (i) asynchronous versus synchronous versus multisynchronous interactions; (ii) anonymous versus disclosed identity of participating stakeholders; (iii) individual-based interaction versus group interactions; (iv) push versus pull mode of knowledge delivery; (v) open participation versus members-only participation; (vi) supporting dynamic versus static knowledge content; and (vii) manifesting informal and temporary coupling versus long-term dedicated relationship between stakeholders.

The abovementioned range of knowledge-sharing mediums and the kind of knowledge-sharing modalities can serve as design considerations for designing knowledge-sharing frameworks.

6.4   Healthcare Knowledge Sharing: Prevailing Practices

Healthcare knowledge sharing, in knowledge management terms, is quite prevalent amongst healthcare shareholders. To characterize healthcare knowledge-sharing practices formally, we adapt Nonaka's two-dimensional knowledge creation model [16] to realize a novel three-dimensional knowledge-sharing practice model (shown in Figure 6.2): the three dimensions are (1) the source knowledge modality, (2) the target knowledge modality, and (3) the stakeholders. The third dimension, i.e. the stakeholders, is in response to the perceived dichotomy in the knowledge needs and knowledge-sharing practices of healthcare practitioners and patients. We explain below the knowledge-sharing practice for each cell of the knowledge-sharing practice model using the legend stakeholder–source–target.

6.4.1   Practitioner's Perspective of Knowledge Sharing

Put simply, the practitioner's perspective of healthcare knowledge sharing aims to improve patient care and health outcomes by bridging the knowledge gaps with relevant and up-to-date knowledge. In this case, knowledge sharing entails (a) disseminating published evidence (i.e. the explicit aspects of healthcare knowledge), (b) sharing experiences, insights, know how, etc. of specialists (i.e. the tacit aspects of healthcare knowledge), and (c) formulating communities of practice around specific healthcare topics.

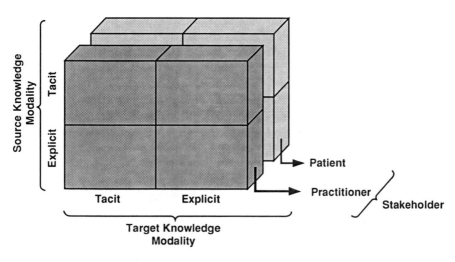

FIGURE 6.2. The three-dimensional model of healthcare knowledge-sharing practices.

6.4.1.1   Practitioner–Tacit Knowledge–Tacit Knowledge Sharing

Healthcare practitioners are routinely confronted with knowledge gaps, whether due to the lag in relevant evidence being published in the medical literature, the lack of published evidence for an unusually complex clinical problem, or simply inaccessibility to knowledge resources. A practitioner's tacit knowledge, i.e. clinical experiences, insights, judgments, and intuitive problem-solving skills, is a well-recognized alternative to evidence-based knowledge [20]. Sharing the tacit knowledge of healthcare experts, via *socialization* [16], can assist fellow practitioners in terms of providing them practical insights into *what solution will work, why it will work, and how to make it work* [20].

Collaboration, though at times informal and ad hoc, is a common activity in discharging healthcare, such that practitioners converge to solve a complex clinical problem collaboratively [14]. The knowledge-sharing medium of an online discussion forum serves as an apt collaborative learning environment for *experience-mediated knowledge sharing* between practitioners bound by a common objective or interest [22]. Online discussion forums provide a virtual meeting space for healthcare practitioners to engage in problem-specific discussions that lead to the explication and sharing of tacit knowledge [27]. The workings are as follows: (1) a practitioner seeks a solution/advice to a clinical problem by presenting it to the discussion forum; (2) practitioners with an interest and expertise in the advertised topic respond by providing their knowledge about the problem; (3) a debate ensues between practitioners, during which they share experiences, negotiate viewpoints, relate theory to practice, and finally conclude a peer-validated solution; (4) the validated solution encapsulating the tacit knowledge of specialist practitioners is shared via the discussion forum to a wider community of practitioners. Although not evidence based, the tacit knowledge being shared has a high trust value because it originates from specialist practitioners and is critiqued (for veracity and quality) by a group of practitioners.

Knowledge sharing through discussion forums has both a problem-solving aspect and learning aspect to it, because the observing practitioners not only learn about a potential solution to a atypical clinical problem, but, as the discussion unfolds, they also observe the tacit problem-solving strategy and reasoning methods employed by specialist practitioners. This knowledge-sharing approach corresponds to Hansen's [28] notion of *personalization*, which entails the provision of one-off problems to professionals with tacit knowledge as a means to communicate effectively with other experts, and Abidi's [20] proposal for tacit knowledge acquisition by challenging experts to solve atypical problems.

6.4.1.2   Practitioner–Tacit Knowledge–Explicit Knowledge Sharing

This knowledge-sharing practice leads to the *externalization* [16] and *codification* of a practitioner's tacit knowledge that is explicated during collaborative problem-solving or critical analysis of evidence and professional practice. The knowledge-sharing exercise can be characterized as *experience-mediated knowledge sharing*, as the knowledge being shared is grounded in the professional experience, intuition, and problem-solving strategies of healthcare practitioners.

There are four prominent manifestations of *practitioner–tacit–explicit* knowledge-sharing practices. (1) The online discussion threads withhold within them highly specialized tacit knowledge. The discussion threads represent the temporal progression of the discussion in terms of topic-specific messages exchanged between practitioners. We posit that the systematic coding, indexing, and storing of discussion threads can result in an explicit knowledge resource that can be subsequently shared between practitioners [29]. It is interesting to note that this codification of tacit knowledge materializes as an indirect consequence of knowledge sharing between practitioners. (2) The formulation of clinical practice guidelines and protocols involves a knowledge-rich dialog between specialist practitioners whereby they share their experiences and negotiate their viewpoints to derive a consensual and explicit knowledge artifact, i.e. a clinical practice guideline. Through knowledge sharing, tacit knowledge is explicated, captured, and codified to realize an explicit knowledge artifact. (3) Online educational programs, seminars, and talk (such as those delivered using WebCT) are a case of tacit to explicit knowledge sharing. In most cases, the tacit knowledge is electronically captured as explicit knowledge and made available together with the educational content (such as slides, notes, papers, etc.). (4) A corollary of such knowledge-sharing practices is the realization of a social network (a social knowledge resource that is based on the communication patterns between individuals during knowledge sharing) that depicts the role and relevance of participating stakeholders with respect to a specific topic [30]. The analysis of the social network leads to the externalization of implicit social knowledge that can be used to identify subject specialists, knowledge brokers, and like-minded peers in order to collaborate and to seek knowledge in the future.

6.4.1.3   Practitioner–Explicit Knowledge–Explicit Knowledge Sharing

This knowledge-sharing practice features a *combination* of explicit healthcare knowledge resources whereby practitioners engage in *artifact-mediated and resource-mediated* knowledge sharing. Knowledge sharing involves the exchange of relevant and validated explicit knowledge artifacts, such as research papers, clinical studies, and guidelines, in response to a mitigating knowledge artifact [31]. Typically, a practitioner may seek pertinent explicit knowledge (say journal articles) in order to critique, review, or validate a published clinical study. Such knowledge-sharing practice typically transpires in systematic review-type exercises, where one research article leads to other related articles. The tangible outcome of such knowledge-sharing exercises is the identification, collation, and sharing of a corpus of salient journal articles that cumulatively forms a body of explicit knowledge around the given topic. Knowledge sharing mediums such as e-mail, Web portals, and P2P networks are typically used for explicit–explicit knowledge sharing.

Explicit–explicit knowledge sharing also supports *resource-mediated knowledge sharing* by leveraging the externalized social knowledge characterizing the stakeholders (i.e. their expertise, access to knowledge resources, and ability/willingness to support other stakeholders (attributing to trust in the stakeholder)) to solicit knowledge directly from or share knowledge with identified knowledge resources.

6.4.1.4   Practitioner–Explicit Knowledge–Tacit Knowledge Sharing

This knowledge-sharing practice is tantamount to the *internalization* of shared explicit healthcare knowledge into the mental models, behaviors, and knowledge constructs of the practitioners, i.e. the translation of shared explicit knowledge (or evidence) into their professional practice. From a knowledge translation perspective, one may regard *internalization* [16] or *codification* [28] as the ultimate objective of healthcare knowledge sharing, i.e. to improve the practice and delivery of healthcare by optimally sharing evidence and, in turn, accordingly adjusting clinical practice to achieve better outcomes. Such a*rtifact-mediated* knowledge sharing is typically achieved through both indirect mediums, such as Web portals and knowledge artifacts, and direct mediums, such as e-mails and online training (such as WebCT).

6.4.2   Patient's Perspective of Knowledge Sharing

Broadly speaking, the patient's perspective of healthcare knowledge sharing aims to educate and empower patients (and their care givers) to understand their health condition and to self-manage their healthcare process. This aim is pursued by facilitating the provision of online patient-specific healthcare knowledge (knowledge that may be generic, personalized to meet individual needs, or mass customized for a patient community) in a proactive and timely manner through patient education and support programs. In this regard, knowledge sharing entails (a) disseminating health maintenance information, i.e. the explicit aspects of healthcare knowledge, (b) sharing personal experiences, insights, resources, etc. between patients (and their care givers), i.e. the tacit aspects of healthcare knowledge, and (c) high-lighting support groups around specific healthcare issues, i.e. the social aspects of healthcare knowledge.

6.4.2.1   Patient–Tacit Knowledge–Tacit Knowledge Sharing

Patient care extends beyond healthcare institutions and practitioners. For chronic illnesses the longitudinal therapeutic regimes and rehabilitation programs demand continuous and proactive patient-level education and community-level support to manage the psychosocial, behavioral, lifestyle, and care planning aspects of the disease. These nonmedical elements of patient care are partly administered by healthcare practitioners through counseling, but largely such issues are addressed through the tacit and experiential knowledge of patient support groups (comprising patients, care givers/families, and public health and healthcare practitioners). Patient support programs provide self-help or mutual support that is deemed more effective because patients who share common experiences, situations, or problems can offer each other a unique perspective that is not available from those who have not shared these experiences [32]. And, in practice it is noted that patients indeed seek out and do benefit from opportunities to share their feelings with others when faced with uncertainty, stress, and pain [33].

Online discussion forums provide a knowledge-sharing environment for patient support by the patients and for the patients [33]. Web portals or e-mails are pre-dominantly used to share a patient's individual tacit and experiential knowledge with a community of patients experiencing similar health challenges and having a common interest. Patient-specific knowledge sharing through discussion forums allows patients/care givers to interact, consult, and collaborate with each other in order to (a) offer psychosocial support to help reduce feelings of isolation, teach coping techniques, societal adjustment, and behavioral changes and (b) provide home-based care in terms of sharing personal experiences, i.e. what works, what does not work, what resources were available, what options were provided, how to deal with different psychosocial issues, and what outcomes were achieved. It is this *socialization* of patient's tacit knowledge that is sought and shared in this experience-mediated knowledge-sharing practice to assist patients in decision making, education, empowerment, and self-management of the disease at the home and community levels.

Online patient support groups can be distinguished as: (i) peer-led groups, which focus on self-help and tend to be informal, where leadership is shared, participation is voluntary, and membership size can vary widely; and (ii) professional-led support groups, which primarily focus on education involving a trained facilitator and are more structured with a limited group size. In either case, active collaboration between the members result in the development of "trusted" relationships and knowledge artifacts (vocabularies, documents, understandings, and shared skills) that address the knowledge needs of the patient community [33].

6.4.2.2 Patient–Tacit Knowledge–Explicit Knowledge Sharing

A significant tenet of patient-specific knowledge sharing is online patient education that entails the provision of healthcare knowledge concerning a variety of issues, such as (i) explanations on the disease and therapeutic procedures, (ii) health maintenance information, (iii) lifestyle and behavioral modification interventions, (iv) psychosocial and emotional support solutions, (v) stress management strategies, and (vi) validated information resources [34]. Patient education is a crucial aspect of managing chronic diseases, since appropriate education can impact modifications in health perceptions and behaviors, which in turn can help to prevent the onset or progression of chronic disease [35,36].

From a knowledge-sharing perspective, patient education entails (a) the externalization of the practitioner's tacit knowledge and experiences in terms of a specification of the knowledge needs of a patient, (b) the mapping of the patient's knowledge needs to corresponding explicit knowledge vis-à-vis patient educational content and interventions, and (c) facilitating the patient's uptake and compliance to the shared knowledge resource in order to empower them to self-manage the disease at the therapeutic, behavioral, and psychosocial levels. The translation of the practitioner's assessment of the patient's knowledge needs to actual actionable healthcare knowledge is the major contribution of this kind of knowledge-sharing activity.

Personalized knowledge sharing, i.e. patient educational interventions that are specifically *tailored* to meet the health needs of an individual patient, has been shown to be better received by patients and, in turn, leads to better outcomes [37,38]. Instead of providing generic healthcare knowledge suitable to a wide range of patients, personalized knowledge sharing is based on the individual assessment (or health profile) of the patient by either a practitioner or a recommender system, and constitutes a combination of patient-specific healthcare knowledge and behavioral-change strategies that are intelligently tailored to meet the unique healthcare needs of the patient.

This knowledge-sharing practice entails *artifact-mediated knowledge sharing*, whereby two different artifacts, i.e. the patient health profile and the health education content, are synergized to realize the knowledge content. Knowledge sharing is largely practiced via a Web portal (in the pull mode of sharing) or direct e-mails (in the push mode of sharing) to the patient.

6.4.2.3 Patient–Explicit Knowledge–Explicit Knowledge Sharing

This is the most common knowledge-sharing practice, as it features *artifact-mediated* and *resource-mediated* knowledge sharing typically in situations when patients search for additional or more validated healthcare knowledge to complement some healthcare knowledge that they may already have. A requirement for patient empowerment is that the patient strives to become better informed by vehemently pursuing additional knowledge to enhance his/her understanding of the disease, the associated therapeutic options, and the criterion for measuring outcomes. Knowledge sharing, in this scenario, entails a *combination* of two explicit healthcare knowledge artifacts: (1) a source knowledge artifact from a healthcare practitioner, a fellow patient, or a publication such as newspaper, magazine, leaflet, or poster; (2) the corresponding target knowledge artifact shared in order to complement the source knowledge artifact. Typically, patient-specific health knowledge resources, such as the Web-based health portals, are used to source additional knowledge.

Resource-mediated knowledge sharing also plays a vital role in identifying relevant and validated knowledge sources: the social knowledge about the predispositions of patient peers and their accumulated knowledge resources helps to seek additional knowledge in a more focused manner. As an outcome of this knowledge-sharing exercise, the patient both identifies knowledge sources and collects knowledge artifacts to form a body of explicit knowledge around a healthcare topic of interest.

6.4.2.4   Patient–Explicit Knowledge–Tacit Knowledge Sharing

Patient-mediated knowledge sharing is about educating and effectuating behavior changes, lifestyle changes, and improving health outcomes as a consequence of sharing and consuming healthcare knowledge. The patient's aspect of this knowledge-sharing practice is primarily about the patient's ability, desire, and motivation for the uptake of the shared knowledge.

Akin to the practitioner's aspect of explicit–tacit knowledge sharing, the patient's perspective of this knowledge-sharing practice entails the patient's *internalization* of shared explicit knowledge to achieve a better quality of life, improved decision-making abilities, better coping of psychosocial distress, and positive changes in behavior. *Artifact-mediated* knowledge sharing is responsible for promoting an improved state of self-determination for patients so that they may take charge of their health and healthcare needs.

It may be noted that patient-mediated knowledge sharing can significantly influence the actual care-delivery process: the recommendations, insights, critiques, and solutions shared by patients hold within them explicit indicators and pointers to their satisfaction pertaining to the outcome or implications of their treatment plans. This vital patient-based feedback, transpired through knowledge sharing, augurs well for streamlining prevailing healthcare knowledge and practices.

6.5   Healthcare Knowledge-Sharing Prospects: The Future Outlook

Patient management, in its entirety, is a complex process that can be investigated from different perspectives. We investigated patient management from a knowledge-sharing perspective, whereby we characterized healthcare knowledge-sharing practices and presented a healthcare knowledge-sharing framework, i.e. LINKS, that identified the determinants of healthcare knowledge sharing for developing healthcare knowledge-sharing programs.

Globally, there is an increasing demand for effective (and even accountable) clinical practices and decisions, efficient clinical pathways, optimal resource utilizations, ostensively improved health outcomes, home-based healthcare, enhanced patient empowerment, and creation of a health-conscious society. Such objectives compel the evolution of current healthcare knowledge-sharing practices from individualistic, subject-specific, ad hoc, and need-driven activities to *a consolidated and concerted knowledge-sharing enterprise that specifically focuses on a clinical case and uses it to instigate proactive and pertinent knowledge-sharing activities leading to the sharing of case-specific knowledge congruent to the needs, interests, background, and orientation of all concerned stakeholders.* As per this future outlook, case-specific knowledge sharing will: (a) attempt to meet the knowledge needs as per the temporal sequence of medical events, judgments, actions, and outcomes within the longitudinal continuum of patient care; (b) involve the appropriate sharing of heterogeneous knowledge modalities to support the various case management activities; (c) proactively prescribe highly personalized health maintenance knowledge, typically in the realm of patient education, based on validated clinical decision-support artifacts (such as clinical practice guidelines or protocols) and dispense the knowledge in keeping with the individual patient's degree of readiness, belief, or disposition to uptake and apply the knowledge in order to achieve a positive health outcome.

Current healthcare knowledge-sharing practices usually involve the sharing of a specific knowledge modality as per the designated knowledge-sharing activity. The limitation of this approach is that any knowledge-sharing request results in only a limited quantum of the total available knowledge to be sourced and shared. Yet, for effective patient management one should demand *holistic* knowledge (i.e. healthcare knowledge that spans across heterogeneous knowledge modalities and orientations, thus encompassing a diversity of opinions, explanations, experiences, judgments, resources, solutions, theoretical models, and knowledge artifacts) pertaining to the clinical case at hand [39].

We posit that the future of healthcare knowledge sharing will be *one-stop knowledge sharing* whereby a stakeholder may issue a single knowledge-sharing request that will instigate multiple simultaneous knowledge-sharing activities (each pursuing a different knowledge modality, stakeholder orientation, and sharing medium for the same topic) leading to the collection of multiple, yet relevant, knowledge artifacts. The knowledge-sharing solution will be carried out in two stages. In stage 1, the assortment of knowledge artifacts will be systematically morphed [40] to yield a holistic knowledge object; in stage 2, the morphed knowledge object will be duly customized to meet the specific needs, interests, and consumption capacity of the user (as shown in Figure 6.3).

The above knowledge-sharing outlook not only predicates the need for more focused case-specific knowledge sharing amongst stakeholders, but it further posits case-specific knowledge sharing as the vehicle to systematically, seamlessly, and dynamically *morph* the hitherto individual knowledge modalities to realize holistic healthcare knowledge pertinent to the knowledge needs at specific stages during the lifetime of patient care [40]. It is foreseen that the ability to share holistic and

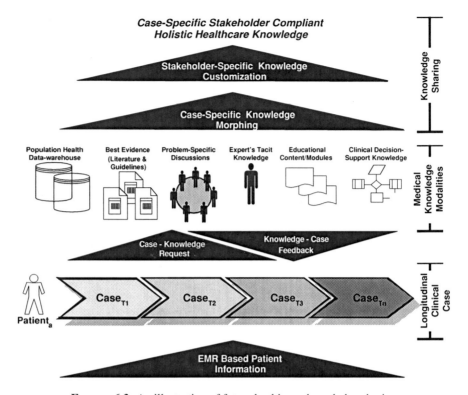

FIGURE 6.3. An illustration of future healthcare knowledge sharing.

customized healthcare knowledge around a particular topic will have a profound impact towards enriching the body of knowledge and enhancing the knowledge quotient of healthcare stakeholders.

Postscript. The future outlook for healthcare knowledge sharing is interesting, yet challenging, and calls for developing innovative knowledge-management-based strategies, techniques, and frameworks.

References

1. Zack MH. Developing a knowledge strategy. *Calif Manage Rev* 1999;41(3):125–145.
2. Steinheider B, Al-Hawamdeh S. Team coordination, communication and knowledge sharing in SMEs and large organizations. *J Inf Knowl Manage* 2004;3(3):223–232.
3. Bieber M, Im I, Rice R, Goldman-Segall R, Stohr E, Hiltz SR, et al. Towards knowledge-sharing and learning in virtual professional communities. In: *35th Annual Hawaii IEEE International Conference on System Sciences*, 2002.
4. Lee CK, Al-Hawamdeh S. Factors impacting knowledge sharing. *J Inf Knowl Manage* 2002;1(1):49–56.
5. Majchrzak A, Rice R, King N, Malhotra A, Ba S. Computer-mediated inter-organizational knowledge-sharing: insights from a virtual team innovating using a collaborative tool. *Inf Resourc Manage J* 2000;13(1): 44–53.

6. Kang M, Byun HP. Framework for a Web-based knowledge construction support system. *Educ Technol* 2001;(July):48–53.

7. Ryu S, Ho SH, Han I. Knowledge sharing behavior of physicians in hospitals. *Expert Syst Appl* 2003;25:113–122.

8. Jadad AR, Haynes RB, Hunt D, Browman RB. The Internet and evidence-based decision-making: a needed synergy for efficient knowledge management in health care. *J Can Med Assoc* 2000;162:362–365.

9. Montani S, Bellazzi R. Supporting decisions in medical applications: the knowledge management perspective. *Int J Med Inform* 2002;68:79–90.

10. Jackson JR. The urgent call for knowledge management in medicine. *Physician Exec* 2000;26:28–31.

11. Jadad AR. Promoting partnerships: challenges for the Internet age. *Br Med J* 1999;319:761–764.

12. Ho K, Chockalingam A, Best A, Walsh G. Technology-enabled knowledge translation: building a framework for collaboration. *Can Med Assoc J* 2003;168:710–711.

13. Eysenbach G, Powell J, Englesakis M, Rizo C, Stern A. Health related virtual communities and electronic support groups: systematic review of the effects of online peer to peer interactions. *Br Med J* 2004;328:1166–70.

14. Safran C, Jones P, Rind D, Bush B, Cytryn K, Patel V. Electronic communication and collaboration in a health care practice. *Artif Intell Med* 1998;12:137–152.

15. Dirks KT, Ferrin D. The role of trust in organizational settings. *Organ Sci* 2001;12:450–467.

16. Nonaka I, Takeuchi H. *The knowledge creating company*. New York: Oxford University Press; 1995.

17. Wyatt JC. Management of explicit and tacit knowledge. *J R Soc Med* 2001;94:6–9.

18. Patel BL, Arocha JF, Kaufman DR. Expertise and tacit knowledge in medicine. In: Sternberg RJ, Horvath JA, editors, *Tacit knowledge in professional practice—researcher and practitioner perspectives*. Mahwah, NJ: Lawrence Erlbaum Associates; 1999.

19. McAdam R, McCreedy S. A critique of knowledge management: using a social constructionist model. *New Technol Work Employ* 2000;15(2):155–168.

20. Abidi SSR, Cheah Y-N, Curran J. A knowledge creation info-structure to acquire and crystallize the tacit knowledge of healthcare experts. *IEEE Trans Inf Technol Biomed* 2005;9(2):193–204.

21. Yu-NC. Abidi SSR. The role of information technology in the explication and crystallization of tacit healthcare knowledge. *Health Inform J* 2001;7(3–4):158–167.

22. Curran-Smith J, Abidi SSR, Forgeron P. Towards a collaborative training environment for children's pain management: leveraging an online discussion forum. *Health Inform J* 2005;11(1):31–43.

23. Pear J, Crone-Todd D. A social constructivist approach to computer mediated instruction. *Comput Educ* 2002;38:221–231.

24. Augusto JC. Temporal reasoning for decision support in medicine. *Artif Intell Med* 2005;33:1–24.

25. Shahar Y. Timing is everything: temporal reasoning and temporal data maintenance in medicine. In: *Proceedings of Seventh Joint European Conference on Artificial Intelligence in Medicine and Medical Decision Making (AIMDM'99)*, Aalborg, Denmark. Springer Verlag; 1999, pp. 30–46.

26. Kahn M. Modeling time in medical decision-support programs. *Med Decis Making* 1991;11(4):249–264.

27. Billings D. Online communities of professional practice. *J Nurs Educ* 2003;42(8):335–336.
28. Hansen MR, Nohria N, Tiernye T. What's your strategy for managing knowledge. In: Cortada JW, Woods JA, editors, *The knowledge management yearbook 2000–2001, part two*. Boston: CWL Publishing Enterprises, Butterworth-Heiniman; 2000.
29. Abidi, SSR, Finley GA, Milios E, Shepherd M, Zitner D. Knowledge management in pediatric pain: mapping online expert discussions to medical literature. In: *11th World Congress on Medical Informatics (MEDINFO'2004)*, San Francisco, 7–11 September 2004.
30. Wenger EC, Snyder WM. Communities of practice: the organizational frontier. *Harvard Bus Rev* 2000;78:139–145.
31. Abidi SSR, Kershaw M, Milios E. Augmenting GEM-encoded clinical practice guidelines with relevant best-evidence autonomously retrieved from MEDLINE. *Health Inform J* 2005;11(2):95–110.
32. Finfgeld D. Therapeutic groups online: the good, the bad, and the unknown. *Issues Mental Health Nurs* 2000;21:241–255.
33. Barrera M, Glasgow RE, McKay HG, Boles SM, Feil EG. Do Internet-based support interventions change perceptions of social support? An experimental trial of approaches for supporting diabetes self-management. *Am J Community Psychol* 2002;30(5):637–654.
34. Gray RE, Fitch M. Cancer self-help groups are here to stay: issues and challenges for health professionals. *J Palliative Care* 2001;17(1):53–58.
35. Nguyen HQ, Carrieri-Kohlman V, Rankin SH, Slaughter R, Stulbarg MS. Internet-based patient education and support interventions: a review of evaluation studies and directions for future research. *Comput Biol Med* 2004;34:95–112.
36. Scherrer-Bannerman A, Fofonoff D, Minshall D, Downie S, Brown M, Leslie F. Web-based education and support for patients on the cardiac surgery waiting list. *J Telemed Telecare* 2000;6:S72–S74.
37. Gustafson DH, Hawkins R, Boberg E, Pingree S, Serlin RE, Graziano F. Impact of a patient-centered, computer-based health information/support system. *Am J Prevent Med* 1999;16(1):1–9.
38. Kreuter MW, Oswald DL, Bull FC, Clark EM. Are tailored health education materials always more effective than non-tailored materials? *Health Educ Res* 2000;15:305–315.
39. Pantazi S, Arocha J, Moer J. Case-based medical informatics. *BMC Med Inform Decision Making* 2004;4:19–42.
40. Abidi SSR. Medical knowledge morphing: towards case-specific integration of heterogeneous medical knowledge resources. In: *18th IEEE International Symposium on Computer-Based Medical Systems*, Dublin, 23–24 June 2005.

7
Healthcare Knowledge Management: Incorporating the Tools, Technologies, Strategies, and Process of Knowledge Management to Effect Superior Healthcare Delivery

NILMINI WICKRAMASINGHE

Abstract

As medical science advances and the applications of information and communications technologies to healthcare operations diffuse, more and more data and information begin to permeate healthcare databases and repositories. However, given the voluminous nature of these disparate data assets, it is no longer possible for healthcare providers to process these data without the aid of sophisticated tools and technologies. The goal of knowledge management is to provide the decision maker with appropriate tools, technologies, strategies, and processes to turn data and information into valuable knowledge assets. This chapter discusses the benefits to the healthcare arena of incorporating these tools and techniques in order to make healthcare delivery more effective and efficient, and thereby maximize the full potential of all healthcare knowledge assets. To ensure a successful knowledge management initiative in a healthcare setting, the chapter proffers the knowledge management infrastructure framework and intelligence continuum model.

The benefits of these techniques lie not only in the ability to make explicit the elements of these knowledge assets, and in so doing enable their full potential to be realized, but also to provide a systematic and robust approach to structuring the conceptualization of knowledge assets across a range of healthcare environments, as the case study data presented demonstrate.

7.1 Introduction

Knowledge management (KM) is an emerging management technique that is aimed at solving the current business challenges to increase efficiency and efficacy of core business processes and simultaneously incorporating continuous innovation. The premise for the need for KM is based on a paradigm shift in the business environment where knowledge is central to organizational performance [1,2].

KM offers organizations many tools, techniques, and strategies to apply to their existing business processes. Healthcare is an information-rich industry that offers a unique opportunity to analyze extremely large and complex data sets. The collection of data permeates all areas of the healthcare industry and, when coupled with the new trends in evidence-based medicine and electronic medical record systems, it is imperative that the healthcare industry embraces the tools, technologies, strategies, and processes of KM if it is to realize the benefits from all these data assets fully.

The successful application KM hinges on the development of a sound KM infrastructure (KMI) and the systematic and continuous application of specific steps supported by various technologies. This serves to underscore the dynamic nature of KM where the extant knowledge base is always being updated. The KMI framework not only helps organizations to structure their knowledge assets, but also makes explicit the numerous implicit knowledge assets currently evident in healthcare [3], while the intelligence continuum (IC) provides the key tools and technologies to facilitate superior healthcare delivery [4]. Taken together, the KMI and IC can enable healthcare to realize its value proposition of delivering effective and efficient value-added healthcare services.

7.2   Knowledge Management

"Land, labor, and capital now pale in comparison to knowledge as the critical asset to be managed in today's knowledge economy." Peter F. Drucker [2, p. 47].

The nations that lead the world in this century will be those who can shift from being industrial economies, based upon the production of manufactured goods, to those that possess the capacity to produce and utilize knowledge successfully. The focus of the many nations' economies has shifted first to information-intensive industries, such as financial services and logistics, and now toward innovation-driven industries, such as computer software and biotechnology, where competitive advantage lies mostly in the innovative use of human resources. This represents a move from an era of standardization to an era of innovation where knowledge, its creation, and management hold the key to success [1,2,5].

KM is a key approach to helping solve current business problems that are faced by organizations today, such as competitiveness and the need to innovate. The premise for KM is based on a paradigm shift in the business environment where knowledge is central to organizational performance [6,7]. In essence, KM not only involves the production of information, but also the capture of data at the source, the transmission and analysis of this data, and the communication of information based on or derived from the data to those who can act on it [8]. Thus, data and information represent critical raw assets in the generation of knowledge, whereas successful KM initiatives require a tripartite view, namely the incorporation of people, processes, and technologies [9].

Broadly speaking, KM involves four key steps of creating/generating knowledge, representing/storing knowledge, accessing/using/reusing knowledge, and disseminating/transferring knowledge [8,10–12]. Knowledge creation, generally accepted as the first step for any KM endeavor, requires an understanding of the knowledge construct as well as its people and technology dimensions. Given that knowledge creation is the first step in any KM initiative, it naturally has a significant impact on the other consequent KM steps, thus making the identification of and facilitating of knowledge creation a key focal point for any organization wanting to leverage its knowledge potential fully.

Knowledge, however, is not a simple construct. Specifically, knowledge can exist as an object, in essentially two forms: explicit or factual knowledge and tacit or "know-how" [13,14]. It is well established that although both types of knowledge are important, tacit knowledge is more difficult to identify and thus manage [15,16]. Of equal importance, though perhaps less well defined, knowledge also has a subjective component and can be viewed as an ongoing phenomenon, being shaped by social practices of communities [17]. The objective elements of knowledge can be thought of as primarily having an impact on process, whereas the subjective elements typically impact innovation [9]. Enabling and enhancing both effective and efficient processes and the functions of supporting and fostering innovation are key concerns of KM.

Organizational knowledge is not static; rather, it changes and evolves during the lifetime of an organization. What is more, it is possible to transform one form of knowledge into another, i.e. transform tacit knowledge into explicit and vice versa [12]. This process of transforming one form of knowledge into another is known as the knowledge spiral [15]. Naturally, this does not imply that one form of knowledge is necessarily transformed 100% into another form of knowledge. According to Nonaka [15]: (1) Socialization, or tacit to tacit knowledge transformation, usually occurs through apprenticeship-type relations where the teacher or master passes on the skill to the apprentice. (2) Combination, or explicit to explicit knowledge transformation, usually occurs via formal learning of facts. (3) Externalization, or tacit to explicit knowledge transformation, usually occurs when there is an articulation of nuances; e.g. if an expert surgeon is questioned as to why he performs a particular surgical procedure in a certain manner, by his articulation of the steps the tacit knowledge becomes explicit. (4) Internalization, or explicit to tacit knowledge transformation, usually occurs when explicit knowledge is internalized and can then be used to broaden, reframe, and extend one's tacit knowledge. Integral to these transformations of knowledge through the knowledge spiral is that new knowledge is being continuously created [15], and this can potentially bring many benefits to organizations. What becomes important, then, for any organization in today's knowledge economy is to maximize the full potential of all its knowledge assets and successfully make all germane knowledge explicit so that it can be used effectively and efficiently by all people within the organization as required [12].

Healthcare is an industry currently facing major challenges at a global level [4,18]. This industry has yet to embrace KM. Yet, KM appears to provide several viable possibilities to address the current crisis faced by global healthcare in the areas of access, quality, and value [4]. In healthcare, one of the most critical knowledge transformations to effect is that of tacit to explicit, i.e. externalization, so that the healthcare organization can best leverage its knowledge potential to realize the healthcare value proposition [19]. Integral to such a process is the establishment of a robust KMI and the adoption of key tools and techniques. This is achieved by the application of the KMI and IC models.

7.3   Establishing a Knowledge Management Infrastructure

The most valuable resources available to any organization are human skills, expertise, and relationships. KM is about capitalizing on these precious assets [20]. Most companies do not capitalize on the wealth of expertise in the form of knowledge scattered across their levels [21]. Information centers, market intelligence, and learning are converging to form KM functions. KM offers organizations many strategies, techniques, and tools to apply to their existing business processes so that they are able to grow and effectively utilize their knowledge assets. The KMI not only forms the foundation for enabling and fostering KM, continuous learning, and sustaining an organizational memory [2], but also provides the foundations for actualizing the four key steps of KM, namely creating/generating knowledge, representing/storing knowledge, accessing/using/reusing knowledge, and disseminating/transferring knowledge (discussed in Section 7.2). An organization's entire "know-how," including new knowledge, can only be created for optimization if an effective KMI is established. Specifically, the KMI consists of social and technical tools and techniques, including hardware and software, that should be established so that knowledge can be created from any new events or activities on a continual basis. In addition, the KMI will have a repository of knowledge, systems to distribute the knowledge to the members of the organization, and a facilitator system for the creation of new knowledge. Thus, a knowledge-based infrastructure will foster the creation of knowledge and provide an integrated system to share and diffuse the knowledge within the organization [22], as well as support for continual creation and generation of new knowledge [9]. The KMI depicted in Figure 7.1 contains the five essential elements of organizational memory, human asset infrastructure, knowledge transfer network, business intelligence infrastructure, and infrastructure for collaboration that, together, must be present for any KM initiative to succeed.

7.3.1   Elements of the Knowledge Management Infrastructure

From Figure 7.1 it is possible to identify the five key elements that, together, make up the KMI. It can be seen that these elements support the socio-technical perspective of KM, in that they consist of people, process, and technological aspects [12]. We will now examine each of them in more detail.

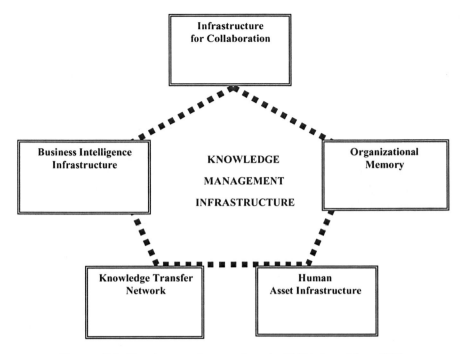

FIGURE 7.1. Key elements that constitute the KMI (adapted from [23]).

7.3.1.1   Infrastructure for Collaboration

The key to competitive advantage and improving customer satisfaction lies in the ability of organizations to form learning alliances; these are strategic partnerships based on a business environment that encourages mutual (and reflective) learning between partners [24]. Organizations can utilize their strategy framework to identify partners and collaborators for enhancing their value chain.

7.3.1.2   Organizational Memory

Organizational memory is concerned with the storing and subsequent accessing and replenishing of an organization's "know-how" that is recorded in documents or in its people [24]. However, a key component of KM not addressed in the construct of organizational memory is the subjective aspect [9]. Knowledge as a subjective component primarily refers to an ongoing phenomenon of exchange where knowledge is being shaped by social practices of communities [18], in the tradition of a Hegelian/Kantian perspective, where the importance of divergence of meaning is essential to support the "sense-making" processes of knowledge creation [25].

Organizational memory keeps a record of knowledge resources and locations. Recorded information, whether in human-readable or electronic form or in the memories of staff, is an important embodiment of an organization's knowledge and intellectual capital. Thus, strong organizational memory systems ensure the access of information or knowledge throughout the company to everyone at any time [26].

7.3.1.3   Human Asset Infrastructure

This deals with the participation and willingness of people. Today, organizations have to attract and motivate the best people: to reward, recognize, train, educate, and improve them [27] so that the highly skilled and more independent workers can exploit technologies to create knowledge in learning organizations [27]. The human asset infrastructure, then, helps to identify and utilize the special skills of people who can create greater business value if they and their inherent skills and experiences are managed to make explicit use of their knowledge.

7.3.1.4   Knowledge Transfer Network

This element is concerned with the dissemination of knowledge and information. Unless there is a strong communication infrastructure in place, people are not able to communicate effectively and thus are unable to transfer knowledge effectively. An appropriate communications infrastructure includes, but is not limited to, the Internet and intranets for creating the knowledge transfer network, as well as discussion rooms and bulletin boards for meetings and for displaying information.

7.3.1.5   Business Intelligence Infrastructure

In an intelligent enterprise, various information systems are integrated with knowledge-gathering and analyzing tools for data analysis and dynamic end-user querying of a variety of enterprise data sources [28]. Business intelligence infrastructures have customers, suppliers, and other partners embedded into single integrated system. Customers will view their own purchasing habits, and suppliers will see the demand pattern which may help them to offer volume discounts, etc. This information can help all customers, suppliers, and enterprises to analyze data and provide them with the competitive advantage. The intelligence of a company is not only available to internal users, but can also even be leveraged by selling it to others, such as consumers, who may be interested in this type of informational intelligence.

7.3.2   The Intelligence Continuum

The IC consists of a collection of key tools, techniques, and processes of the knowledge economy, i.e. including data mining, business intelligence/analytics, and KM which are applied to a generic system of people, process, and technology in a systematic and ordered fashion [4,18,29,30]. Taken together they represent a very powerful system for refining the data raw material stored in data marts

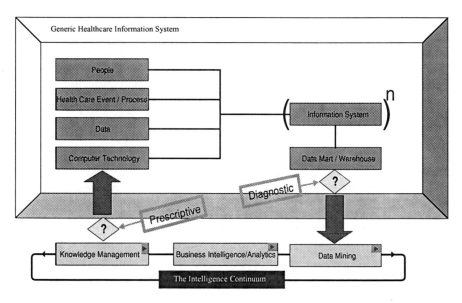

FIGURE 7.2. Application of the IC on the generic healthcare system.

and/or data warehouses, thereby maximizing the value and utility of these data assets for any organization [31–36]. As depicted in Figure 7.2, the IC is applied to the output of the generic healthcare information system. Once applied, the results become part of the data set that are reintroduced into the system and combined with the other inputs of people, processes, and technology to develop an improvement continuum. Thus, the IC includes the generation of data, the analysis of these data to provide a "diagnosis," and the reintroduction into the cycle as a "prescriptive" solution. In this way, the next iteration, or "future state," always represents the enhancement of the extant knowledge base of the previous iteration. For the IC to be truly effective, however, the KMI must already be in place so that all data, information, and knowledge assets are explicit and the technologies of the IC can be applied to them in a systematic and methodical fashion.

7.4 Case Study

This case study focuses on a well-renowned Spine Unit in the Midwest of the US. It is possible to define this environment as a cure environment, since the primary goal of this Spine Unit is to return patients to normal life activities. The following serves to furnish the key elements from this environment as they pertain to KM, its benefits, and applications in this setting. An exploratory case study research was adopted to enable the generation of rich data in a nonrestrictive manner. Information was gathered from several sources, including semi-structured interviews, the collecting of germane documents and memos, numerous site visits, and the direct observation of various procedures, thus enabling triangulation among different data sources [37]. Rigorous coding and extensive thematic analysis was conducted to analyze the qualitative data gathered [38,39]. Each of the points listed was confirmed by multiple interviews, written documentation, and passive observation, thus ensuring the highest level of reliability possible for qualitative research [39].

7.4.1   Background for Case

In the US, the healthcare industry is in a state of flux [40–43].

The rate of the rise in healthcare costs has been variable. The shocking increases experienced in the early 1990s, has slowed in the mid- and late 1990s, but there is no guarantee that they will continue to do so [44, pp. xvii].

In other market places, buyers are sensitive to the price of the product and undertake cost–benefit analysis.

In the medical market place, however, the buyers and users of medical services and technologies have been relatively insensitive to the cost of these services ... The traditional financing and reimbursement policies of the healthcare industry are felt to be largely responsible for this price insensitivity, inhibiting the forces of competitive supply and demand economics [40, pp. 80].

As a result, there is increased pressure on providers of medical care to develop ways to control and mange costs, as well as to increase productivity without compromising quality. In an attempt to stem the escalating costs of healthcare, managed care has emerged. It is aimed at creating value through competition in order to combat "... an extremely wasteful and inefficient system that has been bathed in cost-increasing incentives for over 50 years" [45, p. 40]. The intended result is to provide adequate quality healthcare and yet minimize, or at least reduce, costs.

Managed care organizations (MCOs) contract with individuals, employers, and other purchasers to provide comprehensive healthcare services to people who enroll in their health plans. The essential difference between MCOs and more traditional types of medical care is connected with the distribution of financial risk among the purchaser of healthcare, the provider of the care, and the insurer [46].

MCOs typically reduce this financial risk for the purchaser of healthcare insurance by guaranteeing a comprehensive range of services at a fixed price to them. To do this of course, the MCO must keep the use of healthcare resources within a budget; thus making critical a focus on managing medical care [18].

This then represents a radical change to the traditional healthcare environment, where quality irrespective of cost was the goal. The new goal is cost-effective quality care, and thus also demands a more competitive healthcare environment.

7.4.2   Spine Care

Nearly everyone experiences back or neck pain at some time during their life. Pain or disability can be caused by injuries sustained at home or work, while involved in sports or recreation, during accidents or falls, or from medical conditions, such as arthritis, osteoarthritis, or osteoporosis. The Spine Unit is part of a large multispecialty group practice and academic medical center located in the Midwest of the US. This center is actually made up of surgeons and medical staff from the Department of Neurology and Neurosurgery and the Department of Orthopedics. A cooperation of the surgeons of these two departments has led to the Spine Unit, where more than 9000 patients with spinal problems are treated annually. The multidisciplinary team in this setting consists of experienced spine surgeons, well-trained psychologists, physical therapists, operating room personnel, and laboratory pathology experts. The multidisciplinary team works with well-established proven protocols. Naturally, with back and neck complaints the process cannot be the same for every patient; rather, it is dependent on the specific complaint the patient has.

7.4.3   Technologies

In order for the Spine Unit to achieve its goal of providing high-quality treatment to patients suffering from various back and neck complaints, many key factors must be addressed concerning both the clinical and practice management issues. Technologies of various types play a key role in enabling effective and efficient high-quality treatments at the center. The clinical technologies include the laboratory and radiology facilities to enable the best possible detection of the specific complaint, as well as the technologies to support the treating of this complaint, especially if surgery is the course of action, e.g. the use of image-guided spinal navigation to facilitate the accuracy, precision, and safety of spinal instrumentation and reduction in operative time, or laparoscopic or endoscopic procedures to minimize invasive spinal surgery. On the practice management side, the technologies include the hospital management information system (HMIS) in place. Table 7.1 describes the systems that comprise the HMIS.

7.4.4   Structure

The spine is a very complex part of the human anatomy. Bones and nerves play a central role in the well-functioning back and neck. Given the inherent complexity with the spine, it is understandable that, for high-class spine care, a multidisciplinary team made up of neurology, neurosurgery, and orthopedics is central to the care of spine patients. In addition to these disciplines, it is also important to incorporate other disciplines, such as physical therapy, pain management, and psychiatry. Thus, what we can see is that, in spine care, the use of multidisciplinary teams is critical to the cure process.

7.4.5   Knowledge Management in the Spine Unit

Modern medicine generates huge amounts of heterogeneous data on a daily basis. For example, medical data may contain SPECT images, signals like EKG, clinical

TABLE 7.1. Systems comprising HMIS.

System	Description
Hospital information systems (HISs)	Provide integrative medical and clinical information support services using a variety of computer services that are linked with high-speed networks.
Expert systems (ESs)	Provide expert consultation to end user for solving specialized and complex problems.
Case management systems (CMSs)	Evolved recently as a result of a growing trend of integrating health service delivery both vertically (coordinating clinical care across providers, i.e. between surgeons and physical therapy) and horizontally (linking institution providing the same types of treatment).
	Another feature of these systems is that they enable case mix applications and thus provide the capability and flexibility of integrating financial and clinical data. The benefits of this cannot be understated.
Health database management systems (HDBMSs)	Have been used extensively in some hospital settings. HDBMS refer to a repository of logically organized facts and figures which query facilities. A typical example of such an HDBMS is the automated patient record system. These systems also enable data mining and other data analysis techniques to be used with the help of OLAP (on-line analytic processes) features, so that it will be able to analyze cumulative treatments and thus update, revise, or adjust practice protocols as required. This will, of course, ensure the Spine Unit maintains its high standard of offering best possible services to its patients.
Group decision support systems (GDSSs)	Involve the use of interactive, computer-based systems that facilitate the search for solutions to semi-structured and unstructured problems shared by groups. Once again, these systems will benefit the quality of the patient treatment by supporting decision-making processes regarding patient treatments made within the Spine Unit.

information like temperature, cholesterol levels, etc., as well as the physician's interpretation. Added to all of this are the daily mountains of data accumulated from a healthcare organization's administrative systems. Those who deal with such data understand that there is a widening gap between data collection and data comprehension and analysis. These data represent raw assets that need to be converted into knowledge via information. Technologies play a significant role in facilitating the transformation of raw data assets into knowledge. This is done in many ways, from including application of data-mining tools, to just providing a structure and context for apparently disparate data elements so that they can be viewed as a whole within a specific context, typically a case scenario; this, in turn, then supports critical decision making [47]. Integral to any sound KM strategy within a healthcare organization is the transformation of these data and information assets into germane knowledge [48]. However, in order to do this both effectively and systematically it is necessary to have an organizing structured approach.

The HMIS in place at the Spine Unit helps physicians as well as administrators to address this problem by enabling these raw data assets to be transformed into information and knowledge. At the clinical level, for example, the HMIS helps in early detection of diseases from historical databases of symptoms and diagnosis, thus providing an early warning system that leads to a much more effective quality treatment. At the hospital administration level, for example, the HMIS helps in tracking certain kinds of anomalies, which may reveal areas of improvement and may help the realignment of certain kinds of resources (e.g. equipment, personnel, etc.). The major reason for the specific HMIS in place is to support delivery of quality healthcare in a cost-effective manner. These systems are considered to be very sophisticated systems in the current healthcare market. The systems uses National Committee for Quality Assurance standards and data gathered by the Spine Unit, i.e. findings from key medical journals such as *The New England Journal of Medicine* or *Journal of American Medicine*, as well as data generated and analyzed from the center's own database of patient history. These standards are continually updated and revised as new findings become available.

The systems, therefore, not only enable the physicians to perform their work more effectively and efficiently and render high-quality services to their patients, but also provide them with care parameters. This helps to enforce practice guidelines; in addition, it provides peer data on providers which enables benchmarking for specific treatments in terms of costs, length of stay, and other key variables to be calculated. The systems also enable the center to understand the occurrence of outliers, i.e. physicians' practice patterns can be studied to understand why they are outliers and then, if necessary, to change inappropriate behavior and thereby support effective and efficient delivery of healthcare. Physicians play an active role with defining the criteria and characteristics of the functions of the systems. This is an example of knowledge creating/renewal aspects enabled and supported by the system. In addition, the systems facilitate the sharing of knowledge, enabling discourse and discussion between physicians and other members of the multidisciplinary team. Thus, in an ad hoc fashion, the HMISs are supporting the four key knowledge transformations of combination, internalization, externalization, and socialization. However, without a structured systematic approach, i.e. given the ad hoc nature of these knowledge transformations, it is reasonable to expect that the Spine Unit is not fully maximizing the potential of these knowledge assets. We assert that the full potential of these knowledge assets can be realized through the establishment of a KMI.

7.5   Discussion

From the data presented on the Spine Unit in Section 7.4, it is possible to observe that the Spine Unit has a significant investment in technology, both at the clinical and practice management levels. On the clinical side there are various technologies that facilitate speedy detection and then enable the subsequent cure to be effective and efficient, thereby ensuring a high standard of quality treatment is experienced by the patient. On the practice management side the HMISs are crucial. When the Spine Unit is analyzed through the lens of KM, the relevant technologies become those on the practice management level, namely the technologies that make up the HMIS. These various technology systems (which make

TABLE 7.2. Relevant case elements in terms of the KMI model.

KMI element	Case study element
Infrastructure for collaboration	Primarily via the HIS: the system provides the forum for the exchanging of patient data and medical information between members of the multidisciplinary team. Also the GDSS: this provides the opportunity to share and discuss treatment options amongst members of the multidisciplinary team in an efficient and effective fashion. For example, when looking at a patient who had spinal fusion: neurosurgeons and orthopedic surgeons have the infrastructure to exchange key information and data easily in an organized and systematic fashion regarding the best procedure to follow and how to proceed on such a procedure. Such interactions support the knowledge transformations, in particular externalization.
Organizational memory	HDBMS: the database stores large volumes of data pertaining to treatments, key protocols, and statistics regarding cure options, as well as lessons learnt pertaining to various cure strategies.
Human asset infrastructure	Multidisciplinary spine care team: the combination of highly trained specialists from neurology, neurosurgery, and orthopedics, as well as psychologists, physical therapists, operating room personnel, and lab/radiology experts, are all vital to ensuring a proper cure outcome.
Knowledge transfer network	Primarily via the GDSS: the creation of new knowledge, as well as the possibilities to discuss and debate appropriate cure strategies to various cases, is enabled and facilitated. Also via HIS: the ability to access complete medical records and thereby develop a clear understanding of the patients' true history is supported via the HIS; in addition, it is possible to access the latest medical findings via this system. Once again, key knowledge transformations are supported in a systematic and structured fashion, including combination and externalization.
Business intelligence infrastructure	CMS: the case mix data and information stored on this system, as well as the ability of the system to link both vertically and horizontally, enables integration across the Spine Unit, resulting in supporting the business infrastructure.

up the generic healthcare information system of the Spine Unit and are described in Table 7.1) form the collection of key data and information and then, through various interactions of members of the multidisciplinary team with these technologies, protocols, and treatment, patterns are changed or developed; that is, through the interactions of both people and technologies, these raw data and informational assets are transformed into knowledge assets. Table 7.2 identifies each relevant case element in terms of the KMI framework presented earlier.

What can be seen, then, is a very heavy investment in the business intelligence infrastructure, i.e. HMISs which are facilitating the knowledge transfer, maintaining the organizational memory, and enabling the collaboration of the multidisciplinary team in a very effective and efficient fashion. The Spine Unit has highly trained specialists who are encouraged always to keep at the cutting edge of new techniques for achieving better results and higher quality outcomes, with a strong emphasis on continuous improvement, they impart and exchange the knowledge and skills gained via interacting with the GDSS and the HIS components of the HMIS.

One can see from Table 7.2 that, in this cure setting, the KMI is established and sustained through the technologies in place. By explicitly identifying the components of the KMI in the Spine Unit case study, it is possible to make explicit the knowledge assets currently in place, thereby facilitating better management of these knowledge assets, as well as maintaining and updating the KMI itself, as it becomes possible to identify key knowledge transformations in a systematic fashion.

Technologies are continuously changing, and when new technologies are added to the Spine Unit it will then also be possible to evaluate their role in sustaining and supporting the existing KMI. Furthermore, by making explicit the elements within the KMI as they occur in the case study, it is possible to get a feel for the relative complexity of various tasks and processes that are evidenced in the Spine Unit and thus be able to evaluate these to identify whether modifications are required or how best to support them. Therefore, it is not only possible to identify elements of the KMI within the Spine Unit, but by doing so one can ensure that the KM processes that occur are supported and enhanced so that the primary goal of cure for the patient is indeed realized.

In addition, the KMI facilitates the knowledge transformations of the knowledge spiral, which in turn serve to increase the extant knowledge base of the organization, thus enabling the spine unit to maximize the full potential of its knowledge assets. Moreover, once such a KMI is established it is then possible to apply the IC to the data and information stored and generated throughout the healthcare setting so that superior healthcare decisions can be made, as the following example from the orthopedic operating room highlights [4].

The orthopedic operating room represents an ideal environment for the application of a continuous improvement cycle that is dependent on the IC. For those patients with advanced degeneration of their hips and knees, arthroplasty of the knee and hip represents an opportunity to regain their function. Before the operation ever begins in the operating room, there are a large number of interdependent individual processes that must be completed. Each process requires data input and produces a data output, such as patient history, diagnostic test, and consultations.

From the surgeon's and hospital's perspective, they are on a continuous cycle. The interaction between these data elements is not always maximized in terms of operating room scheduling and completion of the procedure. Moreover, as the population ages and a patient's functional expectations continue to increase with their advanced knowledge of medical issues, reconstructive orthopedic surgeons are being presented with an increasing patient population requiring hip and knee arthroplasty. Simultaneously, the implants are becoming more sophisticated, and thus more expensive. In turn, the surgeons are experiencing little change in system capacity, but are being told to improve efficiency and output, improve procedure time, and eliminate redundancy. However, the system legacy is for insufficient room designs that have not been updated with the introduction of new equipment, poor integration of the equipment, inefficient scheduling, and time-consuming procedure preparation. Although there are many barriers to re-engineering the operating room, such as the complex choreography of the perioperative processes, a dearth of data, and the difficulty of aligning incentives, it is indeed possible to effect significant improvements through the application of the IC.

The entire process of getting a patient to the operating room for a surgical procedure can be represented by three distinct phases: preoperative, intraopertive, and postoperative. In turn, each of these phases can be further subdivided into the individual, yet interdependent, processes that represent each step on the surgical trajectory. As each of the individual processes is often dependent on a previous event, the capture of event and process data in a data warehouse is necessary. The diagnostic evaluation of these data, and the reengineering of each of the deficient processes, will then lead to increased efficiency. For example, many patients are allergic to the penicillin family of antibiotics that are often administered preoperatively in order to minimize the risk of infection.

For those patients who are allergic, a substitute drug requires a 45 min monitored administration time as opposed to the much shorter administration time of the default agent. Since the antibiotic is only effective when administered prior to starting the procedure, this often means that a delay is experienced. When identified in the preoperative phase, these patients should be prepared earlier on the day of surgery and the medication administered in sufficient time such that the schedule is not delayed. This prescriptive reengineering has directly resulted from mining of the data in the information system in conjunction with an examination of the business processes and their flows. By scrutinizing the delivery of care and each individual process, increased efficiency and improved quality should be realized while maximizing value. For knee and hip arthroplasty, there are over 432 discrete processes that can be evaluated and reengineered as necessary through the application of the IC [49].

7.6   Conclusions

Healthcare globally is facing many challenges, including escalating costs and more pressures to deliver high-quality, effective, and efficient care. By nurturing KM and making the knowledge assets explicit, healthcare organizations will be more suitably equipped to meet these challenges, since knowledge holds the key to developing better practice management techniques, and data and information are so necessary in disease management and evidence-based medicine. The case study data presented depicted the complexity of the service delivery process, driven by the complexity of the issues being dealt with by the teams, which in turn requires that many disciplines create and share knowledge to enable the delivery of a high quality of care. Thus, the need for shared knowledge is a fundamental requirement. The KMI was presented and used to structure these disparate knowledge assets as explicit and integrated within a larger system, i.e. the generic healthcare information system, that allowed analysis of the extent of the KMI for the Spine

Unit. Further, such a framework in particular supports in a systematic and structured fashion all four key knowledge transformations identified by Nonaka [15], in particular that of externalization (tacit to explicit). The application of the IC to this generic healthcare information system ensures that maximization of appropriate and germane knowledge assets occurs and a superior future state will be realized.

On analyzing the case data with the KMI framework and IC model, the benefits to healthcare of embracing KM become clearly apparent. Given the challenges faced by healthcare organizations today, the importance of KM, understanding the means available to support KM, and explicitly developing and designing an appropriate healthcare information system using the KMI framework and then applying to this the IC model is, indeed, of strategic significance, especially as it serves to facilitate the realization of the value proposition for healthcare.

References

1. Drucker P. *Post-capitalist society*. New York: Harper Collins; 1993.
2. Drucker P. Beyond the information revolution. *Atl Mon* 1999;(October):47–57.
3. Wickramasinghe N, Davison G. Making explicit the implicit knowledge assets in healthcare. *Healthcare Manage Sci* 2004;17(3):185–196.
4. Wickramasinghe N, Schaffer J. Creating knowledge-driven healthcare processes with the intelligence continuum. *Int J Electron Healthcare* 2006; in press.
5. Bukowitz WR, Williams RL. New metrics for hidden assets. *J Strateg Perform Measure* 1997;1(1):12–18.
6. Swan J, Scarbrough H, Preston J. Knowledge management—the next fad to forget people? In: *Proceedings of the 7th European Conference in Information Systems*; 1999.
7. Newell S, Robertson M, Scarbrough H, Swan J. *Managing knowledge work*. New York: Palgrave; 2002.
8. Davenport T, Prusak L. *Working knowledge*. Boston: Harvard Business School Press; 1998.
9. Wickramasinghe N. Do we practice what we preach: are knowledge management systems in practice truly reflective of knowledge management systems in theory? *Bus Process Manage J* 2003;9(3):295–316.
10. Markus L. Toward a theory of knowledge reuse: types of knowledge reuse situations and factors in reuse success. *J Manage Inf Syst* 2001;18(1):57–93.
11. Alavi M, Leidner D. Review: knowledge management and knowledge management systems: conceptual foundations and research issues. *MIS Q* 2001;25(1):107–136.
12. Wickramasinghe N. Knowledge creation: a meta-framework. *Int J Innov Learn* 2006; in press.
13. Polanyi M. *Personal knowledge: towards a post-critical philosophy*. Chicago: University Press; 1958.
14. Polanyi M. *The tacit dimension*. London: Routledge and Kegan Paul; 1966.
15. Nonaka I. A dynamic theory of organizational knowledge creation. *Organ Sci* 1994;5:14–37.
16. Nonaka I, Nishiguchi T. *Knowledge emergence*. Oxford: Oxford University Press; 2001.
17. Boland R, Tenkasi R. Perspective making perspective taking. *Organ Sci* 1995;6:350–372.

18. Wickramasinghe N, Silvers JB. IS/IT the prescription to enable medical group practices to manage managed care. *Health Care Manage Sci* 2003;6:75–86.
19. Wickramasinghe N, Schaffer J, Fadllal A. Actualizing the knowledge spiral through data mining—a clinical example. In: *MedInfo*, 7–11 September 2004.
20. Duffy J. The KM technology infrastructure. *Inf Manage J* 2000;34(2):62–66.
21. Duffy J. The tools and technologies needed for knowledge management. *Inf Manage J* 2001;35(1):64–67.
22. Srikantaiah TK. *Knowledge management for information professional*. ASIS Monograph Series. Information Today, Inc.; 2000.
23. Wickramasinghe N, Sharma S. A framework for building a learning organization in the 21st century. *Int J Innov Learn* 2006; in press.
24. Holt GD, Love P, Li H. The learning organization: toward a paradigm for mutually beneficial strategic construction alliances. *Int J Proj Manage* 2000;18(6):415–421.
25. Wickramasinghe N, Mills G. Integrating e-commerce and knowledge management—what does the Kaiser experience really tell us? *Int J Account Inf Syst* 2001;3(2):83–98.
26. Croasdell DC. IT's role in organizational memory and learning. *Inf Syst Manage* 2001;18(1):8–11.
27. Ellinger AD, Watkins KE, Bostrom RP. Managers as facilitators of learning in learning organizations. *Hum Resource Dev Q* 1999;10(2):105–125.
28. Hammond C. The intelligent enterprise. *InfoWorld* 2001;23(6):45–46.
29. Wickramasinghe N, Fadlalla A. An integrative framework for HIPAA-compliant I*IQ healthcare information systems. *Int J Health Care Qual Assur* 2004;17(2):65–74.
30. Wickramasinghe N, Lichtenstein S. Supporting knowledge creation with e-mail. *Int J Innov Learn* 2005; in press.
31. Geisler E. *The metrics of science and technology*. Westport, CT: Greenwood Press; 2000.
32. Geisler E. *Creating value with science and technology*. Westport, CT: Quorum Books; 2001.
33. Geisler, E. The metrics of technology evaluation: where we stand and where we should go from here. *Int J Technol Manage* 2002;24(4):341–374.
34. Geisler E. Mapping the knowledge-base of management of medical technology. *Int J Healthcare Technol Manage* 1999;1(1):3–10.
35. Geisler E, Wickramasinghe N. *Knowledge management: concepts and cases*. M. E. Sharpe Publishers; 2006, in press.
36. Kostoff R, Geisler E. Strategic management and implementation of textual data mining in government organizations. *Technol Anal Strateg Manage* 1999;11(4):493–525.
37. Eisenhardt K. Building theories from case study research. *Acad Manage Rev* 1989;14: 532–550.
38. Kavale S. *Interviews: an introduction to qualitative research interviewing*. Thousand Oaks: Sage; 1996.
39. Boyatzis R. *Transforming qualitative information thematic analysis and code development*. Thousand Oaks: Sage Publications; 1998.
40. Applegate L, Mason R, Thorpe D. Design of a management support system for hospital strategic planning. *J Med Syst* 1986;10(1):79–94.
41. Chandra R, Knickrehm M, Miller A. Healthcare's IT mistake. *McKinsey Q* 1995;5.
42. Malhotra, Y. 2000. Knowledge management & new organizational form. In: Malhotra Y, editor, *Knowledge management and virtual organizations*. Hershey: Idea Group Publishing; 1995.
43. Wolper L. *Healthcare administration*. Maryland: Aspen Publication; 1995.

44. Kongstvedt P. The managed healthcare handbook, Maryland: Aspen Publication; 1997.
45. Enthoven A. The history and principles of managed competition. *Health Aff* 1993;25–48.
46. Knight W. *Managed care: what it is and how it works.* Maryland: Aspen Publication; 1998.
47. Wickramasinghe N, Fadlalla A, Geisler E, Schaffer J. Knowledge management and data mining: strategic imperatives for healthcare. In: *3rd Hospital of the Future Conference*, Warwick, UK, 2003.
48. Sharma S, Wickramasinghe N, Gupta J. Knowledge management in healthcare. In: Wickramasinghe N, Gupta JND, Sharma SK, editors, *Creating knowledge-based healthcare organizations.* USA: Idea Group Publishing; 2004, pp. 1–13.
49. Schaffer J, Steiner, E, Krebs, K, Hahn, R. Orthopedic operating room of the future. unpublished data; 2004.

8
The Hidden Power of Social Networks and Knowledge Sharing in Healthcare

JAY LIEBOWITZ

Abstract

Social networking has been shown to lead to effective collaboration, innovation, and knowledge sharing. In the healthcare field, knowledge flows and knowledge gaps in healthcare providers can be identified by social network analysis. Social network analysis should be used as part of the knowledge audit process. This will better inform the knowledge management strategy of the organization.

8.1   Introduction

The biomedical computation community is complex. According to Noy et al. [1], there are hundreds of different knowledge bases (e.g. Gene Ontology, SNOMED-CT), multiple metadata formats (e.g. caBIO), many primary databases (e.g. GenBank, MEDLINE), multiple languages for representing data structures (e.g. DICOM, MAGE-ML), numerous vocabularies (e.g. UMLS, SNOMED-RT), and various ontologies (Protégé tools [2]). At the same time, a great need exists for sharing knowledge among physicians and other healthcare workers [3]. This is exemplified by Dr Feied's keynote address at the 2004 Annual Medical Informatics and Emergency Medicine Conference, when he stated:

> You should work to reduce institutional dependence on specialized personnel with "secret knowledge" that allows them to complete tasks nobody else can perform. If the unit secretary is the only one who knows how to place or cancel an order, every coffee break can put a congested department further behind.

A number of studies have looked at knowledge-sharing behaviors in the health profession. One study [4] examined knowledge-sharing behaviors of physicians in hospitals. There were 286 physicians in 28 types of subunits in 13 hospitals who were part of the study. Using the theory of reasoned action and the theory of planned behavior, it was found that a physician's perceived social pressure to perform or not to perform the knowledge-sharing behavior ("social norm") has the strongest total effect (direct plus indirect) on his/her behavioral intentions to share knowledge. Attitude (the degree to which a physician has a favorable or unfavorable evaluation of performing the knowledge sharing behavior) and perceived behavioral control (perceived ease or difficulty of performing the knowledge sharing behavior) were found to have significant effects on the physician's knowledge-sharing behavior. From the study, it was suggested that hospital management should pay more attention to creating an environment where physicians can have positive subjective norms and attitudes towards knowledge sharing. Also, those responsible for knowledge management systems should make more effort to enhance the accessibility of physicians to workplace communications.

Gabbay and le May [5], in their ethnographic study of knowledge management in primary care in the UK, highlight the potential advantage of exploiting existing formal and informal networking as a key to conveying evidence to clinicians. Olsson Neve [6], from Stockholm University, also looked at knowledge sharing in the primary care sector and found similar conclusions.

Atkinson and Gold [7], in their Delphi study of PreventionEffects.net, found that a knowledge management system would facilitate knowledge transfer. The study respondents wanted a knowledge management system that was user friendly (92.86%), fit the content to user needs (85.71%), and included descriptors that indicate what kind of information and standards of evidence went into a report (82.14%).

Anderson [8] identified the structure of the referral and consultation networks that link 24 physicians in a group practice. Anderson studied the effect of the physician's location in the network on their use of the hospital information system. Through the use of social network analysis (a technique for mapping relationships between actors), Anderson identified influential individuals or opinion leaders who are critical in the introduction of new information technology. Relationships among healthcare providers, departments within healthcare organizations, and other organizations were also analyzed. Cravey et al. [9] used socio-spatial knowledge networks for chronic disease prevention and found knowledge network nodes that were strong, reluctant, latent, isolated, and irrelevant.

Even pharmaceutical companies are learning from success and failure, as discussed by Zimmermann [10]. They are making the most of knowledge management from drug development to delivery. For example, Spirig Pharma AG is pushing knowledge to individuals based on their current projects and interests. Pfizer is using a knowledge management system to store product data and make it accessible to the sales force in the field.

Dambita et al. [12] conducted a knowledge audit using social network analysis in the Division of Health Sciences Informatics at Johns Hopkins University School of Medicine. The focus of the knowledge audit study was to make recommendations to the Division on how to improve knowledge management.

8.2 Social Network Analysis

In order to assess knowledge sharing patterns in healthcare better, social network analysis is a technique that could be used to a great extent. Cross and Parker [11] indicate that networks of informal relationships have a critical influence on work and innovation. Research shows that appropriate connectivity in well-managed networks within organizations can have a substantial impact on performance, learning, and innovation [11].

Social network analysis involves mapping relationships/ties (links/arcs) between actors/nodes (individuals/units) in order to determine knowledge flows. There are six main steps to conducting a social network analysis [11]:

1. Identify a strategically important group.
2. Assess meaningful and actionable relationships.
3. Visually analyze the results.
4. Quantitatively analyze the results.
5. Create meaningful feedback sessions.
6. Assess progress and effectiveness.

Social network analysis software, such as NetMiner and Netdraw, help in quantitatively and visually analyzing the results. For example, Figure 8.1 shows a network diagram by department based on the type of knowledge that is requested and conveyed.

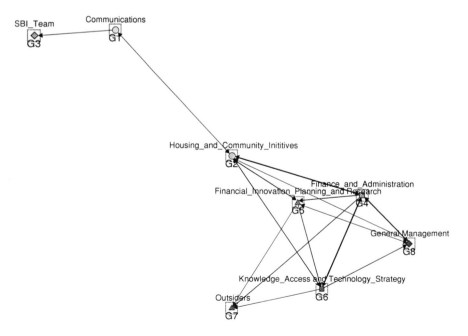

FIGURE 8.1. Network diagram: subject matter expertise (department).

Through determining centrality (in-degree, out-degree, betweenness, closeness, etc.), knowledge flows can be mapped using social network analysis to determine knowledge sources and sinks. Brokerage measures can also be determined, such as who are the coordinators (i.e. people who broker connections within the same group), gatekeepers (people who broker connections between their own group and another), and liaisons (those who broker connections between two different groups). Social network analysis can uncover the central connectors, boundary spanners, information brokers, and peripheral specialists. Social groups and positions in groups can be visualized by considering the strength of connections between individuals (proximity data).

8.2.1   Organizational Issues Affecting Knowledge Sharing Among Physicians and Other Healthcare Professionals

Bali et al. [13] state that the main reason for a lack of a comprehensive healthcare knowledge management system in organizations is the failure of healthcare stakeholders in properly creating a conducive organizational culture. Part of building an organizational culture that accepts knowledge sharing as everyday practice is the notion of knowledge exchange. According to Johannessen et al. [14] and Whittaker and van Beveren [15], four conditions must be met for a knowledge exchange to happen:

- *Accessibility.* The opportunity must exist to make an exchange.
- *Anticipation.* The parties in the exchange must anticipate the creation of value.
- *Motivation.* Parties must be motivated and feel that the exchange will provide them with benefits.
- *Capability.* The parties have the capability to execute the exchange.

Often times, the motivation may be lacking as a central ingredient for knowledge exchange and knowledge sharing. In some cases, the physician may act as a "knowledge czar" and the caste system may inhibit knowledge exchanges from taking place. Some organizations, like The World Bank, have included learning and knowledge-sharing proficiencies as part of the employee's annual job performance appraisal. Some other organizations base promotions partly on knowledge-sharing activities.

However, the training of physicians is typically through a master–apprentice relationship, where mentoring is the key mechanism for knowledge exchanges. Thus, a culture for knowledge sharing, through the mentoring activities, should be embedded within the physician's value system. Additionally, as the age of specialization continues to become more niche-like, it becomes more paramount to seek out others for advice, which again should contribute towards building a knowledge-sharing culture.

Part of the confusion may be this blending of roles and responsibilities among healthcare professionals. For example, physician assistants provide healthcare services under the supervision of physicians—according to the US Department of Labor Occupational Outlook Handbook (www.bls.gov). In 47 states and the District of Columbia, physician assistants, however, may prescribe medications, which used to be the auspices of the physician. According to the *Occupational Outlook Handbook*, the duties of physician assistants are determined by the supervising physician and by state law. The responsibilities of nurse practitioners have also increased throughout the years. According to the *Occupational Outlook Handbook*, nurse practitioners provide basic, primary healthcare and they diagnose and treat common acute illnesses and injuries. Nurse practitioners also can prescribe medications, but certification and licensing requirements vary by state.

The differentiation between the physicians and other related healthcare practitioners has blurred over recent years. This may cause some discomfort and annoyance among various healthcare professionals, as roles and responsibilities are changing somewhat. This could cause some people to hold back their knowledge and could lessen knowledge sharing from taking place.

Knowledge management can be an integrative mechanism to cut across functional silos. In the healthcare field, like most disciplines, functional silos are pervasive; and often, one hand doesn't know what the other is doing. A classic example of this case is getting reimbursed for health claims. How many times has the health claim reimbursement that you receive as an insured been incorrect and later edited to the proper amount? Likewise, how many times have hospitals incorrectly billed health insurance companies for medical supplies, tests, and other items? Part of the reason for these occurrences is due to the lack of information and communication among interested parties, who are often departmentalized and "siloed." Knowledge management can form the bridges between these isolated islands of knowledge. However, again, there must be incentives and motivation for doing so. Motivation should exist, however, such as improving the quality of care, improving patient safety, reducing litigation, enhancing worker productivity and effectiveness, and improving cost efficiencies. Senior leadership must communicate their vision for such goals to their employees, and the employees must feel empowered to act towards contributing to these goals.

Knowledge management efforts may fail from an organizational point of view because the knowledge management strategy and resulting implementation plan may not be aligned with the organization's strategic goals. Proper strategic alignment is critical towards achieving knowledge management success in any healthcare organization. According to Liebowitz [16,17], organizations typically undertake knowledge management initiatives for the following reasons:

Adaptability/agility

- anticipate potential market opportunities for new products/services;
- rapidly commercialize new innovations;
- adapt quickly to unanticipated changes;
- anticipate surprises and crises;
- quickly adapt the organization's goals and objectives to industry/market changes;

- decrease market response times;
- be responsive to new market demands;
- learn, decide, and adapt faster than the competition.

Creativity

- innovate new products/services;
- identify new business opportunities;
- learn not to reinvent the wheel;
- quickly access and build on experience and ideas to fuel innovation.

Institutional memory building

- attract and retain employees;
- retain expertise of personnel;
- capture and share best practices.

Organizational internal *effectiveness*

- coordinate the development efforts of different units;
- increase the sense of belonging and community among employees in the organization;
- avoid overlapping development of corporate initiatives;
- streamline the organization's internal processes;
- reduce redundancy of information and knowledge;
- improve profits, grow revenues;
- shorten product development cycles;
- provide training, corporate learning;
- accelerate the transfer and use of existing know-how;
- improve communication and coordination across company units (i.e. reduce stovepiping).

Organizational external *effectiveness*

- reach to new information about the industry and market;
- increase customer satisfaction;
- support e-business initiatives;
- manage customer relationships;
- deliver competitive intelligence;
- enhance supply-chain management;
- improve strategic alliances.

   If healthcare organizations and healthcare professionals can benefit from these factors, as well as improving patient safety and care, knowledge management can have a key role to play towards achieving "mission success."

8.2.2   Linking Social Network Analysis for Improving Knowledge Sharing in Healthcare

To erode some of these organizational issues relating to knowledge sharing among healthcare professionals and healthcare organizations, social network analysis can help identify where the knowledge gaps are occurring in the knowledge exchanges among healthcare individuals and units. By applying social network analysis, social groups and positions in groups can be visualized by considering the strength of connections between individuals (proximity data). Social network analysis and knowledge sharing/knowledge management techniques (e.g. online communities of practice, lessons learned/best practice systems, expertise locators, and others) can enhance the organizational learning environment.

Social network analysis can also identify the sources and sinks of knowledge, and determine where the barriers might exist for smooth knowledge flows. Different types of knowledge applied by healthcare professionals could be examined, such as context knowledge, expert process knowledge, general process knowledge, relationship knowledge, and strategic knowledge. By applying social network analysis to each of these types of knowledge, an informed opinion could be generated on how the different types of knowledge are permeating the organization. Social network analysis could also examine the healthcare organization's employees by tenure in the organization in order to see whether the junior-level employees are in communication with the senior-level employees. Additionally, intra- and inter-department communications flows could be analyzed to see distinct patterns of interactions. Through social network analysis, individuals in the "power" positions could be identified based upon knowledge flows, and individuals could also be represented as isolates, transmitters, receivers, and carriers. These analyses will then provide the data to develop improved ways to share knowledge and communicate better between healthcare individuals and units.

8.3   Summary

Social network analysis is becoming more pervasive in various applications. For example, the Web site www.thefacebook.com allows university students to form social networks, and www.linkedin.com allows social networks to form among people with related organizational interests. Social network analysis has been used in applications ranging from determining collaboration among executives in a multinational firm after a merger has taken place, to determining knowledge flows and gaps in an information technology division at a major international bank. Social network analysis should be part of the knowledge manager's toolkit to assess knowledge-sharing techniques and communications within their organization better. In the healthcare field, as things continue to become more specialized, the silo effect can be a likely occurrence. This creates a greater need for applying knowledge management processes, systems, and tools to improve collaboration and communication among healthcare professionals and organizations.

Social network analysis can help in this endeavor, and, in the years to come, social network analysis will continue to be used and embraced within the healthcare profession.

References

1. Noy N, Rubin D, Musen M. Making biomedical ontologies and ontology repositories work. *IEEE Intell Syst* 2004;19(6).
2. Crubezy M, O'Connor M, Buckeridge DL, Pincus Z, Musen, MA. Ontology-centered syndromic surveillance for bioterrorism, *IEEE Intel Syst*, 2005;20:(26–35).
3. Chen H. *Medical informatics: knowledge management and data mining in biomedicine.* Springer-Verlag; 2005.
4. Ryu S, Ho SH, Han I. Knowledge sharing behavior of physicians in hospitals. *Expert Syst Appl* 2003;25(1):113–122.
5. Gabbay J, le May A. Ethnographic study of knowledge management in primary care. *Br Med J* 2004;329(7473):1013.
6. Olsson Neve T. Knowledge sharing in primary care. In: *Promote IT 2002 Conference Proceedings*, Sweden, 22–24 April 2002.
7. Atkinson NL, Gold RS. Online research to guide knowledge management planning. *Health Educ Res* 2001;16(6):747–764.
8. Anderson J. Evaluation in health informatics: social network analysis. *Comput Biol Med* 2002;32(3).
9. Cravey A, Washburn S, Gesler W, Arcury T, Skelly A. Socio-spatial knowledge networks in chronic disease prevention. *Soc Sci Med J* 2001;52(12).
10. Zimmermann K. Learning from success and failure. *KMWorld* 2003;12(9).
11. Cross R, Parker A. *The hidden power of social networks.* Cambridge, MA: Harvard Business School Publishing; 2004.
12. Dambita N, Gold J, Ghazinouri R, Malik R, Meinsler J. Knowledge audit study for DHSI. White paper, Knowledge Management Course, Columbia, MD; 2005.
13. Bali R, Dwivedi A, Naguib R. Issues in clinical knowledge management: revisiting healthcare management. In: Bali R, editor, *Clinical knowledge management: opportunities and challenges.* Hershey, PA: Idea Group Publishing; 2005.
14. Johannessen J, Olaisen J, Olsen B. Aspects of a systemic philosophy of knowledge: from social facts to data, information, and knowledge. *Kybernetes* 2002;31(7–8).
15. Whittaker J, van Beveren J. Social capital, an important ingredient to effective knowledge sharing: Meditute, a case study. In: Bali R, editor, *Clinical knowledge management: opportunities and challenges.* Hershey, PA: Idea Group Publishing; 2005.
16. Liebowitz J. *Addressing the human capital crisis in the federal government: a knowledge management perspective.* Elsevier/Butterworth-Heinemann; 2004.
17. Liebowitz J. *Strategic intelligence: Business intelligence, competitive intelligence, and knowledge management.* Auerbach Publishing; 2006.

9
Constructing Healthcare Knowledge

ZHICHANG ZHU

Abstract

Healthcare knowledge is social constructs and the management of it is essentially context specific, constructive processes via which concerned actors interact with each other so as to accomplish socio-cognitive changes. Critical factors shaping these processes include social structure, institutional logic, and political action. The socio-cognitive construction of healthcare knowledge underlies broad ranges of healthcare phenomena, issues, and programs, from designing healthcare technology to reforming healthcare service.

9.1   Introduction

In this chapter we take as the point of departure that healthcare knowledge is social constructs and that knowledge creation, consumption, and management are essentially social processes [1,2]. In particular, we adopt a socio-cognitive perspective that conceives the construction of knowledge as accomplishing changes not only in technical, but also, and primarily, in cognitive and social fronts [3,4]. We aim to enlarge our conceptual scope for looking at healthcare knowledge management beyond a purely technology perspective whilst still take into account the important effect of technology. We introduce readers to the critical factors involved in knowledge construction: social structure, institutional logic, and political action. Drawing upon recent researches in technology development, social movement, and institutional entrepreneurship studies, with this chapter we wish to explore a holistic, pragmatic, and hence realistic approach to the knowledge construction process, i.e. to understand how socio-cognitive changes are accomplished via purposive actions by concerned actors who hold varying interests and frames of reference. We present two case studies to illustrate how such an approach can help to generate new insights upon how new healthcare technology is created and how healthcare services are reformed.

9.2   Healthcare Knowledge as Social Constructs

How should a National Health Service (NHS) be managed and delivered? How does one choose between competing designs of healthcare technology when safety and efficacy effects are ambiguous and uncertain? Are obesity, binge drinking, and heavy smoking health or social problems? Should people with such problems receive NHS treatment with equal opportunities as those without such problems do? Are these really "problems" to be solved after all, or simply personal choices of life style which individual citizens are entitled to and which democratic polities must protect? Who should make these decisions: doctors, patients, managers or politicians, and how? These kinds of issue increasingly occupy the center stage of knowledge discourse upon healthcare services, particularly in Western, developed economies. Settlements and compromises, not necessary convictions or consensus, from such discourses constitute what we claim as healthcare knowledge based on which healthcare services are organized, financed, designed, consumed, and evaluated, affecting what healthcare to deliver, with what means, how, by, and to whom.

Technology plays an important role in the construction of healthcare knowledge. It is well documented, for example, that, with the spread and popularity of the Internet usage in society, doctors found themselves no longer the only source or authority of medical knowledge: patients were becoming increasingly well informed and knowledgeable, better prepared, and willing to participate in and influence decisions concerning the treatments and cares they receive. WebMD (www.webmd.com), an online healthcare company, currently receives 20 million visitors every month for consumer-focused healthcare information that helps them to take an active part in managing their own health. Non-for-profit organizations (NPOs) greatly facilitate healthcare knowledge construction, too. Cochrane Collaboration (www.cochrane.org), an international NPO, for example, provides up-to-date analysis about the effects of healthcare services readily available worldwide through the Internet, enabling healthcare consumers to discuss, review, design, and disseminate treatments and cares that suit them. As patients become more and better knowledgeable about healthcare due to increased availability of information and communication technology, they are, more than ever before, demanding and willing to enter into dialogues and decisions. As a result, healthcare knowledge is generated and consumed increasingly through a sharing relationship between doctors and patients rather than the once-dominant doctor-centered process. In short, the social construction of healthcare knowledge becomes more apparent, conscious, and widely spread.

While the impacts of technology are in no doubt, it is critical to note that such impacts are taking place in historically situated contexts, both temporally and spatially. They are likely to differ across times and spaces, due to ideological, cultural, social, institutional, and political circumstances. This also applies in healthcare discourses. A mother from Hong Kong would be horrified to watch a Singaporean doctor pouring cold water onto her baby who got fever; we did not call patients consumers 20 years ago; and it remains a strange idea in China that fathers are entitled to maternal leave. The settlements and practices generated from healthcare policy discourses and healthcare knowledge claims are hence context specific, shaped by socio-cognitive factors. For a systemic understanding of these shaping factors, and hence of the social construction of healthcare knowledge, in the following we introduce a few useful analytical constructs: social structure, institutional logic, and political action.

9.3   Social Structure

Social structure denotes in this chapter the actors who are involved in the knowledge construction process, as well as the relationships between those actors. Studying social structure is critical for the understanding of knowledge construction, since, after all, knowledge is created by social actors who are embedded in a world of norms, values, beliefs, experiences, expectations, and relationships. A useful tool for investigating social structure is "stakeholder analysis" [5]. While recognizing that different empirical situations implicate different sets of stakeholders, as well as relationships, we propose a generic healthcare stakeholder model for readers to kick-off their learning and analyzing process. We begin with considering four key stakeholder groups: consumers, providers, agencies, and sponsors.

Consumers. These are patients and prospective patients who consume healthcare services. Significant features of contemporary healthcare consumers deserving particular consideration are consumer diversity and the consumers' increasingly active roles. Over the past decades, we have witnessed a long-term, stable pattern of social change in Western, developed societies. "This shows up in population statistics as shorter marriages, more divorces, smaller households, later date of first marriages, increased number of single mothers, increased mobility, and increased number of women and children in poverty" [6]. At the same time, as a direct consequence of increased immigration, the population becomes more diverse by ethnic group, culture, and language. As democracy and decentralization trends deepen, consumption patterns and consumer behaviors are changing. Services and products, in the healthcare domain, as in other areas of consumption, are expected to adjust to fragmented, individual consumer needs rather than gear toward the no-longer-existing homogeneous need of a single, large population. Mass media nurture and reinforce the awareness and assertions of diversity and customization. Consumers are also differing in accessing education and information, in the ability to negotiate and utilize healthcare knowledge. Overall, however, consumers are becoming more demanding and willing to enter into dialogue and negotiation, participate, and influence decisions concerning their own care and treatment.

Providers. Under this group we put together doctors, nurses, and other healthcare professionals, public as well as private hospitals, pharmaceutical and medical equipment companies, other medical service suppliers, healthcare research institutes, and so on. Apparently, providers, differentiated because of division of labor, need to corporate with each other in order to provide appropriate services for consumers. On the other hand, competition abounds: the interests and demands of these providers are no less diverse than those of consumers. What healthcare duties, opportunities, and resources are allocated to which groups, and how, are generating different and even conflicting viewpoints and suggestions, all based on distinctive disciplinary knowledge and professional experiences, in addition to vested interests, that are particularly appealing to different service providers. Disagreements are likely continuing to exist, too, between frontline professionals and backend management upon how services and performance is to be conducted and evaluated, especially during the "reforms" that, nowadays, appear to be taking place anywhere and everywhere all over the world.

Agencies. These are the government and sublevel governmental bodies, plus "independent" administrative/research institutions, that are granted authority and responsibility to evaluate, approve, regulate, and fund medically necessary health-care provisions. They are accountable to the public for ensuring that high-quality services are available when required, and are responsible for ongoing system-wide review and coordination. We qualify these agencies, including the government, as stakeholders in order to stress the point that they are not necessarily neutral guarantors of public interest. Rather, these agencies have their own inherently vested interests. This is because agencies are peopled and the people belong to and control these agencies are no less interest-aware and interest -seeking than other stakeholders. After all, "agency problems" are not confined to hired corporation executives only. In a sense, the vested interests of agencies in representative democratic polities are more determining and opportunistic than in autocratic systems. There is no lack of evidence that agencies please and manipulate other stakeholders in order to benefit themselves, e.g. burying "bad news" and economizing information in order to stay in power. In addition to this, various agencies have divergent experiences, expertise, and frames of reference, and they believe, honestly to different extents, that their specific knowledge, rather than that of other agencies, serves the public best.

Sponsors. These are the general public, taxpayers, particularly voters, who select the government, and hence also the agencies to manage the healthcare services on their behalves, and who ultimately finance the NHSs. It is self-evident that the analysis of healthcare consumers is equally applicable to sponsors. Nevertheless, one additional dimension is relevant to sponsors, i.e. sponsors are also concerned with the relationships between healthcare and other public services they want to receive and pay for, e.g. childcare, education, pension, police, and transportation. In the real world, where resources are scarce, decisions have to be made and relevant knowledge is needed upon the relationships and priorities between these services. Given that sponsors are further differentiated by wealth, life style, family situation (e.g. the number of children, old age, and working people), etc., they have different rankings of priority among healthcare and other public services and benefits, which will in turn influence their beliefs, knowledge, and decisions about what constitutes proper healthcare service and how it is to be fairly and efficiently organized, financed, and provided.

In the above, we briefly introduced four groups of key stakeholders which constitute the social structure insofar as healthcare service is concerned. Several points deserve our attention.

First, stakeholder is an analytical concept that concerns the roles that actors play. In the empirical world, an actor is likely to play more than one role, e.g. a patient as a consumer is at the same time a sponsor if s/he is a taxpayer, and perhaps also working in a healthcare agency, hence assuming a further third role. Thus, stakeholders' interests, expectations, and knowledge claims can well be as overlapping as competing, full of divergence, and compromising.

Second, the above analysis is only a preliminary starting point; further sublevel analysis is usually needed in empirical situations so as to take into account the vast differences within each of the stakeholder groups. In some circumstances, it should be noted, the nature of the problem at hand may dictate that the relationships, interactions, and power plays between stakeholders within one group be more fierce and crucial than those among stakeholder groups.

Third, the criticality of different stakeholders may not be the same across cases and situations. In some circumstances, the government wields sufficient power to accomplish change programs, whilst in others the healthcare providers are able to insert stronger influences, and sponsors are likely to be listened to more carefully when a general election is approaching. In cases of long-term illness or healing, consumers could be fairly knowledgeable and actively involved in designing treatments, whereas during the early stage of a healthcare technology design, a patient's role can be largely confined to being a research subject, muted into the background of decision making.

Fourth, stakeholders need to, as they did and are doing, interact with each other, formally and informally, consciously or unconsciously, via multiple channels, so that the provision and consumption of healthcare services can be realized. It is also through such interactions that healthcare knowledge is continuously constructed and reconstructed. Isolated from the interaction between stakeholders, detached from "moments of truth," healthcare knowledge ceases to be effective, useful, or even meaningful.

Then, why is stakeholder analysis, and hence the investigation of social structure, important? Viewed from a socio-cognitive, constructivist perspective, this is because knowledge is created by social actors who assume varying interests and hold heterogeneous experiences, expertise, expectations, and frames of reference. In other words, different stakeholders are likely to contribute to the construction of healthcare knowledge differently, in content, manner, and purpose, partly due to diverse interests and positions in power structure, and partly due to the diverse training they received and the experiences/expertise they have accumulated. Because of the diversities in past experiences, development paths, and cognitive frames among stakeholders, it is difficult, if not impossible, to erect all-agreed and all-embracing criteria for evaluating knowledge claims objectively, even if stakeholders strive to do so; thus, knowledge is, in the end, negotiated and settled rather than discovered and validated. Investigating who is involve in, what roles they play, what interests they assume, what expertise they possess, what frames they adopt, what resources they mobilize, and what relationships they are creating and imbedded in is, thus, a prerequisite for a fuller understanding of how knowledge is constructed.

Finally, stakeholders and their relationships are changing. This is significant, since changes in social structures will inevitably lead to changes in healthcare services. For example, a more diverse and assertive population sooner or later demands customized rather than homogeneous healthcare services, for the benefits of individuals as well as the efficiency of the society. The central problem we need to explore and are looking at is that the latter, due changes do not occur automatically in a deterministic, "natural" manner, since any such change will shake the status quo, disrupt the extant configurations of interests, resources and power, confront cognitive barriers and tensions, and hence encounter divergent reactions and strategies.

9.4   Institutional Logic

Institutional logics are organizing principles guiding social actions, and refer to a set of belief systems and associated practices [7].

There are institutional logics at various levels of social organization and in different social domains: societies, industries, organizational fields and populations, ethnic groups, professionals groups, etc. [8]. "The market," for example, is a well-known institutional logic via which social actors conduct, coordinate, and govern activities in the economic realm. Doctor-centered medical professionalism used to be a widely held institutional logic guiding the provision of healthcare services. Churches, the army, commercial firms, and families follow distinctive institutional logics to organize and maintain their unique relationships and practices respectively. Even inside the same industry, "logics" tend to be varying: the microchip producer Intel is not operating in the same way as the PC provider Dell. On the other hand, the "logics" of the microchip arms of Intel, Samsung, and Siemens resemble each other, so too do those of Dell, Gateway, and Lenovo.

As principles, beliefs, and value systems, institutional logics are human devices. Once being created, reinforced, and taken for granted, i.e. institutionalized, however, institutional logics tend to take on lives of their own, obtain fact-like status, gain law-like capabilities and efficacy, and underlie and shape social relations and practices [9].

From a knowledge construction point of view, we stress the following four features of institutional logics: stability, heterogeneity, dominant logic, and complementarity.

Stability. Institutional logics are relatively stable, held by social actors, able to pattern actors' conduct, with traceable consequences. With institutional logics, actors know how they should act and how other actors are likely to act under a broad spectrum of circumstances. The "wheel" of social understanding, expectation, contract, and guidance has already taken shape, molded by institutional logics, no need to be reinvented every time. As such, institutional logics provide legitimacy, set standards, supply codes of practice, reduce uncertainty, facilitate reasonable action, smoothen intended interaction, nurture social coherence, and increase societal efficiency [10]. Institutional logics do change, as we discuss below, but no society or social domain, healthcare service included, can operate properly without stable institutional logics. Stability is close to inertia, however. As a set of values, belief systems, and associated practices, institutional logics can become deeply ingrained, resistant to change initiatives. It is difficult to "switch" from one institutional logic to another overnight at will. The problematics of the market-oriented reforms that occurred in the planned economies in the former Soviet Union and Eastern European countries underscore this point. In this sense, actors are "embedded" in institutional logics. Doctors used to believe they were the only source and authority of healthcare knowledge; citizens in Western, developed societies, as well as former communist countries, took as granted comprehensive healthcare service from the state for free. These dearly held beliefs and taken-for-granted principles remain strong and deeply entrenched, despite the wide-ranging changes that have occurred.

Heterogeneity. Different institutional logics are usually coexisting and competing with each other within a social domain. All organizational fields, industries, and societies consist of heterogeneous institutional logics [11,12]. In modern economic history, for example, no society has been fully or purely coordinated by the "market", or by a "plan". No homogeneous value or belief system can be found within national or regional borders, not even under bloody dictatorships. Because of heterogeneity, there are always tensions, ruptures, and competitions among institutional logics, such as those between the "market" and "plan" in an economy, between diversification and focusing strategies in corporate management, between personal agency and social solidarity in citizenship education, between employee loyalty and labor mobility in human resource management, etc. In one sense, the coexistence of competing institutional logics gives rise to uncertainty, incoherence, and hence inefficiency. On the other hand, however, it is the availability of competing institutional logics that generates possibilities for managerial agency, policy choice, innovation, and reform [8]. It is proposed that coexistence of heterogeneous institutional logics enables "adaptive efficiency" [13], from which organizations and the society have much to gain [14]. That China's economic reform has proceeded more smoothly and successfully than those of the former Soviet Union and Eastern European countries is partly due to the fact that the "plan" as an institutional logic was far less strong, effective, overwhelming, or completed in China and that other institutional logics, such as "financial federationalism—Chinese style," had been allowed to exist [15].

Dominant logic. Owing to heterogeneity, actors within communities hold different logics, and all social domains, healthcare service included, can be characterized by competing institutional logics to some degree. But coexisting and competing logics are not equal, in that, with identifiable eras or equilibrium points over time, a dominant institutional logic exists and others are subordinated [16]. Otherwise, codes of practices become confusing, values and beliefs uprooted, social coherence lost, and institutional logics cease to be effective. "Actors within a field recognise the dominance of one institutional logic during times what we can characterized as relative stability, even though all actors may not agree with that dominant logic" [7]. A dominant logic does not eliminate competing ones, only subordinate them. During times of change and reform, heterogeneous institutional logics compete for dominance, e.g. "market" competes with "plan" in an economy, medical professionalism competes with business principles in healthcare provision. But a domain and/or society must return to a new point of relative stability with one institutional logic emerging as dominant so that change or reform can be consolidated. From this perspective, change and reform are a process of moving from the dominance of one institutional logic to another [17]. Such moves may never be completed or total; nevertheless, they occur; different logics continue to coexist and compete with each other, but under new dominant–subordinate relationships [16]. Viewed from this perspective, the creation of new knowledge as accomplishment of socio-cognitive changes is a process during which concerned actors settle the dominance between competing institutional logics.

Complementarity. There are complementarities between institutional logics across different domains [9,16], as well as between institutional logics and social structures [7]. In economics, two variables are regarded complements when the increase of one introduces increase of the other. Butter and bread are complementary within a region or population, because an increase in bread consumption pushes up the demand for butter (in contrast, bread and rice are not complementary; rather, they are substitutive, because an increase in the consumption of one reduces the other). This explains why a more diverse and assertive population equipped with newly available information and communication technologies leads to increasingly fragmented healthcare demands which can only be satisfied by customized healthcare services that are provided better through a sharing partnership between patients and healthcare professionals. Industries and public services, such as healthcare systems, usually develop, over time, logics and designs that "parallel" with those prevailing in the wider society [9]. Properly materialized, complementarities give rise to systems effects, with the whole being more than the sum of the parts [18]. Failures to materialize complementarities, on the other hand, result in misfits between a domain's dominant logic and that of the society, between dominant institutional logic and social structure, giving rise to dissatisfaction, tension, disruption, and inefficiency.

In social domains, complementarities are unlikely occur automatically, even though they are necessary, particularly when changes are in order. There are usually gaps between the necessity and reality of complementarities, which is mainly due to vested interest (stakeholders benefit from complementary change initiatives differently), structural legacies (stakeholders vested with the status quo hold more actionable resources than those who favor changes), and cognitive barriers (how to materialize complementarities is difficult to comprehend and work out). In some circumstances, for example, a particular stakeholder group may hold the power to alter aspects of social structure, e.g. the government in the UK may use its legislation power to grant healthcare agencies more power by one stroke. But such direct command and control over the change of dominance in and of institutional logics is not possible due to institutional inertia. The development of a new dominant logic that is complementary with the altered social structure must thus be worked out over time among all stakeholders [7,12]. To overcome misalignments between social structure and institutional logic, to work out a dominant logic, and hence to materialize necessary complementarities, purposive, dedicated, and systemic political actions are needed [19].

9.5   Political Action

In the above, we posit that knowledge construction is essentially a social accomplishment involving socio-cognitive changes in both social structure and institutional logics, that changes in social structure and institutional logics must be complementary, and that the realization of such complementarities demands proper political actions. The next question is what political actions are in order, i.e. what do actors do so as to accomplish socio-cognitive changes and hence settle knowledge claims. In this regard, much can be learnt from recent researches in technology development [20–22], social movement [23,24], and institutional entrepreneurship [25,26] studies, where the following actions are commonly and consistently stressed.

Problematizing. Owing to inherent ambiguity and uncertainty, the real function, form, and benefit of an innovation that embodies intended knowledge are unknown at the present. To gain conceived superiority of the innovation over others, to secure a chance to start, actors need to problematize stakeholders' present understandings, framing their future situations and needs as problems to which the proposed innovation is to provide the solution. Innovation, and hence knowledge construction, is thus as much about manufacturing problems as solving them [27]. This is significant, because it is through situation/issue framing and articulation that institutional logics are devised and proposed.

Deliberating. To choose from different and competing proposals and designs, concerned stakeholders need, via deliberation, to evaluate and compare options of various kinds, based on their respective experiences, aspirations, and expectations. It is through deliberation that underlying institutional logics are put into competition, the outcome of which will determine which institutional logic gains dominance whilst others subordinated. The settlement upon a dominant logic does not mean that all stakeholders agree with or are convinced by that logic, but simply that actors become aware of the dominance of that logic and recognize that violating the logic will invite sanctions unless that dominance is uprooted [7].

Mobilizing. To gain support, endorsement, and acquiescence, actors need to motivate cooperation of other stakeholders by taking their interests and circumstances into account, providing them with common meaning, identity, and commitment [28], offering shared psychological ownership [29], by the means of social [26] and political skills [30], and, if necessary, modifying and compromising the innovation and knowledge itself [31,32]. In the end, erecting dominant logic and constructing knowledge is about persuasion and negotiation, and hence depends on the competitive advantage generated from the power, resources, and skills of competing coalitions [33].

Institutionalizing. This is done by rationalizing, formalizing, legislating and diffusing favorable standards, codes, protocols, criteria, routines, and beliefs so that the intended dominant logic and knowledge claim become settled and stable, and obtain regulative might and legitimacy [34]. It is through such actions and processes that new meaning gets externalized then internalized, new order established, social domains and organizational fields recomposed, changes and reforms consolidated, innovation accomplished, and knowledge constituted. With institutionalization, a round of the knowledge construction cycle completes.

Successful political action demands "institutional entrepreneurship" [25,26,35] that is pragmatic in nature. It cannot be centrally planned or linearly executed, due to novelty and uncertainty, but is always in a state of comprehending, adjusting, brokering, promising, and improvising. Furthermore, it is intrinsically relational, since it is about compromising, sharing, motivating, allaying, working with, and leading others. In seeking dominance for a favored logic and to constitute intended knowledge, actors need to reflect continuously on their own against emerging contingencies, and prepare to embrace logics and knowledge of others if necessary. In social domains, during the social construction process, pragmatic attitude and maneuvre are a necessity.

In the following, we borrow two case studies to illustrate the explanation power of our constructivist, socio-cognitive approach to knowledge creation and management. Both cases are in the domain of healthcare service and concerned with healthcare knowledge. One is about designing a socio-psychological healthcare technology [3,34], and the other is an efficiency-oriented healthcare reform [7].

9.6   Designing Cochlear Implants

A cochlear implant is a surgically implanted electronic device that provides the profoundly deaf patient with a sensation of sound. Until the 1980s, human implantation research and practice using human subjects, especially involving electrical simulation, was considered to be morally and scientifically unacceptable, and any researcher who became involved did so at their own professional risk. This was because the mechanism by which the human ear functioned was poorly understood. It is also because of a lack of testing, comparison, and reporting standards, making it difficult to assess and compare different approaches.

The new technology later gained requisite legitimacy because of certain serendipitous events. In particular, regulatory and funding agencies in the US, such as the National Institutes of Health (NIH) and the Food and Drug Administration (FDA), who played a major role in sanctioning the safety and efficacy of medical devices through approval processes, decided to support cochlear implant work as a result of unrelated research activities on neural cortex simulation initiated in Europe. Consequently, cochlear implant technology had developed rapidly within a short period of merely several years and became an acceptable clinical practice so that a consensus development conference had to be held in 1988 by the NIH and the FDA in order to resolve a debate between advocates of single- and multiple-channel cochlear implants.

Seen through a social structure perspective, around the development of cochlear implant technology there were research institutes, commercial companies, regulative agencies, and research universities (universities that received funding and authority from agencies to evaluate competing approaches). It is interesting to note that the differences in design logics did not lie, and the battle for legitimacy was not fought, among stakeholders as homogeneous groups. Rather, they were between different coalitions of members across these groups, such as between the coalition of a pioneering researcher William House with 3M Corporation on one side and the coalition of another pioneering researcher, Graem Clark, with Nucleus Corporation on the other. There were by 1980 approximately seven such coalitions or groups. Each was equally qualified and dedicated, but each had to begin with their distinctive past experiences, starting assumptions, and future expectations and pursue a different research and clinical approach, since, at this early stage of technology-in-the-making, nothing else existed but divergent beliefs about what was feasible or at least worth attempting.

Given the limited state of knowledge regarding hearing, House–3M believed, based on inductive studies upon clinical experiments, that cochlear implant research should begin with a simple device, as it would present the least potential for neuro-physiological harm to patients, which satisfies the NIH–FDA concern of safety, while providing researchers valuable knowledge required for future improvement. This belief led House–3M to develop single-channel technology, which uses a single electrode implanted at a relatively shallow depth into the cochlea, designed to provide profoundly deaf patients with a perception of environmental cues rather than the ability to discriminate between spoken words. Consequently, those who pursued the single-channel approach believed that the ability to perceive environmental cues should be the appropriate measure of cochlear implant efficacy.

Other researchers held contrasting assumptions about cochlear implant efficacy and safety. They believed that normal hearing could only be replicated with multiple electrodes, each inserted deep into the cochlea so that different frequency signals could be delivered at different spots in the cochlea. The deeper insertion of multiple electrodes might eventually provide patients with the ability to understand speech. For multi-channel advocates, such as the Clark–Nucleus coalition, the ability to recognize speech, as opposed to environmental cues, was the primary function of cochlear implants and, therefore, the appropriate measure of efficacy. These coalitions also rejected the likelihood of cochlea damage by multi-channel devices, largely because of the lack of sufficient evidence. Instead, they saw more harm in what they considered to be an inferior single-channel technology. What was of greater safety concern to them was the potential future damage when patients with single-channel devices sought to replace their implants with multi-channel devices.

Seen from a socio-cognitive perspective, this is an "institutional battlefield," a situation where competing logics coexist and fight for dominance. Because of the uncertainty and ambiguity associated with technology development, it is not possible to ex ante determine the success or failure of any particular trajectory, i.e. single- or multi-channel design in this case. Furthermore, several evaluation routines existed, each tautological with the specific path and approach that the different coalitions pursued. To settle for a dominant logic and constitute a favorable knowledge claim, political actions came into play, so that a particular evaluation routine and criterion was applied and the others were selected away. The battle for a settlement is political in nature since, no matter how formalized or neutral minded, the NIH and FDA evaluation and approval process cannot mask the fact that what was measured and how it was measured was subject to interpretation due to these regulative stakeholders not possessing the prerequisite knowledge to determine an acceptable evaluation scheme. The resolution of acceptable measures of efficacy and safety depended largely on the congruence of the beliefs between researcher–company coalitions and NIH–FDA administrators.

In searching for a favorable settlement, i.e. to obtain the dominance of their cognitive frame and design logic, House–3M proposed measuring a patient's ability to understand environment sounds (the monosyllable trochee spondee test) and the resultant improvement in quality of life. In contrast, Clark–Nucleus employed and promoted tests that measured a patient's ability to perceive speech and tracked improvements in speech recognition over time. Consequently, each development approach led to the development and usage of its own unique evaluation routines, which selectively reinforced and perpetuated the advantages of their respective design logics.

Further, 3M proposed to the FDA as a guideline for pre-market approval application (PMAA) that a minimum of 100 patients be required for establishing efficacy. This number was based on clinical experience with the 3M–House single-channel device at that time. 3M organized technical seminars on safety issues for FDA staff so as to mobilize support. If the 3M proposal was accepted, then Nucleus would be in a disadvantageous position, since by that time it had clinical data on only 43 patients. To prevent this eventuality, Nucleus audiologists visited the FDA and argued that sample size should be a function of the actual performance of each device, the claims each manufacturer wanted to make about its device, and the statistical approach adopted to support such claims. During the deliberation between designs, the different coalitions sought and were each able to find, endorsements from evaluation-relevant bodies such as the American Association of Otolaryngology and the University of Iowa, which received evaluation authority from the NIH–FDA.

From the vantage point of 3M, proponents of multi-channel technology had overstated their benefits and minimized the risks. On the other side, multi-channel proponents alleged that 3M exaggerated the performance of single-channel devices. It is, however, not clear who, if anyone, was exaggerating most. The claims simply reflected the beliefs and evaluation routines that each coalition had adopted and promoted. Rather than being persuaded by "objective" evaluations, which were impossible and unavailable, controversy was more likely to lead researchers to become even more entrenched in their own frame and practice. Here, we observe that the struggle to define safety and efficacy, and then measure it, illustrates how researchers projected their own beliefs onto cochlear implants and attempted to influence each other, including regulators. The evaluation routines adopted by researchers were congruent with their beliefs about cochlear implants. These routines, in turn, further reinforced researchers' beliefs [3].

The FDA eventually agreed with Nucleus, by not specifying the number of patients required for a PMAA, based on the reason that overly emphasizing big sample size would, in the face of uncertainty and ambiguity, put more patients at risk. Instead, the FDA would leave the minimum sample size flexible so that clinical investigators could tailor their studies to collect sufficient data to achieve statistically valid results.

Initially, the FDA had felt comfortable granting approvals to single-channel technology, since the simplicity of such a design facilitated their evaluation process and because single-channel devices possessed at that time the best potential to demonstrate device safety. Accordingly, in the early 1980s, single-channel implants dominated clinical practice. However, once single-channel devices had been able to demonstrate safety of cochlear implants as a class of products, the FDA shifted its focus to efficacy, emphasizing the ability to provide speech discrimination. In 1988, the NIH–FDA consensus development conference established funding and regulatory guidelines that favored multi-channel technology. This was a double blow to the single-channel coalitions, since the "consensus" practically institutionalized the multi-channel design as the dominant logic. Since then, the number of multi-channel cochlear implants has steadily increased whilst single-channel implants have continuously declined.

It should be noted that, despite failing to obtain a dominant position, House–3M researchers "continued advocating the single-channel path" [3]. A battle might have ended with temporarily prevailing knowledge constructed around the multi-channel cochlear implants. The war, however, appears far from over, as new comparative evidence has emerged afterwards that is inconsistent with the belief that single-channel devices are too simplistic to provide speech recognition. It is thus too early to rule out a new round of de-settling of the dominant logic and prevailing knowledge about cochlear implants. Whether it will happen and how it will develop are of course uncertain, depending, again, at least partly on the political wills and skills of concerned actors.

9.7   Reforming the Alberta Healthcare System

In the mid 1990s, the provincial government in Alberta, Canada, announced its new strategy for healthcare provision and introduced legislation to guide the implementation process. Up to that time, similar to other healthcare systems throughout the Western world, the provision of healthcare in Alberta was organized around a medical professional model with physicians actively involved in planning and governing hospitals and other healthcare facilities, and qualities of services were assessed through a strong reliance on medical opinion. Physicians were the only gatekeepers to healthcare services and the primary source of healthcare knowledge, at all levels. The logic of medical professionalism held institutional dominance, and the Alberta healthcare domain was relatively stable until then, despite years of calling for rationalization of services, implementation of new delivery strategies, and reduction of overall public expenditures.

In 1993, a new provincial government was elected based on the promise of efficiency. As part of its cost-cutting reform initiative announced in 1994, the government replaced more than 200 hospital boards, public health boards, and nursing home agencies with 17 regional health authorities (RHAs). These RHAs were given authority over all health providers within their geographic region, except for physicians, who continued to be employed on a fee-for-service basis and negotiated directly with the government. Structural changes occurred virtually overnight, as hospitals and other healthcare providers lost their legal identity and all their assets, and government-appointed board members took over the responsibility of managing healthcare resources for a designated geographic area. Around this reform initiative, all the key stakeholders presented: consumers, providers, agencies, and sponsors, with the key battles fought between the government (the key agency) and the physicians (the key provider). The powers and relationships among stakeholders changed dramatically via the government's political action: RHA board members were appointed based primarily on their prior business experience and support for health reforms, rather than their experience and expertise in healthcare. Indeed, physicians were not allowed to become RHA board members.

From the government's point of view, the change was an exercise of decentralization, giving more responsibilities to local RHAs for increasing efficiency. From the perspective of physicians and individual hospitals, however, the result was a centralization of power in the hands of RHAs that would harm healthcare services. The reform program thus can be seen as a powerful actor's attempt to move the healthcare domain from the dominance of one, the "old", institutional logic of medical professionalism, to another, the "new," institutional logic of business-like healthcare. Now the government had successfully used its power to alter the basic social structure in its favor by excluding physicians from controlling positions in RHAs. In order to materialize the complementarities between the altered structure and the guiding principle, intended practice, and belief system, a new dominance must be settled between the two competing logics, and the healthcare economics logic had to prevail if the reform was to succeed.

For this, the government began to articulate and publicize "consumer relationship" as the appropriate model for providing healthcare services, and stress the importance of "market forces" in determining appropriate healthcare delivery and quality. A new language was adopted and promoted which included the development of health policy through a "business planning model," organizing the healthcare domain to "focus on efficiency and effectiveness," and developing new strategies to ensure that services were delivered by the "lowest-cost provider." The government increasingly relied on a popular rhetoric, replacing the word "medical patient" with "healthcare consumer," indicating its confidence upon a more knowledgeable and demanding public, making clear its commitment and determination to the intended reform.

Gradually, with identifiable people appointed as RHA members to make decisions on behalf of communities in a "business-like" way, a change in other key stakeholders' views emerged and became apparent: other than physicians, key stakeholders began to accept the altered structure and the associated logic of business-like healthcare provision. Instead of arguing against the basic principles of market-oriented healthcare reform, these stakeholders converged to discuss how the inevitable changes would affect them, and how they would need to respond. A powerful coalition between agencies, consumers, and sponsors was thus taking shape to endorse the dominance of the government's intended institutional logic. A change in and of belief systems and the reconstruction of knowledge about how healthcare service should be provided were under way.

There is no evidence, however, that one key stakeholder, the physicians, agreed with the institutional logic of business-like healthcare based primarily on healthcare economics and market force. Not only did physicians feel that their views were ignored, but they also saw themselves as excluded from the major arenas of decision making and governance, and saw their interests being threatened by the institutionalization of new criteria/routines for evaluating the transformed system. Physicians wanted to maintain their role as leaders of healthcare governance, the gatekeeper of healthcare services, and the authority of healthcare knowledge. They were pragmatic and prepared to accept the already-in-place RHA boards, but only if they could gain a significant degree of control over them. They organized and entered into a multiphase public relations campaign to re-establish their role in the new system, and made their view clear that the doctor–patient relationship should remain central in the restructured domain. Physicians claimed that only through a reliance on medical professionalism, not the market mechanism, could the public be assured of high-quality healthcare. They attempted to use their remaining power to maintain dominance of the medical institutional logic, in spite of the domain's new structure.

With a successful public relations campaign, physicians were able to show public support for their claims of a deteriorating healthcare system under the new government. As a result, extra government funding to reduce surgical waiting lists was promised, and physicians were able to negotiate a satisfactory fee schedule. In the end, physicians remain committed to a competing institutional logic against the government and want to show they also hold the power to act. They settled into a position where they could maintain their own institutional logic, while working within the transformed structure of the domain. With all other stakeholders (i.e. consumers, agencies, sponsors) lined up into a powerful coalition, the structure and the dominant institutional logic of the healthcare domain changed, but the previously dominant logic of medical professionalism is subdued rather than eliminated. Given the distribution of power between the two powerful stakeholders, i.e. the government and the physicians, a sense of uneasy truce between their competing logics may be the best characterization of stability for the Alberta healthcare domain, with the government's market-oriented change program being consolidated and compatible healthcare knowledge claim constituted.

9.8 Conclusions

In this chapter, we explored a socio-cognitive approach to healthcare knowledge construction which focuses attention on social structure, institutional logic, and political actions. We discussed some significant features of these critical factors that shape the condition, process, and outcome of knowledge construction, and introduced some useful concepts and methods. We did this by drawing from recent studies in technology development, social movement, and institutional entrepreneurship. With this approach, we intend to move beyond a purely technology perspective toward healthcare knowledge management. We believe that the proposed constructivist approach is interesting, appropriate, and useful to all those concerned with healthcare services, be they consumers, providers, agencies, or sponsors, particularly in an era when healthcare needs become fragmented, the population becomes assertive, and reforms are in order. Knowledge management is much more than, and essentially not about, structuring detached "knowledge" and putting it into computers. It is not the exclusive domain of managers and technicians either. It instead involves primarily changes in social structures, value and belief systems, frames of reference, and working practices. Its efficacy and value can only be realized at "moments of truth," i.e. the involvement of and interactions between concerned parties, in our words stakeholders, involvements, and interactions that are essentially social, cognitive, and political in nature.

With the two case studies, we try to show the explanation and analytical power of our approach toward a wide range of knowledge construction phenomena, tasks, issues, and processes, from healthcare technology development to healthcare service reform. All this is what we wish the readers to think about and put into healthcare knowledge management practice.

References

1. Berger PL, Luckman T. *The social construction of reality*. London: Penguin Press; 1966.
2. Latour B, Woolgar S. *Laboratory life*. Beverly Hills, CA: Sage; 1979.
3. Garud R, Rappa MA. A socio-cognitive model of technology evolution: the case of cochlear implants. *Organ Sci* 1994;5(3):344–362.
4. Nakamori Y, Zhu Z. Exploring a sociological underpinning for the i system. *Int J Knowl Syst Sci* 2004;1(1):1–8.
5. Freeman RE. *Strategic management: a stakeholder approach*. Boston: Pitman; 1984.
6. Edgren L. Health customer diversity and its implications. *J Syst Sci Syst Eng* in press.
7. Reay T, Hinings CR. The recomposition of an organizational field: health care in Alberta. *Organ Stud* 2005;26(3):351–384.
8. Whittington R. Putting Giddens into action: social systems and managerial agency. *J Manage Stud* 1992;29(6):693–712.

9. Douglas M. *How institutions think*. Syracuse, NY: Syracuse University Press; 1986.
10. Beckert J. Agency, entrepreneurs, and institutional change. The role of strategic choice and institutionalised practices in organisations. *Organ Stud* 1999;20(5):777–799.
11. Friedland R, Alford RR. Bringing society back in: symbols, practices, and institutional contradictions. In: Powell WW, DiMaggio PJ, editors, *The new institutionalism in organisational analysis*. Chicago: Chicago University Press; 1991, pp. 232–263.
12. Greenwood R, Hinings CR. Understanding radical organisational change: bringing together the old and the new institutionalism. *Acad Manage Rev* 1996;21:1022–1054.
13. North DC. The contribution of the new institutional economics to an understanding of the transition problem. In: *WIDER Annual Lectures 1*, Helsinki, 1997. UNU World Institute for Development Economics Research (UNU/WIDER).
14. Aoki M. *Information, corporate governance, and institutional diversity*. New York: Oxford University Press; 1995/2000.
15. Zhu Z. Reform without a theory: why does it work in China? *Organ Stud* in press.
16. Thornton PH, Ocasio W. Institutional logics and the historical contingency of power in organisations: executive succession in the higher education publishing industry, 1958–1990. *Am J Sociol* 1999;105:801–843.
17. Hoffman AJ. Institutional evolution and change: environmentalism and the US chemical industry. *Acad Manage J* 1999;42(4):351–371.
18. Roberts J. *The modern firm*. Oxford: Oxford University Press; 2004.
19. Seo M-G, Creed WED. Institutional contradictions, praxis, and institutional change: a dialectical perspective. *Acad Manage Rev* 2002;27(1):222–247.
20. Bijker WE, Hughes TP, Pinch TJ. *The social construction of technological systems*. Cambridge, MA: MIT Press; 1987.
21. Orlikowski WJ. The duality of technology: rethinking the concept of technology in organisations. *Organ Sci* 1992;3(3):398–427.
22. Rosenkopf L, Tushman ML. On the co-evolution of organisation and technology. In: Baum J, Singh J, editors, *Evolution dynamics of organisation*. New York: Oxford University Press; 1993.
23. McAdam D, McCarthy JD, Zald MN, editors. *Comparative perspectives on social movements*. Cambridge: Cambridge University Press; 1996.
24. Rao H, Morrill C, Zald MN. Power plays: how social movements and collective action create new organisational forms. In: Staw BM, Sutton RI, editors, *Research in organisational behaviour*, vol. 20. New York: Elsevier Science; 2000, pp. 237–281.
25. DiMaggio PJ. Interest and agency in institutional theory. In: Zucker LG, editor, *Institutional patterns and organisations: cultural and environment*. Cambridge, MA: Ballinger; 1988, pp. 3–22.
26. Fligstein N. Social skill and institutional theory. *Am Behav Sci* 1997;40(4):397–405.
27. Munir KA, Jones M. Discontinuity and after: the social dynamics of technology evolution and dominance. *Organ Stud* 2004;25(4):561–581.
28. Tushman ML, Rosenkopf L. On the organisational determinants of technological change: towards a sociology of technological evolution. In: Staw B, Cummings L, editors, *Research in organisational behaviour*, vol. 14. Greenwich, CT: JAI Press; 1992, pp. 311–347.
29. Kostova T. Transnational transfer of strategic organisational practices: A contextual perspective. *Acad Manage Rev* 1999;24(2):308–324.
30. Hardy C. Understanding power: bringing about strategic change. *Br J Manage* 1996;7:3–16.

31. Christensen C. *The innovator's dilemma: when new technologies cause great firms to fail*. Boston, MA: Harvard Business School Press; 1997.
32. Hargadon AB, Douglas Y. When innovations meet institutions: Edison and the design of the electric light. *Admin Sci Q* 2001;46:476–501.
33. Cyert RM, March JG. *A behavioural theory of the firm*. Englewood Cliffs, NJ: Prentice Hall; 1963.
34. Garud R, Ahlstrom D. Researchers' roles in negotiating the institutional fabric of technologies. *Am Behav Sci* 1997;40(4):523–538.
35. Selznick P. *Leadership in administration*. New York: Harper and Row; 1957.

10
Narratives in Healthcare

CHU KEONG LEE AND SCHUBERT FOO

Abstract

In this chapter, the narrative is defined and the elements of the narrative are elucidated. Three lenses through which one can view the role of narratives in healthcare are discussed. First, organizational narratives help to foster social capital in the organization and, therefore, contribute to the people aspect of the knowledge management initiative in the organization. Second, the recuperative and relationship building roles of illness narratives are described. Third, narratives from the practice of narrative medicine are explored. The chapter concludes by proposing four requirements for narratives to be effective, namely, effective listening skills, the availability of time and place for storytelling, and the codification of narratives.

Keywords   narrative; typology of narratives; storytelling

10.1   Introduction

Jean-Dominique Bauby was the editor-in-chief of the French *Elle* magazine. On 8 December 1995, he was struck with a massive stroke which damaged his brain stem, leaving him with the "locked-in syndrome." He was paralyzed from head to toe and could only communicate by blinking his left eye. With the help of a speech therapist, who introduced him to an alphabet in which the letters were ordered according to their frequencies in the French language, he dictated the book *The Diving-Bell and The Butterfly* to Claude Mandibel at Room 119 in the Naval Hospital at Berck-sur-Mer on the coast of the French Channel, where he was warded. In his book, Bauby described his initial hopes that he would very quickly recover his movement and speech. He filled his roving mind "with a thousand projects: a novel, travel, a play, marketing a fruit cocktail of his own invention," projects which he would undertake once he had regained his ability to walk and speak. Alas, as time progressed, he realized that this was not to be. He wrote about the devastation and despair upon discovering that he was a quadriplegic and would have to be confined to the wheelchair for the rest of his life. He described the vacillation of his emotions over the sudden dependence on others for even the simplest of tasks, the amusement and pleasure one day of having someone bathe him and wipe his bottom, only to feel unbearable gloom and sadness the next day about the same thing. He painfully wrote about the sadness when he thought of the little pleasures in which he participated before the stroke. Bauby's account about his experience of the "locked-in syndrome" in his book is an example of a narrative in the context of healthcare [1].

What exactly is a narrative? Several definitions that have been put forward are listed below:

• A narrative is a spoken or written account of connected events [2].
• A narrative is a verse or prose accounting of an event or sequence of events, real or invented [3].
• A narrative is a representation of past events in any medium: narratives can be oral, written, filmed, or drawn [4].

A few elements of narratives can be gleaned from the definitions. A narrative: (1) can be a spoken, written, filmed, or drawn account; (2) it can be in verse or prose; (3) it can be used to represent real or fictional events. Greenhalgh and Hurwitz [5] added four more features to this list: (1) narratives have a beginning, several intervening events, and an ending; (2) narratives incorporate both the viewpoints of the narrator and the listener; (3) narratives are concerned with individuals, how they feel, and how others feel about them; (4) narratives are absorbing and memorable, and they engage the listener and invite him to interpret the account, i.e. to "live through" them. Narratives are such an essential part of human nature that Fisher [6] has used the term *homo narrans* to label human beings. To need to narrate is part of the universal human trait of needing to be understood, and needing to be in communication even if only from the margins [7].

There are at least three lenses through which we can view narratives in the world of healthcare. First, there are organizational stories. These are stories whose main purpose is to create and strengthen social capital, and in doing so to contribute to the success of the organization's knowledge management initiative [8]. Second, there are illness narratives. These are stories people tell about their subjective experience of illness. Illness narratives have become a major literary genre. They are a source of knowledge about the disruptive nature of illness and their therapeutic potential has been recognized [9]. It must be clarified at this point that "medical sociologists distinguish between disease (the diagnostic entity) and illness (the way that disease is perceived, enacted, responded to by a person, in relationships with others)" [10]. Third, there are stories that are told by physicians that practice medicine with narrative competence [11]. Many authors use the term "narrative" interchangeably with the term "story". In this article, I, too, have adopted this stance. Indeed, Frank [12] has noted that it is more natural to say "let me tell you a story" rather than "let me tell you a narrative."

10.2   Organizational Stories

Stories build social capital because they are told with three possible objectives, i.e. to reaffirm, to create, or to redirect the relationship within which the story is told. In fact, the story itself, which is an act of telling, is the relationship. Stories are told with (and not just to) listeners. The listeners in a storytelling session are not incidental to the act of storytelling; they are a critical element of it, as the stories that are told reaffirm what the participants of a storytelling session mean to each other and how they relate to each other [12].

Cohen and Prusak [8] suggested several ways in which stories build and support social capital in the organization: (1) stories convey the norms, values, attitudes, and behaviors that define social groups more fully than any other types of communication; (2) stories are memorable and contain lessons that can be applied directly to real life as they "show by example" [8, p. 112]; (3) storytelling sessions are social events which help to connect people and define them as members of a social group; (4) stories recount past events and bond people together; (5) stories help people to frame their thinking and allow them to bring reality into an abstract discussion.

In addition, they suggested a taxonomy of stories, stressing that the categories they propose are not watertight and that any one story can belong to one or more categories. *Organizational myths* are stories that define the organizational culture. These stories are fundamental to the organization in the sense that they encode how the organization views itself and its relationship with the world, describe the priorities of the organization, and explain how things work and get accomplished around the organization. These stories center on the founders, or on critical events that the organization has faced in the past. An example of an organizational myth that centers on the founder is the one that David Packard, one of the co-founders of the Hewlett-Packard Corporation, related in his book *The HP Way* [13]. In the book, Packard related the story where he was walking around the shop floor with the manager of that unit. During his walk, he stopped to watch a machinist make a plastic mold die with great care and reached out to touch the carefully polished die with his finger. The machinist exclaimed, "Get your finger off my die!", to which his manager replied, "Do you know who this is?" The machinist countered, "I don't care." Packard stressed that the machinist was not taken to task for this incident. Instead, he was commended for being proud of his work. This story illustrates the fundamental aspects of the organizational culture at Hewlett-Packard: (1) a strong belief that each person in the organization and the job he does is important; (2) individuals are to be treated with consideration and respect; (3) little details make the difference between an average and a great product. The stories Robert Watson tells in his book about the management philosophy at the Salvation Army repeatedly lay down the order of priority in the Army's unique way of meeting human needs called "holistic ministry," i.e. soup, then soap, then salvation [14].

Hero stories are stories that tell of successes and triumphs over great trials and difficulties, usually owing to the courage, persistence, determination, and fortitude of one individual. These stories also tell of heroic gambles. Hero stories seek to inspire the listener. The story of Helen Keller is such a story [15]. It tells of Helen, who was born with the sense of hearing and of sight, catching a fever at 19 months of age, and subsequently becoming an impossibly difficult deaf–blind child. It tells also of her courage in the face of adversity that allowed her to overcome the odds through perseverance and the help of a dedicated Irish–American teacher named Anne Sullivan. Despite the odds stacked against her, Helen managed to accomplish much in life, graduating from Radcliffe College cum laude, becoming a successful writer, and an active fund raiser for the American Foundation for the Blind. The stoical attitude that she adopted made her a heroic role model for many. She has become a timeless icon and the single disabled person that Americans can name.

Many hero stories were told during the severe acute respiratory syndrome (SARS) outbreak in 2003. One such story had to do with Carlo Urbani, a 46-year-old physician and infectious disease specialist working with the World Health Organization. Dr Urbani was an Italian physician who, at 22, left his hometown of Maiolati Spontini to work in Africa. In 1999, he accepted the Nobel Peace Prize on behalf of Médicins sans Frontières, an international humanitarian group dedicated to providing medical care to victims of political violence or natural disasters. In 2003, he was called to the Vietnam–French hospital in Hanoi as an epidemiological expert. It was in Hanoi that he alerted the world to SARS. Without his early warnings of the importance of infection control safeguards and the need for heightened global surveillance of SARS, the outbreak could have been far worse. He started treating Vietnam's only index patient, a Chinese–American businessman who brought the disease into Vietnam after having visited Shanghai and Hong Kong, on February 28. By March 11 he realized he himself had been infected with the disease. He succumbed to SARS in Bangkok on March 29. As a memorial to Dr Urbani, colleagues from around the world have proposed naming the SARS virus after him [16]. This is a story of a fallen hero. Owing to the nature of healthcare, which has much to do with caring, curing, saving, helping, healing, and relieving, it is naturally replete with hero stories.

Failure stories caution the listener against certain acts, as these offend the organizational culture. They define the out-of-bound markers in the organization and, therefore, contain the dos and don'ts that one must know to function effectively in the organization. Failure stories are, therefore, a part of one's organizational navigation knowledge. *War stories* are stories of disasters. These stories have a connecting experience and they build social capital. These two story types were frequently recounted during the Singapore National Kidney Foundation (NKF) controversy when it was revealed that the NKF Chief Executive Officer (CEO) earned in excess of half a million Singapore dollars a year and flew first class when he traveled at NKF's expense. This flew in the face of the NKF's culture of transparency, accountability, and prudence. The war stories that followed shortly after were on the public outcry against NKF by canceling their monthly donations, on the setting up of an online petition calling for the CEO's resignation, and on the call for greater transparency by charitable organizations in general.

Stories of the future are stories that can unite organizational members towards a goal for which they can strive. These stories are used by charismatic leaders to draw people into a cooperative effort, gelling them into a community in the process.

Such stories create a collaborative culture by drawing organizational members together and showing them what they can achieve if they work together. Several articles have been written predicting what the hospital of the future would be like. Some trends that can be expected are increased pressure to contain cost, increased integration and alliances among healthcare providers, increased use of information and telecommunication technologies, and increased adoption of breakthrough technologies [17]. In explaining these trends to his colleagues, the CEO of a hospital that paints a picture of his hospital 10 years on and describes the steps he plans to take to achieve that vision during a speech he makes in an annual staff dinner, say, would be telling a story of the future.

10.3   Illness Narratives

Illness narratives refer to the reflective and insightful autobiographical accounts of illness. They are not merely chronicles of events, but can also provide valuable insights into how patienthood, brought upon by the assault of illness, is experienced as a disruption of selfhood. The very act of narration itself is an important way of making sense of the illness, of restoring personhood and connectedness, and of reclaiming the illness experience [9]. When life is hard, such as the demoralization that one experiences when afflicted with an illness, stories can also provide the narrators some distance from their illness. Stories have a recuperative role and can be used to recuperate persons, relationships, and communities. Stories have a relationship-building role, and listening to a story outside of a relationship is meaningless. Those who tell stories are most concerned about being heard, wondering if they will find others who will answer their call for a relationship [12]. Illness narratives celebrate the subjectivity and uniqueness of the illness experience, which is often objectified and depersonalized by the healthcare system.

Illness narratives are typically organized in a chronological plot style, starting with the time before the illness, the onset of illness, the crisis point, and the resolution of the crisis. Therefore, the questioning technique used can follow a lineal sequence: past-present-future [9].

General practices offer physician and patient the opportunity to exchange stories for over half a lifetime. The narratives allow general practitioners to form special relationships with three cohorts of patients, namely those of the same gender and approximately the same age, those of approximately the same age as the physician's parents, and those approximately the same age as the doctor's children. Patients in the first group progress through life along with their physicians, and a common cultural context holds them together. Patients in the second group face the same problems with deteriorating health as the physician's own parents, and their common struggle provides the context for the relationship. Patients in the third group grow up along with the physician's own children, and their common passage through the most exciting and complex transitions of their lives binds physician and patient. The narratives shared over a prolonged time allow strong bonds to be formed, engendering trust and effective care [18].

Illness narratives have also appeared on the World Wide Web. McLellan [19] wrote about the long series of postings on Gabe Catalfo's experience with acute lymphocytic leukemia, written by his father, Phil Catalfo, on Whole Earth 'Lectronic Link (WELL), a conferencing system that started in 1985. This is a unique work compared with traditional illness narratives like poems and short stories (e.g. Bauby's *The Diving-Bell and The Butterfly*), because whereas traditional narrative forms are complete and finished, Phil's postings about his son's experience is an ongoing and unfinished account of Gabe's experience. This account, which has been written as a chronicle of daily events, has enabled healthcare professionals to understand patients' and their families' experiences of illness better. Another major difference is its involvement of the readers. In electronic narratives, the readers are not the same as the silent and unseen buyers of a book. The readers become active participants in the telling by:

- being concerned in asking about how father and son are coping;
- acting as learners, seeking clarification on what has been posted;
- acting as a source of advice and information, e.g. the poster that told Catalfo about a health information service available to the public;
- acting as a source of emotional support for the Catalfo family, sending messages of encouragement, cheer, and congratulations when the treatment went well;
- acting as volunteer researchers.

In addition to the day-to-day treatment and coping issues, the illness narratives posted provide insights into the meaning of the illness for the father as well as for the family, and encompass the total experience of the illness, not just the progression of the disease. Online illness narratives (OINs) have several unique features. First, they are unfinished. In a sense they are always "work-in-progress." Second, OINs are collaboratively constructed by the voices of many discussants along the way. Third, they are interactive in nature and the readers are not silent; rather, they become active participants in the telling of the story, and they exert their influence on the story in different ways. Therefore, the authorship of an OIN is unclear. Fourth, they are told in real time with a limited time perspective. Last, there is a certain rawness and emotional power in the postings that allow the actual experience to be told closer than through any other genre. Participants of OINs benefit by gaining access to experts in many areas, and because the narrative is multi-authored, they get to see many perspectives on any single issue; but the downside is the lack of a formal mechanism for review of the postings [19].

10.4   Narratives from the Practice of Narrative Medicine

These narratives are a product of the practice of medicine enhanced with narrative competence. An important idea is that people who are experiencing illness require physicians that are not just medically competent, i.e. physicians that can understand their disease and prescribe the appropriate medication and treatment, but also (and perhaps more important) physicians that can accompany them through their illness, understand their plight, and empathize with them. Narratives are seen as the vehicle that will allow for authentic engagements. Charon [11] has identified four central narrative situations in which physicians play a part: physician and patient, physician and self, physician and colleagues, and physician and society. Physician–patient narratives are used to bridge physician and patient, allowing the physician to join his patient in illness. They are told in words, gestures, and silences. Besides being therapeutic in themselves, these narratives allow the physician to enter into the world of his patients. Groopman [20] stressed that this melding of minds is important so that a clinical compass can be built. The physician needs to probe not just the patient's body, but also his spirit, to consider not just the patient's physical repair, but also his psychological and emotional repair. This requires open dialogue; this requires the magic of the narrative. Clinical decisions cannot be made algorithmically, as each person experiences his illness differently, has very different risk profiles, and is willing to give up different things to continue living.

Physician–self narratives are the reflections and self-examination of contemplative physicians when they attempt to make sense of their own emotional responses to patients. Reflection also allows physicians to understand the patient's story better and enables them to navigate the uncertainty and devastation of illness better. Physician–society narratives allow physicians to have frank and honest conversations with society about the imperfections of the medical system, the limits of medical knowledge, and the fragility of life. It can be said that Groopman [20] achieves both these narrative types in his book, *Second Opinions*. In the book, he reflects on the complexity of medical decision making. At the same time, he has a conversation with society about reality in the world of medicine, a world many wish to be perfect, but which is far from being so: a world where even the best physicians sometimes give bad advice and make serious mistakes.

Physician–colleague narratives are knowledge-sharing episodes in which a physician participates with his colleagues, who may be other physicians or nurses, social workers, etc. These narratives build social capital and collegiality, and allow physicians to celebrate their roles in the healthcare system. In addition, knowledge sharing prevents reinvention of the wheel, spreads best practices, provides opportunities for peer learning, and provides a ready sounding board to air new ideas [11].

10.5 The Critical Complements to Narratives

Narratives alone, no matter how well told, are insufficient. At least four other requirements are necessary for narratives to be effective in healthcare. Effective listening skills, the availability of time and place, and the codification of narratives are all necessary to ensure that the narratives are heard and preserved.

As it is important to hear out those who tell stories of their illness, and to answer their call for a relationship, listening skills are of paramount importance. Physicians must learn how to listen to their patients to convert the patient's story into a diagnosis and a treatment plan, and nurses must learn the art of history taking in a new way, in a way that privileges the patient's voice and in a way that listens out for meaning rather than just facts. Nichols and Stevens [21] listed six bad listening habits uncovered by research at the University of Minnesota. They found these habits to be almost universal, and used as a rationalization for not listening, even when the listener knows and admits he should be listening. First, the habit of faking attention. Listeners who fake attention deceive themselves and frequently get caught. Second, the habit of "I-get-the-facts" listening. These listeners miss the point of listening, which is rarely "to get the facts," but rather "to understand the idea," "to grasp the meaning and significance," or "to look with me rather than at me." Third, the habit of avoiding difficult listening. Listening perforce takes energy and requires mental exertion. In addition, listening to the experience of illness is difficult and draining.

Fourth, the habit of prematurely dismissing a subject as uninteresting. Here, the listener equates "interesting" to "valuable." What is required is a change of attitude to views of even the most ordinary person as one who has some ideas to offer and from whom I want to take for myself those ideas of his. Fifth, the habit of criticizing delivery and physical appearance. This habit causes the listener to focus on the physical aspects (i.e. the clothes, accessories, or hairstyle worn by the speaker) or the speech (i.e. the foreign accent or "twang"). Instead of listening intently to the content, the listener gets distracted by mentally criticizing the physical appearance or delivery of the content, adopting an attitude that "a person who talks like that cannot have anything worth listening to." Last, the habit of yielding easily to distractions that compete with the person talking refers to a lack of willingness to proactively shut out the distractions that inevitably interrupt many narratives, e.g. by closing the door, moving closer to the person talking, or mentally shutting out the distractions when all other measures prove futile. These habits have a serious consequence. They cause the listener, and in the case of healthcare, the physician, to lose the opportunity to learn something from what is being said by the patient.

The etymology of the traditional style of the Chinese character to listen (Ting1) (Figure 10.1) clearly conveys the essential elements of listening and depicts listening as a complex and involved task. The radicals " 耳" (Er3, meaning ear) and "王" (Wang2, meaning emperor) on the left, remind the listener to listen to the speaker as if he were listening to the emperor. The importance of giving full concentration is depicted by the radicals " 十" (Shi2, meaning ten or full) and "目" (Mu4, meaning sight or eye). The elements of empathy and whole-heartedness are represented in the radicals " 一心" (Yi1 Xin1, meaning with one heart). Some narratives, e.g. pain narratives, are more difficult to understand and, therefore, will require more effort on the part of the listener. They are especially difficult to understand because of their lack of coherence and structure, and because they are typically poured out in a haphazard way. In order to understand the narrative, physicians not only need to listen to the exact words used and the order in which they were uttered, but also match these with the body language involved.

The importance of time and place is evident. As Heath [18] so clearly puts it, "Stories can only be told if people have time to talk and time to listen and to hear. The richer the narrative, the more time is needed." The time element of narrative was

FIGURE **10.1.** Traditional Chinese character for the verb "listen."

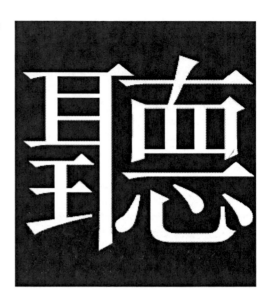

also highlighted by Bayliss [22]. He stressed that both physicians and patients need time for narratives: the physician needs time to listen, and the patients to deliver. He bemoaned the current situation where physicians are required to see more patients in less time, stating that it is not in the best interest of either party to do this, as it lessens the intellectual satisfaction of understanding narratives. A lack of time and opportunity has been frequently cited as being a barrier to knowledge sharing [23], which is most effectively achieved through "a convincing narrative delivered with elegance and passion" [24]. A frequent intrusion to narrative episodes is that created by technology. Telephones, facsimile machines, and portable digital assistants have invaded the workplace, disrupting many narrative episodes with patients. It may be useful (or even necessary) for healthcare organizations to consider providing "Zen gardens," or places of peace. These are "islands of non-technology" where people can concentrate, think, read, write, or have a conversation uninterrupted by technology [25].

Nonaka and Konno [26] have stressed the importance of "ba" (which translates approximately to "place" in English) as a shared space for human interaction (and narration is a form of human interaction) where knowledge can be created and shared. A "ba" can be physical, virtual, or even mental. In healthcare, an example of "ba" is nursing presence, which is seen to play an important role in the process of healing. Nursing presence has to do with "mutual openness with the other, entering the world of the other to see the objective from his or her standpoint, and coexisting for some moments in time and space", and is

an intersubjective encounter between a nurse and a patient in which the nurse encounters the patient as a unique human being in a unique situation and chooses to spend her/himself on the patient's behalf. The antecedents to presence are the nurse's decision to immerse

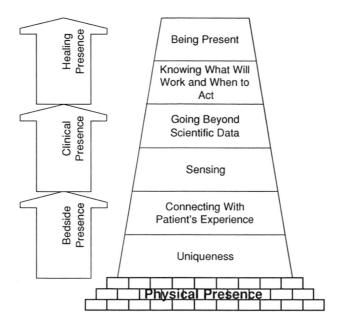

FIGURE 10.2. Godkin's [28] model of healing presence.

him/herself in the patient's situation and the patient's willingness to let the nurse into that
lived experience [27].

One way in which the nurse can "enter the world of the patient" to "immerse
himself in the patient's situation" is through the use of narratives. The patient lets
the nurse enter his lived experience through the use of narratives. Narratives allow
nurses to establish a relationship with the patients and be sensitive to their needs, to
treat the patient as a person and not as a case amenable to technological solutions.
Godkin [28] worked on six features necessary for attaining nursing presence
identified by Doona et al. [29], and proposed a model of nursing presence comprising three layers of six hierarchical levels (Figure 10.2). In Godkin's model, the
lower levels support the higher ones and, therefore, must be in existence before
the higher ones. It will be argued that narratives are a critical aspect of each of the
three layers. The first layer, bedside presence, requires physical presence, and in
essence conforms to Nonaka and Konno's "physical ba." At this layer, narratives
are used to establish rapport through interaction with the patient. In the second
layer, clinical presence, narratives are used to understand the patient's perspective
in order to go beyond the scientific data. The last layer, healing presence, uses
narratives to achieve attunement with each other. Here, the ability to relate closely
to another person, to empathize, will enable a person to know what will work and
when to act for a patient. Healing presence conforms closely with Nonaka and
Konno's "mental ba," i.e. a shared knowledge context [26].

Finally, narratives need to be captured, as codification is the only way the experience of illness can be made permanent for all to learn. This is being done with the Database of Individual Patient Experience (DIPEx; http://www.dipex.org/), a site launched in July 2001 by Ann McPherson and Andrew Herxheimer after their own experiences of illness (breast cancer and knee replacement surgery respectively). They decided to start this patient experience Website (hypertension and prostate cancer were the first two topics) after failing to find others to talk to about their illnesses. Currently, DIPEx is aimed at patients, their caregivers, family, and friends, and also functions as a teaching resource for health professionals. The Website contains interviews with everyday people about their own experiences of serious illnesses, health problems, or health-related matters. Their aim is to cover 100 main illnesses and conditions, as well as areas such as immunization, rare diseases, skin conditions, infertility, and chronic illnesses. The limitation is that the database currently represents the experiences and views of people within the UK. A Website with a similar charter, but on an international scale, is badly needed, as the experience of illness is likely to be influenced by culture. Perhaps the most appropriate organization to champion this effort is the World Health Organization.

10.6   Conclusions

In a healthcare paradigm where there is an increasing call for a more effective use of the organization's knowledge assets to enhance patient safety, avoid waste, reduce wait, and increase quality care [30], and for a more patient-centered approach, narratives can provide a way forward. In this chapter, three types of narrative, namely organizational myths, illness narratives, and narratives from narrative medicine, have been identified. The role that these narratives play in healthcare has been described. Lastly, four requirements before narratives can be truly effective in a healthcare organization have been identified.

References

1. Bauby J-D. *The diving-bell and the butterfly*. London: Fourth Estate; 2002.
2. *The Oxford dictionary of English*, 2nd edition revised.
3. Thomson Gale glossary. Available from: http://www.gale.com/free_resources/glossary/glossary_no.htm.
4. Linde C. Narrative and social tacit knowledge. *J Knowl Manage* 2001;5:160–170.
5. Greenhalgh T, Hurwitz B. Why study narrative? In: Greenhalgh T, Hurwitz B, editors. *Narrative based medicine: dialogue and discourse in clinical practice*. London: BMJ Books; 1998.
6. Fisher WR. Narration as a human communication paradigm: the case of public moral argument. *Commun Monogr* 1984;51:1–22.
7. Mattingly C. *Healing dramas and clinical plots: the narrative structure of experience*. Cambridge, UK: Cambridge University Press; 1998.
8. Cohen D, Prusak L. *In good company: how social capital makes organizations work*. Boston: Harvard Business School Press; 2001.

9. Sakalys JA. Restoring the patient's voice: the therapeutics of illness narratives. *J Holistic Nurs* 2003;21:228–241.

10. Riessman CK. Illness narratives: positioned identities. Available from: http://www.cardiff.ac.uk/encap/hcrc/comet/prog/narratives.pdf.

11. Charon R. Narrative medicine: a model for empathy, reflection, profession and trust. *J Am Med Assoc* 2001;286:1897–1902.

12. Frank AW. The standpoint of the storyteller. *Qual Health Res* 2000;10:354–365.

13. Packard D. *How Bill Hewlett and I built our company*. New York: HarperBusiness; 1995.

14. Watson RA, Brown B. *The most effective organization in the U.S.: leadership secrets of the Salvation Army*. New York: Crown Business; 2001.

15. Keller H. *The story of my life*. New York: W.W. Norton; 2003.

16. Chee YC. Heroes and heroines of the war on SARS. *Singapore Med J* 2003;44:221–228.

17. Geisler E, Vierhout P. The hospital of the future: concepts and directions. In: Geisler E, Krabbendam K, Schuring R, editors. *Technology, health care, and management in the hospital of the future*. Westport, CT: Praeger; 2003.

18. Heath I. Following the story: continuity of care in general practice. In: Greenhalgh T, Hurwitz B, editors. *Narrative based medicine: dialogue and discourse in clinical practice*. London: BMJ Books; 1998.

19. McLellan F. *"A whole other story": the electronic narrative of illness. Lit Med* 1997;16:88–107.

20. Groopman J. *Second opinions: stories of intuition and choice in the changing world of medicine*. New York: Viking; 2000.

21. Nichols RG, Stevens LA. *Are you listening?* New York: McGraw-Hill; 1957.

22. Bayliss R. Pain narratives. In: Greenhalgh T, Hurwitz B, editors. *Narrative based medicine: dialogue and discourse in clinical practice*. London: BMJ Books; 1998.

23. Choo CW. Knowledge management. In: Schement JR, editor. *Encyclopedia of communication and information*. New York: Thomson Gale; 2001.

24. Davenport T, Prusak L. *Working knowledge: how organizations manage what they know*. Boston: Harvard Business School Press; 1998.

25. Myerson J, Ross P. *The creative office*. London: Lawrence King; 1999.

26. Nonaka I, Konno N. The concept of "Ba": building a foundation for knowledge creation. *Calif Manage Rev* 1998,40:40–54.

27. Doona ME, Haggerty LA, Chase SK. Nursing presence: an existential exploration of the concept. *Schol Enquiry Nurs Pract Int J* 1997;11:3–16.

28. Godkin J. Healing presence. *J Holistic Nurs* 1999;19:5–21.

29. Doona ME, Chase SK, Haggerty LA. Nursing presence: as real as a Milky Way bar. *J Holistic Nurs* 1999;17:54–70.

30. Zajac JD. The public hospital of the future. *Med J Aust* 2003;179:250–252.

11
Application Service Provider Technology in the Healthcare Environment

A. MIGUEL CRUZ, DENIS E. RODRÍGUEZ, CAMERON BARR
AND M.C. SANCHEZ

Abstract

With the advancement of medical technology and thus the complexity of the equipment under their care, clinical engineering departments (CEDs) must continue to make use of computerized tools in the management of departmental activities. Researchers at ISPJAE have designed, installed and implemented an Application Service Provider model, at the laboratory level, to offer value added management tools in an online format to CEDs. This completed project to help meet demands across multiple health care organizations and provide a means of access for organizations, which otherwise might not be able to take advantage or readily participate in the benefits of those tools has been well received. Ten (10) hospitals have requested the service and five (5) of those are ready to proceed with the implementation of the ASP. With the proposed centralized system architecture, the model has shown promise in reducing network infrastructure labor and equipment costs, benchmarking of equipment performance indicators and the development of avenues for proper and timely problem reporting. The following is a detailed description of the design process through conception to the implementation of the five (5) main software modules and supporting system architecture.

11.1   Introduction

Today, the use of software tools in clinical engineering departments (CEDs) can be considered commonplace [1,2]. Their use is justified not only by the convenience in performing and managing the day-to-day operations,[1] but also by the advantages within harmonization activities and information exchange between institutions.

The use of computerized systems in CEDs can generally be divided into two main areas:

---

[1] Easy storage and retrieval of amounts of information facilitate data-processing analysis, reducing manual paperwork, etc.

1. Remote diagnostics used by original equipment manufacturers (OEMs) and/or third-party companies in order to monitor and increase service productivity.
2. Computerized systems to support the maintenance and technology management tasks inside the clinical/hospital environment.

The remote diagnostic in the service field environment is usually part of the overall call-managing process. It is based on the strategic use of information and data acquisition methods to identify, isolate, analyze, and ultimately diagnose and evaluate faults within units of equipment or within systems [3].

In turn, the evolution of information technology (IT) solutions in support of both areas has branched into three main paths:

1. Computerized maintenance management system (CMMS).
2. Fully integrated field management systems (FSMS) software.
3. Application service providers (ASPs).

11.1.1   Computerized Maintenance Management System

A few years ago, and currently in many cases, CEDs have relied on CMMSs to maintain information about preventive maintenance activity, equipment inventory, parts, service contracts, and vendor service report, etc. These systems are basically automated databases that enable an organization to track and monitor equipment service requirements and history. The core of a generic CMMS consists of two modules [4]:

• *Equipment inventory records.* Consisting of one record for each device. This record contains information specific to that piece of equipment, such as model, serial number, date of installation, facility, location, and information regarding when it is scheduled for maintenance inspections.
• *Equipment maintenance and repair records.* Contains summary data on each maintenance and repair task that was completed for a given work-order on the equipment.

11.1.2   Fully Integrated Field Management Systems Software

New demands for improved service productivity and efficiency in service quality have forced the use of a new generation of software tools in CEDs. That demand has manifested itself in the form of FSMSs. In contrast to CMMSs, FSMSs provide intelligence for the management and coordination of daily service delivery by providing expanded functionality over and above standard asset management systems. An FSMS offers comprehensive and in-depth automation of data and intelligence related to service tasks, activities, and process, resulting in improved profitability, efficiency, and productivity.

It is estimated that expenditure on FSMSs represents a market of approximately US$100 million. Research indicates that 35% of all purchases in the next year will be among first-time users. However, the remaining 65% will be for upgrading or replacing the existing FSMS [3].

11.1.3   Application Service Providers for Clinical Engineering

The use of the Internet has penetrated almost every aspect of our daily lives. New applications have been developed utilizing the Internet to communicate with medical equipment management information systems. These applications must be supported by ASP technology.

A rigorous definition of the ASP concept is difficult to put forth because it is still a term in its infancy. However, "there is a good amount of consensus that ASP means remotely hosted applications management and onside hosting" [5].

There are two types of ASP that one can see in the marketplace. One is the storage service provider (SSP) model, where everything is going to be stored off-side and the customer will retrieve what is needed on demand. The other is the finance model, where customers have centralized software and storage, and the applications and the storage would be downloaded and used from a central organization as needed, and customers only pay for what is used [5–7].

One area where the benefits arising from the use of ASP can readily be seen is medical image storage, namely in picture archiving and communications systems (PACSs) [5]. Given the amount of storage space required for a single, well-defined picture (i.e. high pixel density), foreseeable storage problems can certainly be anticipated when dealing with potentially hundreds of thousands of them. The most notable and pertinent of these benefits to many organizations in today's political and economic climate is in saved costs.[2] With the use of an ASP, users do not have to acquire the expensive hardware and IT infrastructure (terminal servers, cabling, routers) capable of handling large data traffic. Added savings are realized through eliminating the cost of labor required in maintaining that infrastructure. Users do not have to maintain a backup or a maintenance manager, which improves efficiency of time use related to administration. Industry specialists predict a growth in ASP technology. It is estimated that expenditure represents a market of approximately US$500 million.

Despite the advantages of ASP, the implementation of ASP in the clinical engineering branch has been poor. Before 2002, only a few companies (Genesis Technology Partners LLC, St Croix Systems, Inc., Bio-Tek, etc.) have put CMMS products online through an intermediate group of steps [8].[3] From 2002 to 2004, a growth in the number of companies and products related to the ASP concept

---

[2] The 5-year cost of an IT employee can reach US$500,000. Second, archive and network provisions for redundancy (as required by the Health Insurance Portability and Accountability Act (HIPAA)) will cost as much as a primary archive: US$350,000 to US$400,000 for a 10 terabytes system. The policies for archive disaster recovery (as required by HIPAA) costs run between US$15,000 and US$30,000 a year for a 10 terabytes system.

[3] The use of an application server from Citrix Systems: Citrix metaframe translates input and output for Windows NT applications, allowing these small network applications to interact with the clients using a standard Web browser.

in clinical engineering has been noted. However, the existence of proposals and implementation details of ASP technology in peer-reviewed journals has been nonexistent [9].

Here, we propose an ASP model in order to meet the traditional needs of CEDs involved in the technology management processes of an expanding healthcare system. The insights contained herein are the result of the efforts undertaken at ISPJAE to design, install and implement a working ASP system at the laboratory level. The example provided here could be expanded to other hospital areas.

11.2   Stages in the Development of Application Service Providers for Clinical Engineering

To begin planning for the proposed ASP model, four different stages should be considered:

1. Defining strategic ASP management goals.
2. Identifying and setting operational needs.
3. The ASP design and development.
4. The ASP implementation and validation.

11.2.1   Defining Strategic Application Service Provider Information Management Goals

In the international arena, the US, Canada, and the EU have a considerable impact on technology management standards. As an integral part of the ongoing effort to improve and sustain the quality of patient care within these respective healthcare systems, there exist various standards and accreditation groups dedicated to associated subjects.[4] All three jurisdictions have governmental organizations which stipulate that some form of licensure be obtained for any medical device being manufactured, or imported and distributed, based on the level of risk to the operator or patient. This certification is in the form of a medical device license for the product and an establishment license for the producing or distributing organization. In the US, the Food and Drug Administration (FDA) is the issuer. In Canada, the Therapeutic Product Directorate (TPD) branch of Health Canada deals with licensure. Within the EU, each member state has an appointed "competent authority" that acts as a regulator, which in turn ensures a product's compliance with either the Medical Device Directive or the In Vitro Diagnostic Medical Device Directive [10]. All of them have provisions concerning the practice of a manufacture's monitoring of the performance of their products in the field, and for the reporting of problems and adverse incidents involving those products by the end-user facilities and manufacturers.

In the US, the Joint Commission on Accreditation of Healthcare Organizations (JCAHO) is the most comprehensive and widely accepted authority concerning

---

[4] ANSI/AAMI, NFPA, UL, OSHA.

quality assurance in a clinical setting. The pertinent medical device portions are stated in the Environment of Care section of the JCAHO manual for hospitals.

Analogous to the mandate of the JCAHO is that of the Canadian Council on Health Services Accreditation (CCHSA), which is Canada's national third-party assessment body for healthcare facilities. The CCHSA aids these facilities in self-assessment, quality improvement, and management activities, and then provides surveillance with recommendations for the future. Focusing on the end-user level of the medical device life cycle, the CCHSA has laid out a set of criteria. Again, these criteria are found in the Environment section of their standard, which promotes the utilization of appropriate equipment maintenance, tracking, and education programs.

On the other hand, the Member States of the EU have agreed that their standardization and certification activities are to be handled by the CEN (European Standardization Organization) and ISO. The European Cooperation for Accreditation (EA) also has the mandate of assessing and accrediting the companies, laboratories, and agencies that provide third-party audits concerning accreditation and certification for companies against the appropriate standards. The EA is involved in the healthcare sector, and through consultation with different national groups in the Member States' healthcare systems. A number of other groups are involved in varying capacities.

Having briefly touched upon the makeup of the regulatory environment of these three influential nationals, the common theme of constant quality improvement and adequate processes for the safe use and tracking of equipment, and proper maintenance and problem reporting can be seen. For our purpose of formulating the strategic goals of an implemented ASP system, reference is made to the above-mentioned Environment of Care section of the Accreditation Manual for Hospitals [11]. The contents are seen as a reasonable representation of good practice in the clinical setting. The appropriate criteria state that:

- EC.1.6 (2.6): the hospital develops and implements a medical equipment management plan;
- EC 2.10.3: the medical equipment is maintained, tested and inspected as follows:
  a current, accurate and separate inventory of all equipment identified in the equipment plan regardless of ownership;
  performance and safety testing of all equipment identified in the management plan prior to initial use;
  maintenance of all equipment on the inventory consistent with maintenance strategies to minimize physical and clinical risks.

Combining these fundamental elements in the JCAHO manual with the regulatory information above, it was determined that hospitals need to identify and implement processes for:

1. Selecting and acquiring equipment.
2. Establishing of medical device nomenclature.

3. Establishing risks criteria for identifying, evaluating, and taking an inventory of equipment to be included in the program before the equipment is used.
4. Monitoring and acting on equipment hazard notices and recalls.
5. Monitoring and reporting incidents in which a medical device is connected to the death, serious injury, or illness of any individual as required.
6. Reporting and investigating equipment management problems, failures, and use errors.
7. Establishing maintenance strategies for all equipment in the inventory.
8. Establishing intervals for inspecting, testing, and maintaining appropriate equipment in the inventory.
9. Reporting annually and evaluation of the equipment management plan's objectives, scope, performance, and effectiveness.
10. Developing an equipment orientation and education program for (a) staff responsible for equipment maintenance and (b) operators of said equipment.

These processes form the principle basis for the formulation of the ASP information management goals. Using them in conjunction with a model for technology management in healthcare institutions based on system theory from a previous publication [12], one can envision the potential benefits from the centralized nature of the ASP model, and thus those benefits form the following specific goals:

• Standardizing and harmonizing of information processes across independent hospital, multiple counties, and/or healthcare ministries.
• Compliance with the stringency of the appropriate standards and regulations.
• Improving ability of hospital administrators, technicians, and users to meet increasingly rigorous accreditation requirements related to medical equipment.
• Improving senior manager efficiency by giving them access to standardized performance statistics, previous implementations, etc., thus decreasing implementation time and costs.
• Performance comparison between institutions (benchmarking).
• Increasing the technician satisfaction by providing them the information needed to perform daily tasks accurately, effectively, and efficiently.

11.2.2   Identifying and Setting Operational Needs

A "translation" of each strategic goal into a description of one or several operational needs was performed at the outset of this stage of development. Here, the intent is to outline those interpretations that are specific and fundamental to the successful offering of the management system in an online format, and not to go over operational needs of current CED maintenance management tools.

Given the various levels of connectivity of potential users, clients should have the ASP accessible through the Web in three different ways (see Figure 11.1):

1. For large hospitals: connected to a direct leased line through their hospital information system (HIS). This option requires a copy of the database located

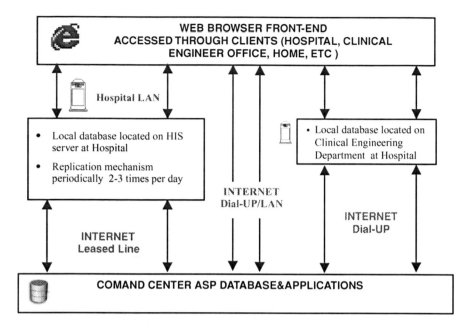

FIGURE 11.1. Data access possibilities for users of ASP.

on the HIS server and a replication procedure two or three times per day to keep the ASP database at the command center updated.

2. For large hospitals, governmental organizations, regulatory bodies, universities, and independent users who wish to connect, the second option is to connect via the Internet using dial-up or through a local-area network directly to the ASP database command center on a continual basis.

3. For smaller hospitals without a network and a limited number of resources, the third option is a dial-up access when needed. This requires a dedicated workstation in the CED. In this way, a manager has access to subsets of a hospital's inventory resident in an ASP database at the command center.

Since some of the above alternatives will indeed make use of dial-up connections, the entire application and data structure will have to be optimized for low-bandwidth access.

Increasing the individual and organizational performance and ability to provide ever-improving patient care is at the heart of the defined management goals. So, an ASP command center is important with regard to client support and access to data. The center will house all of the physical and personnel components that will make possible the offering of technical support for clients, while helping to provide data security (archiving and retrieval) and convenience of maintenance of system architecture and software modules by administrators and technicians.

As discussed previously, harmonization of information is of some import, and so a central coding system and nomenclature for medical devices resident in the ASP database is to be visible to all clients. Additionally, preventive maintenance procedures and checklists by equipment type and models, as well as the typical task time consumption, are also to be readily accessible.

The system should support the capital acquisition, asset management, and regulatory compliance activities that every CED must deal with, irrespective of their size or budget. Capital acquisition and regulatory compliance processes will make use of related data acquired from the progression of the asset management process, and all will benefit from the inclusion of a statistical and data trend analyses capability (with graphical reporting). This will have the added value of allowing accessible benchmarking between institutions. Additionally, hazard monitoring and reporting functions would support regulatory compliance and have a smaller, yet still pertinent, role in the other two processes mentioned and should be a part of the system.

As for the standard maintenance functions that every current CMMS (inventory, maintenance scheduling, work-order status monitoring and updating, etc.) must have, they will find their place in the newly designed system. Again, they, too, must be optimized for low-bandwidth, and thus redesigned and implemented.

11.2.3   The Application Service Provider Design and Development

With the logical progression from healthcare facility requirements to detailed ASP management goals and subsequent operational needs, much thought has been given to the desired software attributes. The following subsections are dedicated to stating the features included in the model, along with some added reasoning and remarks regarding specific functionality. At this point, the focus switches from pre-design lead up to post-design programming and implementation.

11.2.3.1   Application Service Provider Features

Owing to the online nature of the solution, and given connectivity issues in certain regions as discussed previously, the application has not only been optimized for low-bandwidth dial-up connections, but to utilize a true Web-based interface. The data structure has also been designed to be somewhat flexible to make allowances for issues with hospital regions and equipment to allow for customized management of the equipment and assets. This includes the incorporation of multi-currency, language, and calendar capabilities.

As with the FSMS, the ASP model allows for the upload of scheduled task data from test equipment (i.e. electrical safety analyzers) through the Web interface to help make full use of available information.

The last features have more to do with the manner in which the system architecture is set and how clients access the information. A single enterprise database model is the most appropriate selection given the data access and inheritance goals. Inheritance in data entry is of significant importance in the system design, and simply means that users and administrators enter data just one time, in one form to reduce inconsistency and redundancy. And of course, given the nature of the information contained in the database, the application provides a means for assigning

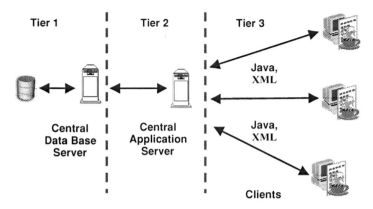

FIGURE 11.2. Three-tier architecture.

different access privileges for multiple levels of users (granting roles). These users access the actual application through connecting to a single or multiple application servers.

11.2.3.2   Platform Architecture

The physical manifestation of the system takes its form in the so-called "three-tier architecture" shown in Figure 11.2, and was foreshadowed above. Intuitively, the singular enterprise database is managed by the database server(s) and makes up Tier 1. Management of the actual application falls to the application server(s) and accounts for Tier 2. All authorized users connect to the application through the true Web-based interface, and all of these connections are considered Tier 3.

Following this schema, Tier 2 requests the connection from Tier 1, making the entire process "transparent" to the user. Separating the application storage and processing medium from that of the database improves processor utilization and speeds up access to information. Management of both is made less complicated, the backup and recovery processes are simpler, and there is a marked reduction in cost of the system implementation. This choice also supports the goal of optimization of the system for low-bandwidth data access.

11.2.3.3   System Description Functions

This ASP model was designed with a modular philosophy and was based in system theory. Modules are independent, but do interact with each other. Here, the entirety of the model has been broken down into the five composite modules.

11.2.3.3.1   The Inventory Module

This module is the core of the entire ASP model. It is comprised of medical equipment recordings and archiving procedures and holds essential data for supporting the functions of the remaining modules. The inventory module was designed to

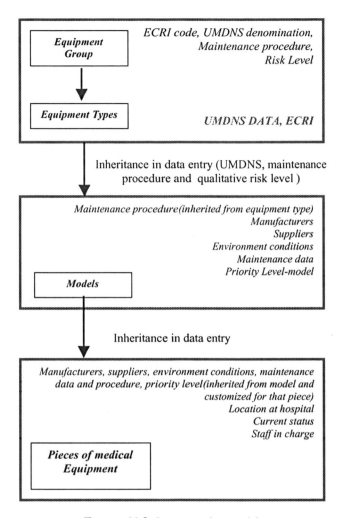

FIGURE 11.3. Inventory data model.

make use of the Universal Medical Device Nomenclature System (UMDNS) developed by the Emergency Care Research Institute (ECRI) [13]. Figure 11.3 shows a graphical representation of the data structure of the module.

On the top level of the structure is the *equipment group*, which is understood as a group of *device types* with the same ECRI maintenance and inspection safety procedure. For every device group a unique code, denomination according to UMDNS, inspection and preventive maintenance (IPM) procedure, technical specialty, and an ECRI risk level are recorded; thus, for every device type the same data are recorded. However, the user does not have to enter the IPM because the inventory module has what is termed "inheritance in data entry." When a user has entered data for a device type, further entries for a device of the same type will inherit the above information from the system. This feature has two important implications: it reduces administration time(s) dramatically, and helps to "reuse data" for new users of the ASP.

The next level down on the structural ladder is devoted to *models*. These models are equipment types (models inherit all data from its group–equipment type) manufactured by an OEM, with a trademark, sold from a specific provider/vendor, with specific information concerning environmental conditions (temperature, humidity, power supply, etc.), maintenance data, and parameters used in setting the priority of the maintenance scheduling. An added feature concerning IPM procedures is the ability to modify equipment type-specific procedure data inherited into a model-specific procedure.

Lastly, the bottom wrung is occupied by the individual *piece of medical equipment*. Attributes of this level will include a unique control number, a location in a specific hospital area, and a status for some specific period of time for each inventoried item. This level inherits all of its composite data from its model–group–equipment-type category; however, the user can customize data related to its maintenance and priority level.

Priority levels for every piece of medical equipment are established by way of numerical parameters associated with its category [14]. That "score" is used in an indicator called the *preventive maintenance index* (PMI), which serves as a non-preemptive service priority order (NPPSO)[5] in a queued work-order discipline [15].

11.2.3.3.2   Inspection and Preventive Maintenance Management

SMACOR 4*Oi* (Figure 11.4) is a module for the overall maintenance and inspection management of medical equipment and was designed with its foundation set in system theory [12]. Overall, the activities involved traditionally in the maintenance and inspection of equipment were considered to be *processes*, and conveniently broken into:

- IPM scheduler
- work-order manager.

The principle function of the *IPM scheduler* process is to timetable all IPM tasks for every medical device included in the equipment inventory. SMACOR 4*Oi* performs this task for both equipment under contractual service arrangements and those under the resident CED responsibility. Key parameters utilized by this process of the module consist of:

- The total time per week for every technician.
- Percentages of clinical engineering department time spent carrying out common tasks for every technician.[6]

---

[5] An NPPSO is when a customer of lower priority (work order) is actually being served and completes his/her service before a customer of higher priority enters the system.

[6] We considered four components of the total time, where cm, μ, ta, and oth are the percentages of the total time spent in corrective maintenance, inspections and preventive

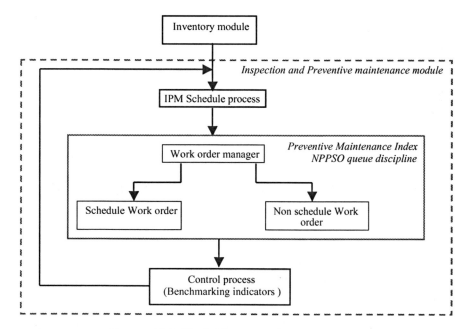

FIGURE 11.4. The IPM processes in SMACOR 4*Oi*.

- Level of training and job titles of every technician assigned to perform their respective IPM tasks.
- Priority level (Px) and PMI.
- Task types, specified in the IPM procedure.
- Standard time by task type per model.
- Supplies needed to perform the IPM procedures.
- IPM cycle and frequency, taking into account the failure rate calculation.

After running the scheduler, one can expect an IPM task scheduling for all pieces of equipment, a workload report for all technicians in a user-specified time period, and a detailing of the supplies needed to perform the IPM tasks.

Primary functions of the *work-order manager* process are to manage documents for both scheduled and nonscheduled maintenance tasks and to keep track of work orders until completion. Typically, requestor name and department, and work-order open, start, and finishing, with the chronology of each, are managed. This process also keeps track of the personnel assigned to accomplish and/or supervise the maintenance tasks. Figures 11.5 and 11.6 show some examples of the main work-order manager forms.

An included design feature of this sub-module is a dispatcher, which uses a queuing model with the above-mentioned NPPSO discipline, and a standardized

---

maintenance, training, and other tasks (contract service management, capital acquisition, etc.) respectively.

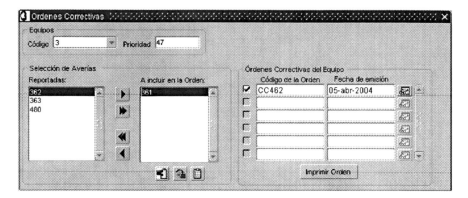

FIGURE 11.5. Work-order dispatcher.

algorithm for both scheduled and nonscheduled work-order generation and count
[14]. In clinical engineering, no work-order manager that applies a dispatcher with
these features has been proposed so far, but this has proven to be a valuable addition
to the system.

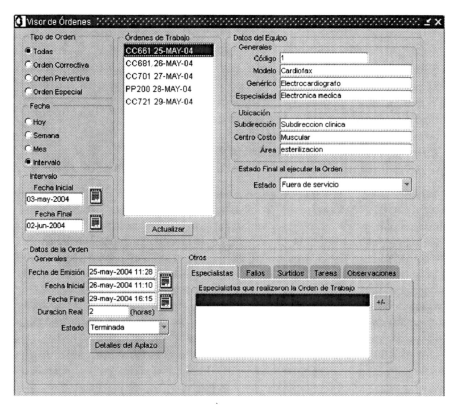

FIGURE 11.6. Form for updating the work orders.

11.2.3.3.3   Contract Service Providers/Vendors Management

Managing and tracking the quality and costs associated with the receipt of service from vendors and contract service providers falls to this sub-module. Basically, this management module aids in the coordination and control of nonbillable warranty work, service performed under a prepaid service contract, and billable services performed under a prepaid service contract but outside of the prepaid terms. The module is supported by means of three subprocesses included in the technology management model presented in Cruz et al. [12]:

- Selection of the service contract provider/vendor.
- Negotiation: to establish the contract clauses, including contract monitoring variables and the final contract agreement.
- Service contract performance evaluation.

Owing to the "pilot project" nature of the present work, only two processes were actually implemented: (1) *selection* and (2) *performance evaluation of the service contract provider/vendor.* Evaluations are executed by analyzing the historical performance of a provider/vendor and determining to what degree the provider may have defaulted upon past service agreements. Variables were therefore established [12] to monitor a service provider so that a contract might be terminated and the provider/vendor changed in the event that a service was deemed "not competitive".

11.2.3.3.4   Capital Acquisition Management

An important feature of the ASP system is capital acquisition management. This is handled by a sub-module of the same name. Intuitively, the application covers the tasks and activities associated with the acquisition of new medical equipment. In the initial design, five subprocesses, included in the aforementioned technology management model, would support the module [12]:

- *Needs assessment.* Reviews all the equipment removal proposals, calls for submissions, processing requests, establishment of selection criteria, committee review, and updating the list to select the best choice service contract provider/vendor.
- *Selection and conformance review.* Selects the best equipment/model and vendor choice with five steps as follows:
  consider regional links;
  relate submissions to existing standards;
  set new standards with minimum requirements;
  final selection;
  evaluation.
- *Funds approval negotiation.* Establishes the contract clauses, including contract monitoring variables and the final contract agreement.
- *Acquisition and installation.* Completes the steps for the acquisition and the installation as established in the above negotiation process.

For the purposes of the current work, only the *Needs assessment* and the *Selection and conformance review* processes have been utilized. The fifth step of the selection and conformance review is programmed to make use of a quantitative method. It allows users that are entering criteria to allocate weights for each and assigns scores for the performance of each alternative [12]. Different stakeholders can make use of the process, and it is this feature that has improved on the limitations reported by the authors in the use of other computerized tools [15]. This process has also proven capable of performing life-cycle cost versus present net value analyses.

11.2.4   The Application Service Provider's Installation and Modules Implementation

Installing and, consequently, implementing the ASP model with all the features described has constituted a large and involved commitment. To complete the installation phase of the project, support staff (database and module administrators) needed to be selected and trained. Owing to the complexity of the selected technology,[7] the services of two IT specialists were retained, i.e. one administrator for each of the first two tiers.

Soon after the establishment of the separate servers was complete, the formal definitions of practical ASP user groups could be specified. Although the combination and modalities of user types could be infinite, the ASP is designed to offer six predetermined user types:

1. *Inventory and maintenance management module administrator.* This type of user has a maximum level of privileges in that module (full control). The typical tasks of the module administrator are updating and deleting inserting operations in the inventory module. She/he can trigger the scheduling algorithm for IPM and the work-order generation for both scheduled and unscheduled tasks. Also, updating, inserting, and querying operations against all work orders, and querying operations against the entire module for preparing custom reports fall within the access of this administrator.
2. *Contract service providers/vendors and/or capital acquisition management module administrator.* This type of user has a maximum level of privileges in their respective module (full control). The typical tasks of the module administrator are open: adding a member, setting the weight of each category (previous opinion of each member of the group), closing the selection process, and performing the recruitment of experts to carry out evaluation processes. Querying operations against the entire module for preparing custom reports is also available to this level.
3. *Clinical engineers or staff engineers.* This category of user has middle-level privileges in all modules. For example, in the inventory module they can only perform querying operations. In the maintenance management module they can perform work-orders updating, but only for their own assignments. Also,

---

[7] ORACLE technology.

querying operations against the entire module for preparing custom reports, and in the contract service providers/vendors management activities they can be part of an evaluation/selection group.

4. *Nurses and medical staff.* These users have a middle–low level of privileges in all modules. For example, in the inventory module they can only perform querying operations. In the maintenance management module they may request maintenance services and perform querying operations against the entire module for the preparation of custom reports. For contract service providers/vendors management they can also be part of an evaluation/selection group.

5. *Institution directors (i.e. managers, etc.).* Typically, these users have low-level privileges in all modules. For all composite modules they can execute querying operations, and in the contract service providers/vendors management module they can be part of an evaluation/selection group.

6. *Guests.* Finally, this user type has minimum-level privileges across all modules. They can only perform querying operations against the entire ASP.

For the actual implementation of the ASP modules, a number of key tasks were to be completed. First, the definition and selection of an implementation workgroup. Usable general common codes, facility names and identification, account numbers, work-order code types, and equipment code types for all users in the ASP had to be specified. Also, the training of an ASP's user groups and the implementation of the respective modules (inventory, maintenance, contract service providers/vendors, and capital acquisition management) given the specific facility or institution required must be concluded. The implementation and use of the last two modules are dependent on whether a request of contract service evaluation/selection or capital acquisition process has been made or is deemed necessary.

Standardization of data entry (Figure 11.7) is key for data reuse for new ASP users. To accomplish this, a unique administrator for every client-institution making use of the ASP enters data into the inventory module.

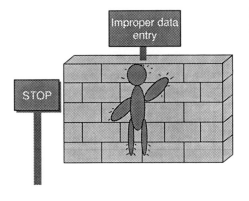

FIGURE 11.7. The most important challenge: a standardized data entry.

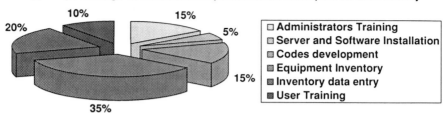

Typical percentage of distribution implementation time spent on each activity

FIGURE 11.8. Typical percentage of distribution time spent on each implementation activity.

A noncentralized inventory data entry schema was tested. Every service department (i.e. cardiology, imaging, etc.) performed their inventory data entry independently; however, less than desirable results were obtained. In spite of the development and utilization of the unique code system, many variations in data entries were observed, and a subsequent move was made to a more centralized format.

Figure 11.8 shows the typical percentage distribution of time spent on each activity. Notice how the equipment inventory, data entry, and training users take more than 50% of the entire time. Administrator training takes a mere 15% at the beginning of the implementation phase. This training has the potential to be spread out over that period, and subsequent to the implementation phase.

The ASP is now being installed at the laboratory level at the ISPJAE University of Havana, Cuba. Ten hospitals have requested the service of the ASP, five of which have proceeded with the implementation phase.

11.3   Conclusions

1. Further work to develop a "noncentralized" data entry schema that will sufficiently diminish deviations from the standard is warranted. This would eliminate work redundancy related to the function of the client-institution ASP administrator.
2. The pilot ASP provides an expanded array of basic and value-added services and improved functionality in an online format and is optimized for low bandwidth. It improves communication abilities between working groups. It has the added potential of contributing to improved patient care through improved management of inventory, maintenance, equipment capital acquisition, and selection–evaluation of service providers.
3. The ASP facilitates information exchange between CEDs, as it promotes the adoption of commonly accepted benchmarking indicators.
4. This solution can be expanded to other hospital areas.

References

1. Glouhova M. International survey on the practice of clinical engineering: mission, structure, personnel and resources. *J Clin Eng* 2000;25(5):205–209.
2. Panousis SG, Malataras P, Patelodimou C, Kolitsi Z, Pallikarakis N. Development of a new clinical engineering management and information system (CLE-MANTIS). *J Clin Eng* 1997;22(5):342–349.
3. Blumberg FD. Service program diagnostics and decision support technology for improving health technology service efficiency and productivity. *Biomed Instrum Technol* 1998;24(1):370–385.
4. Cohen T. Overview of generic computerized maintenance management system. In: Cohen T, editor, *Computerized maintenance management system for clinical engineering*. Arlington: AAMI; 2003.
5. Schuster S. Defining the PACS ASP model. *Med Imag* 2002;(Nov):110–117.
6. Fratt L. Costs and benefits of an ASP e-archive model. *Med Imag* 2001;(Dec):54–58.
7. Klugas G. Web-enabled PACS. *Med Imag* 2000;(Aug):46–50.
8. Hannon D. World wide work orders the online capabilities of CEMS today. *24X7*. 2000;(May):20–22.
9. Keepers of the technology, the clinical engineer's role in healthcare delivery issue. *IEEE Eng Med Biol* 2004;23(3).
10. Quality system requirements for manufacturers: reference guide for manufacturers selling medical devices in Europe, Canada and the United States–2001 version. Industry Canada, Life Sciences Branch.
11. *Accreditation manual for hospital*, vol. 1. Chapter EC: environment of care. New York: JCAHO; 2002.
12. Cruz MA, Rodríguez DE, Sanchez MC. Management of service contracts using an independent service provider (ISP) as support technology. *J Clin Eng* 2002;27(3):202–209.
13. ECRI. Universal medical device nomenclature system. In: *Plymouth meeting*, Emergency Care Research Institute, Philadelphia; 1996.
14. Capuano M, Koritko S. Risk oriented maintenance system. *Biomed Instrum Technol* 1996;30(1):25–35.
15. Sloane BE. Using a decision support system toll for healthcare technology assessments. *IEEE Eng Med Biol Mag* 2004;(May–Jun):42.

12
Secured Electronic Patient Records Content Exploitation

John Puentes, Gouenou Coatrieux and Laurent Lecornu

Abstract

The increasing need for medical information applications to handle varied multimedia data through interoperable systems is continually hindered by incompatible limited platforms, with low or non-existent security. Using the workflow of an imaging service, this chapter describes the structure and protection strategy of a secured specialized electronic patient record which allows exchanging of multimedia medical data in a secured manner. An open multimedia standard adapted to patient record requirements has been applied, combined with security tools. Prospective application scenarios are identified, and the main issues of the approach are discussed.

12.1   Introduction

Understanding how to use patient health data has been permanently evolving during the last 40 years, from detailed healthcare costs on a hospital bill, to the current promise of patient-centered systems. Such an evolution has resulted from both technological progress and mentality changes. Nevertheless, actual applications are mostly proprietary implementations, capable of satisfying medical organizations requirements only in part. Moreover, patient health data systems' escalating complexity offers an action field for multiple competitive solutions that, despite their potential, have not yet been successful in solving the existing issues. Among the multiple questions that we still find remain unanswered are those concerning appropriate design and implementation methodologies, workflow analysis, usability models, how to adapt the electronic patient record (EPR) to uneven geographical distribution of medical experts and population aging, and integration of multimedia data, security, and health data exploitation for other uses than patient follow up. This paper focuses on the interdependencies of the latter three, namely how to make use of multimedia data, in a secured manner, for content exploitation.

The question about whether or not it is necessary to include multimedia data in the EPR is debatable. Legal and medical reasons require the archiving of diagnostic data like medical images and signals, as well as laboratory results and medical prescriptions. However, once the diagnosis has been completed, the physician rarely examines the complete multimedia data set again, except for the consultation reports and the patient history. Alternatively, when patient care implies distant interaction of two or more healthcare actors, collaborative work depends on the availability of multimedia data that are shared in a distributed infrastructure, and later stored for control purposes.

Beyond daily data manipulation for clinical consultation, there is an interest in obtaining other kinds of information processing specific to EPR data in a particular expertise field, e.g. making medical practice and diagnostic support or specialized training possible. Such supplementary utilization of the EPR involves an adapted data organization and the means to protect it. The rest of the chapter is organized as follows. Section 12.2 positions our patient record approach, associated with its functionality and structure. Section 12.3 presents how to protect the proposed patient record content. Section 12.4 identifies some of the applications to alternatively exploit patient data. Issues and perspectives concerning the interaction of the three topics studied are discussed in Section 12.5.

12.2   Multimedia Electronic Patient Record

At the simplest abstract level, the patient record can be considered as a condensed healthcare individual memory, or as part of a collective memory, from which knowledge is obtained. The first concept has been historically carried out using paper records for medical personnel data and information manipulation, and the second has been largely exploited to orient decision making, by means of economic, demographic, and sanitary statistical analysis. The integration of computers in care delivery has enhanced these functionalities, and introduced new issues. Despite the identification and study of paper patient record drawbacks (mainly elevated handling and maintenance costs, data and information redundancy, difficulty reading most of the handwriting, data imprecision and missing data), the adoption of the EPR is not as generalized as expected [1]. Owing to modernization of medical information systems (MISs), a high percentage of patient data and information will be handled by computers, even though balancing all the elements involved in the system design is a very complex task.

12.2.1   Why a Specialized Electronic Patient Record?

Numerous studies have been conducted to define and validate an EPR adapted to medical practice. Recent efforts [2–6] underline the EPR specificity according to the medical speciality, and the need to use semi-structured data. However, significant changes are still necessary to facilitate the adoption of an EPR [7–9].

Currently, component-oriented [10] and document-oriented (www.centc251.org) MIS architectures are promising predominant trends. They both appeal to the idea of a system capable of handling autonomous content objects. As a subset of the EPR, specialized EPR (SEPR) integration to an adapted architecture can be considered as an autonomous content object, capable, up to a certain point, of assuring interoperability across heterogeneous platforms, meeting security requirements, and tailored to facilitate content exploitation. Accordingly, some issues, particularly those related to data sharing and complementary utilization, could be undertaken in a modular and simple manner, underlining the importance of workflow analysis in guiding the technical decisions.

12.2.2 Workflow Analysis

Multiple alternatives have been proposed to organize data within an EPR, mostly influenced by early studies that proposed organizing medical data either chronologically or in a problem-oriented manner, or by combining these two approaches. They have been essentially physician centered and restricted to support medical staff memory, like the original paper records. Considering the previously mentioned issues, this implies revisiting user requirements, particularly through a realistic and iterative field workflow analysis, which is so frequently missing. Figure 12.1 depicts the simplified workflow diagram of our application scenario:

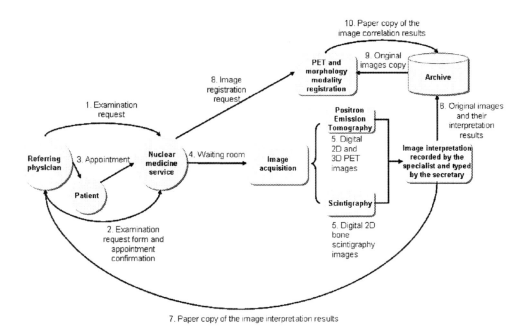

FIGURE 12.1. Simplified workflow of a nuclear medicine service, from the examination request to results archiving.

a nuclear medicine service examination. It identifies activities sequencing and the data concerned. This analysis suggests that the SEPR should be implemented specifically to deal with data exchanged in phases 6, 7, 9 and 10, integrating some of the patient data provided in the examination request form (step 2). Such analysis enables one to design an SEPR, appropriately inserted in the daily practice and resulting from a validated consensus about its functionality. Close work with service physicians and other medical staff at this stage is mandatory, to avoid improper tool design as a consequence of a predominant technological view, disconnected from the actual medical service activity.

12.2.3 The Specialized Electronic Patient Record Structure

The proposed SEPR uses JPEG 2000 [11], an open image-coding standard, rather unknown in the medical domain, which addresses a wide range of image compression applications [12]. It was developed to deal with areas where existing standards fail to produce optimal quality, and offers improved capabilities to domains that normally do not use image compression. Based on a one-dimensional discrete wavelet transform, it compresses single-component (i.e. grayscale) and multicomponent (e.g. color) images. In addition to the basic compression functionality, our work makes use of the standard's JP2 file format, which integrates extensible markup language (XML)-formatted metadata and the coded image, encapsulated in one file. XML metadata can be easily extracted without decoding the image, and is more flexible than predefined content fields. We have adapted this feature to structure and integrate the SEPR to a related set of multicomponent images [13]. For the indicated workflow, the main SEPR tags follow a hierarchy defined by the examination stages (Figure 12.2). Sub-tags' structure and content also depend on workflow analysis. To create the SEPR (Figure 12.3), acquired digital images are lossless compressed using the JPEG 2000 algorithm, which generates the corresponding contiguous code streams. Data input is carried out by filling in an associated form, adapted to obtain the XML data. Finally, the code stream and XML data are integrated in the same JP2 file.

12.2.4 Specialized Electronic Patient Record Usability Scenarios

The SEPR status evolves from its creation, until it is closed (see Section 12.3.2.2). Simultaneously, various usability scenarios are feasible. In essence, they concern data and information manipulation depending on a user's needs and access rights. Five of the most frequent functionalities are:

- SEPR edition (including image processing if required), before closing it definitively.
- Hospital intranet exchanges are frequently required in daily medical practice, even though it is not necessary to exchange all the EPR, just parts of it, depending

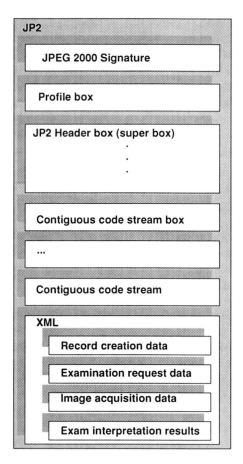

FIGURE 12.2. Organization of the main SEPR tags in the XML box of the JP2 file.

on a physician's objectives. SEPRs can be stored in a central server or distributed in different services.

- Hospital extranet exchanges are more restricted than intranet exchanges, and concern specialists' meetings, second-opinion consultations, or distant diagnosis. In this context, copies of an incomplete SEPR that needs further discussion are transmitted to one or more distant sites, and the diagnostic report stored by the physician responsible.
- Patient mobility consists of the circulation of patients to other regions or countries to look for healthcare. In this scenario, certain information flow should be guaranteed by the patient records. On the other hand, patients' rights to access their medical information imply that independent SEPR storage and access services outside healthcare providers installations should be implemented.
- Content exploitation is the intent to use clinical data in an alternative manner, beyond daily manipulation. In this case, SEPR completeness and structure play a fundamental role.

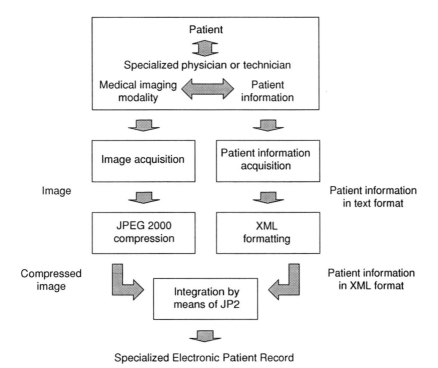

FIGURE 12.3. Generation of the SEPR integrating the acquired images and patient data in one JP2 file.

Any one of these scenarios exposes the transportable SEPR content to potential risks, like unauthorized access. Therefore, in order to exploit the SEPR securely, a security strategy is required.

12.3 Medical Information Security

Whatever the country, medical information security derives from strict ethics and legislative rules, which define the rights and duties of both patient and health professionals. Typically, health professionals are responsible for the data they possess and provide. This imposes three mandatory characteristics (Figure 12.4): confidentiality, availability, and reliability [14, 15]:

- Confidentiality, linked to the medical secrecy, means that only the entitled users, have access to the information.
- Availability is the capacity of an information system to be used by the entitled users in the normal scheduled conditions of access and exercise.
- Reliability deals with both, the confirmation that information has not been modified by unauthorized people (integrity) and that the information belongs to the right patient, being issued from the correct source (authentication).

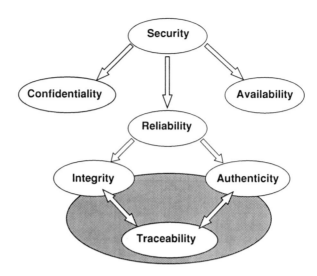

FIGURE 12.4. Relations between medical information security mandatory characteristics.

Hence, an EPR will be reliable only if each one of its elements is certified as reliable. Reliability can be extended with traceability. In that case, we must be able to verify EPR integrity and to authenticate each location where the EPR has been stored, accessed, changed, etc. before it was received. As a result, there is a need for nonrepudiation services (i.e. proof that the EPR was emitted by the claimed entity). Considering that EPR parts are closely connected, because diagnosis is based on available and new acquired data, and that the physician responsibility is enlisted when new data are added to the EPR, an intrinsic link between all data elements should be established to improve EPR reliability. Consequently, EPR handling in an MIS requires a precise content quality validation and control.

12.3.1   Medical Information Systems and Electronic Patient Record Security

When dealing with MISs, a security definition is more difficult to establish, given system complexity, which depends on many features [16], e.g. implemented functionalities, applied technology, infrastructure, institution policies, etc. To cope with such heterogeneity, information assurance models have been proposed [17]. All of them recognize the nonexistence of absolute security, concluding that only some optimized level can be reached. Complementarily, we consider that several security layers have to be distinguished to improve the optimal security degree: the EPR content, the EPR itself, the MIS (storage and processing), and transmission, inherently linking each layer to the others.

Usually, information system security design covers three main steps, according to a predefined security strategy [16, 18]. First, an analysis leads to the identification and evaluation of risks that can damage the system, its functionalities, and especially the medical information being handled. Whatever the approach, risk analysis is mainly concentrated on the sensitiveness of data integrity, confidentiality, and availability. In our case, data are contained by SEPRs. In the second step, security objectives [16] are simultaneously defined and implemented (security policies and procedures design, security tools integration), taking into account system specificities. The third step consists of testing and verifying that the security objectives are satisfied.

Information access control is a good illustration of these concerns [19, 20]. Based on an access control policy and different security tools, it can be deployed with login and password. Nevertheless, the identification process should be replaced by a two-factor authentication, combining two of the following solutions: password, biometrics [21], and smartcard [22]. In the case of an MIS connected to an external network, firewalls should control the access. Specific rules have to be drawn up about how access will be granted from both sides of the firewall [23]. Concerning information communication, most of the existing solutions are based on secure communication channels, like a virtual private network [24].

The EPR security layer is integrated to the previous ones. As a result, the EPR structure has to provide security facilities and attributes to be handled in a secure environment. DICOM (medical.nema.org) integrates this concept, just for medical images, making available a distinctive image identifier which indicates that the image belongs to one patient and is associated with one exam. An image system can be DICOM compliant with several security profiles, related to storage, transmission, and image anonymity. Subsequently, DICOM does not define a security policy, but instead provides security mechanisms to be used in a secure environment.

As a consequence, the EPR structure should provide adapted means and mechanisms to improve security in an MIS, assuming that the EPR has to be exchanged. Besides protecting medical information, requirements also concern tracing its distribution (hospital archival, copy of the record for the patient, data accessed by other services) and use. With interoperability issues being a major concern, EPR content organization has to be securely structured, providing data only to authorized users according to their needs.

12.3.2   Secured Specialized Electronic Patient Record

We propose to protect the medical data by adding to the SEPR structure a set of security attributes processed by security mechanisms of the MIS. For this purpose, the following security layers are taken into account: the healthcare institution, the MIS that allows secured SEPR (SSEPR) handling, and the SSEPR and its content.

Cryptography and watermarking are complementary algorithmic approaches used to define security attributes. Cryptography provides confidentiality through encryption, but also integrity control and nonrepudiation using digital signatures [25]. On the other hand, watermarking (originally proposed for copyright protection of multimedia documents [26]) applied to medical images allows embedding data directly within the host media, by modifying its pixel gray-level values, preserving the image file format [15]. In this way, watermarking facilitates complementary data to be removed and different kinds of information to be put together as a unique entity, i.e. a watermarked image.

12.3.2.1   A Secure Environment

It is assumed that the healthcare institution has defined a security policy, specifying how authorized health professionals access the information. Technically, this authority can be partially denoted by a public key infrastructure (PKI) [27], which provides users with electronic credentials or certificates. These certificates belong only to one entity (a user or a system), and contain its cryptographic public key. Certificates cannot be forged, because they are digitally signed by the certification authority represented by the PKI, i.e. the healthcare institution. Furthermore, a private cryptographic key, exclusively known by one entity, is linked to a certificate. For one particular user, this private key can be stored on a smartcard [22]. When a user requests access to the MIS, the PKI is prompted by the MIS asking for the user credentials. If the authentication is successful, then access is granted. In our approach the MIS acts as an entity, meaning that it is recognized by the PKI and that it possesses its own certificates and cryptographic key pair.

Because, the SEPR may be transferred outside the hospital, a global authority has to be defined and recognized by all healthcare institutions. To support entity authentication, this authority can also be represented by a PKI. The proposed SSEPR structure has been developed in agreement with this constraint.

12.3.2.2   Accessing the Secured Specialized Electronic Patient
Record Content

In the case of the nuclear medicine service, retrieving the patient's SSEPR is based on different unique identification numbers (UINs). These UINs certify the link between the SSEPR and the patient, as well as the exam and the healthcare service it belongs to. Once the SSEPR is retrieved, its information access is controlled by an access control list (ACL) [28], which contains access rules applying the security policy of the institution. Figure 12.5 shows the disposition of the resulting ACLs and digital signatures for the nuclear medicine SSEPR. Given that the SSEPR is exchanged with other systems, several ACLs, each corresponding to an MIS, can be specified. An MIS would only be able to decrypt its own ACL using its private key. When a user access is requested, the MIS identifies and authenticates it through the PKI, and then controls the ACL to ascertain whether the user is authorized to access and exploit the requested SSEPR content. If the user is allowed to access the records, then the last parts of the XML-formatted data are decrypted. Then, an ACL is added each time the SSEPR is transmitted with a content that satisfies the security policies of both communication channel extremities. Successful access requests are recorded by the MIS in the SSEPR.

A complementary security attribute can be used to indicate the actual status of the SSEPR: created, available for authorized edition or consultation, closed, archived, or copy of the original. Once closed, it can no longer be modified.

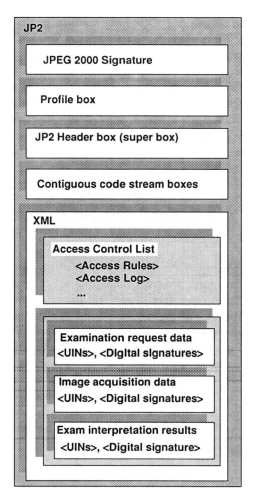

FIGURE 12.5. Encapsulated ACLs and digital signatures in the example SSEPR.

12.3.2.3 Adding Reliable Information to the Secured Specialized Electronic Patient Record

Three different kinds of information are added to the SSEPR: information provided by the physician who has requested the examination, newly acquired data (images in our case), and the medical report. The first two have to be reliable before being included into the SSEPR. A UIN functioning as a data pointer indicates unambiguously the origin and attachment to the same patient. Moreover, data have to be digitally signed by the provider. Once the reliability check is performed, data or their UINs are added to the SSEPR with the corresponding digital signatures, allowing compatible systems to verify that the information has not been changed.

The medical report written by the physician interprets acquired images taking into account existing information. It should be digitally signed by its author, who will not be able to repudiate its content. However, since the report may depend on several data sources, it should integrate all the data UINs that were used. Furthermore, a link must be established between images and the report content. To obtain it in our scheme, digital signatures computed over the report content, as well as the report and images' UINs, are embedded by applying a reversible digital watermarking method to the images. That is, once the watermark is read and removed from the image, the original pixel values are restored, preserving the image quality for the diagnosis.

12.4   Secured Specialized Electronic Patient Record Content Exploitation

The multimedia EPR improves the efficiency of most tasks related to patient data utilization. Placed at the core of the MIS, by the very nature of its functionality, the SEPR content exploitation is de facto done. However, content exploitation needs to be customized, depending on the different kinds of users authorized to employ the MIS. Applications should then ideally provide the appropriate information, to the right user, at the right time. As a consequence, any implemented application is likely to be specialized on a particular task, for a specific user, having access only to part of the SSEPR. This section identifies existing specialized medical content exploitation domains, along with the prospective enhancement that SSEPR application could provide.

12.4.1   Content Exploitation Applications

Besides data storage and visualization applications, the multimedia EPR plays a very significant role in the following contexts:

- clinical management
- medical information sharing
- specialized training
- medical practice and decision support
- knowledge extraction.

All of them, and particularly the last two, are the subject of extended academic and clinical research. Applications concerning the first two are currently used, and technology transfers are expected in the third and fourth.

12.4.1.1   Clinical Management

Applications in this domain are used by healthcare providers to administer and automate the interaction between patients and physicians [29–31]. The main functionalities relate to the input and storage of patient-encounter information, reports generation, and interface with coding and billing software. In healthcare institutions, at an organizational level, the main purpose of these applications is to improve the quality and coordination of medical tasks (global planning, interventions and consultations schedules, stocks and suppliers follow up, resources distribution, etc.). One of the main difficulties in deploying them is to define an adapted usability framework for each user group, medical, and management unit. For example, two or more physicians from different units have access to the examination results, but not necessarily to the complete EPR. On the other hand, the assistant should not have the right to read the examination report, but should be allowed to take care of the administrative part. This implies that system design must take into consideration those requirements. Introduction of an SSEPR can bring more flexibility to solve this issue, although this increases the content protection complexity.

12.4.1.2   Medical Information Sharing

Healthcare structure is intrinsically distributed, consisting of a geographical spread of variable-sized medical centers, from regional hospitals down to individual general practitioners. Although each medical institution is autonomous and devoted to the delivery of particular services, healthcare continuity requires that different medical institutions exchange relevant complementary patient data and operate in a cooperative environment in order to improve the service quality [32]. This implies system interoperability, which can be carried out through the exchange of medical data using open multimedia standards. In our example, image header and pixel values can be extracted from original DICOM images and integrated to the SSEPR, remaining compatible with the original imaging acquisition system [33], while also being available to be transmitted using conventional networks and used in other platforms.

12.4.1.3   Specialized Training

Improved precise and efficient access to specialized training material can be obtained using adapted multimedia EPRs [34]. Study cases are chosen from large image databases, applying retrieval criteria (mirc.rsna.org) [31] like anatomy, diagnosis, or visual similarity. Archived data are selectively available to instructors and students, depending on the training stage. For instance, an oncology lecturer could search a particular lesion visualized in nuclear medicine images, accessing a Web server capable of retrieving the pertinent images and associated patient data, using a limited set of keywords. Given its flexibility, the SSEPR can be adapted to this task, providing the required data, without a patient's identification.

12.4.1.4   Medical Practice and Decision Support

These tools generate supplementary advice or interpretation about a particular case, using explicit knowledge [35]. The recommendations generated are normally associated with a given certainty percentage likelihood, and are based on previous validated diagnoses with identical and similar symptoms, compared with a separate percentage of similar diagnosed cases from the literature. Alternatively, an SSEPR database can be used as a reference, e.g. coupled to case-based reasoning (CBR) or case-based image retrieval (CBIR) tools, combined with rule-based reasoning and a domain knowledge base. The SSEPR should, therefore, be completed following a particular procedure that validates each record only if all relevant fields have been correctly filled in [36]. Relations between record elements are first analyzed by means of rule-based reasoning, which handles common diagnosis. If an unusual case is identified (i.e. it does not follow the rules guideline), then CBR [37] is activated to retrieve a similar one with partially similar record component relations. Sometimes, during the interpretation of an imaging exam, referring physicians encounter complex cases requiring comparison with a previous similar case. CBIR [38] facilitates this procedure using the image description concerned as a query to retrieve records in the SEPR database that contain images with a similar description. SSEPR utilization permits the addition of indexes [39], making interoperability possible with medical practice and decision-support applications.

12.4.1.5   Knowledge Extraction

These applications intend to deduce causal unknown relations from clinical data, focused on specific health problems. Current research efforts look for methodologies and algorithms that are capable of identifying comprehensible knowledge of medical interest in large databases containing measurements, observations, and interpretations [39]. Among the methods studied, we find data mining [40], evidence reasoning [41], and genetic programming [42], with variable results depending on the context application. Yet, for each of them the EPR structure and availability are of prime importance. In this sense, the SSEPR offers the required flexibility to arrange the components involved and make them accessible to authorized knowledge-discovery tools.

12.5   Discussion and Conclusion

The SSEPR provides improved access to protected data that are structured in a flexible manner and which can be adapted to different medical specialities and content exploitation scenarios. It is particularly meant to be the basic information exchange unit in secured synchronous or asynchronous collaborative and multidisciplinary interactions. Additional work is necessary to integrate medical signals, video, and three-dimensional objects. Generalization of the SSEPR to cover most MIS modules depends completely on the exploitation context's scope and security policies.

Notwithstanding the concept advantages, security implementation limits data availability. The main issue concerns security stability through time, given that security policies should follow the changing nature of security attacks, making it obligatory to update protection tools and procedures continuously. Moreover, laws restrict the application of enhanced security technologies, obligating institutions to use technologies that can be disabled by specialists with conventional methods. Another issue relates to accessibility of cryptography keys. Keys can get lost, abruptly preventing one obtaining any of the protected data; or they can change, thus requiring all data be encrypted another time. Image watermarking, inspired by similar ideas to preserve a strong link between security data and protected information, is confronted with the same questions, which become more complex when applied to rich multimedia data sets.

The MISs of the future are supposed to combine multiple databases with medical practice and decision-support systems. They are expected to improve their capabilities, with a demonstrated impact of complementary EPR content exploitation, which is perceived as an appropriate system component in daily practice [43]. Efforts are required to conceive benchmarks capable of assessing the validity of information retrieval technology in clinical situations [44], considering that existing academic research applications are specialized and tested on limited databases. On the other hand, use of true open standards is becoming increasingly important to avoid lack of interoperability between proprietary systems and to avoid backward incompatibility of applications, data storage, and manipulation devices, among others.

References

1. Degoulet P, Fieschi M. Informatisation du dossier patient. In: *Informatique Médicale*, third edition. Paris: Masson; 1998, pp. 119–132.
2. Beuscart-Zéphir MC, Anceaux F, Crinquette V, Renard JM. Integrating users' activity modeling in the design and assesment of hospital electronic patient records: the example of anesthesia. *Int J Med Inform* 2001;64:157–171.
3. Malamateniou F, Vassilacopoulos G. Developing a virtual patient record using XML and Web-based workflow techniques. *Int J Med Inform* 2003;70:131–139.
4. Rassinoux AM, Lovis C, Baud R, Geissbuhler A. XML as standard for communication in a document-based electronic patient record: a 3 years experiment. *Int J Med Inform* 2003;70:109–115.
5. Ueckert F, Goerz M, Ataian M, Tessmann S, Prokosch H-U. Empowerment of patients and communication with healthcare professionals through an electronic health record. *Int J Med Inform* 2003;70:99–108.
6. Law MYY. A model of DICOM-based electronic patient record in radiation therapy. *Comput Med Imag Graphics* 2005;29:125–136.
7. Brown PJ, Warmington V. Data quality probes-exploiting and improving the quality of electronic patient record data and patient care. *Int J Med Inform* 2005;68:91–98.
8. Van Ginneken AM. The computerized patient record: balancing effort and benefit. *Int J Med Info* 2002;65:97–119.
9. Lorence DP, Churchill R. Clinical knowledge management using computerized patient record systems: is the current infrastructure adequate? *IEEE Trans Info Technol Biomed* 2005;9(2):283–288.
10. Van de Velde R, Degoulet P. *Clinical information systems: a component based approach*, first edition. New York: Springer-Verlag; 2003.

11. International Organization for Standardization and International Electrotechnical Commission. *ISO/IEC 15444 1:2000, Information technology—JPEG 2000 image coding system—part 1: core coding system.*

12. Christopoulos C, Skodras A, Ebrahimi T. The JPEG 2000 still image coding system: an overview. *IEEE Trans Consum Electron* 2000;46(4):1103–1127.

13. Montesinos L, Puentes J. Specialized telepathology electronic patient record based on JPEG 2000. In: *Proceedings of 4th International IEEE–EMBS Special Topic Conference on Information Technology Applications in Biomedicine*, 2003; pp. 110–113.

14. Dusserre L, Ducrot H, Allaërt FA. *L'information médicale—l'ordinateur et la loi*, second edition. Cachan: Editions Médicales Internationales; 1999.

15. Coatrieux G, Maître H, Sankur B, Rolland Y, Collorec R. Relevance of watermarking in medical imaging. In: *Proceedings of 3rd International IEEE–EMBS Special Topic Conference on Information Technology Applications in Biomedicine*, 2000; pp. 250–255.

16. CEN/TC251, Env 12924—Security categorisation and protection for healthcare information systems. Technical report, CEN 1997.

17. Schou CD, Frost J, Maconachy WV. Information assurance in biomedical informatics systems. *IEEE Mag Eng Med Biol* 2004;23(1):110–118.

18. Coleman J. Assessing information security risk in healthcare organizations of different scale. *Int Congr Ser* 2004;1268:125–130.

19. El Kalam AA, El Baida R, Balbiani P, Benferhat S, Cuppens F, Deswarte Y, et al. Organization based access control. In: *Proceedings of International IEEE Workshop Policies for Distributed Systems and Networks*, 2003; pp. 120–131.

20. Ferraiolo DF, Sandhu R, Gavrila S, Kuhn DR, Chandramouli R. Proposed NIST standard for role-based access control. *ACM Trans Info Syst Secur* 2001;4(3):224–274.

21. Prabhakar S, Pankanti S, Jain AK. Biometric recognition: security and privacy concerns. *IEEE Secur Priv* 2003;1(2):33–42.

22. Dwivedi A, Bali RK, Belsis MA, Naguib RNG, Every P, Nassar NS. Towards a practical healthcare information security model for healthcare institutions. In: *Proceedings of 4th International IEEE–EMBS Special Topic Conference on Information Technology Applications in Biomedicine*, 2003; pp. 114–117.

23. Zalenski R. Firewall technologies. *IEEE Potentials* 2002;21:24–29.

24. Khanvilkar S, Khokhar A. Virtual private networks: an overview with performance evaluation. *IEEE Mag Commun* 2004;42(10):146–154.

25. Schneier B. *Applied cryptography*, second edition. Paris: International Thomson Publishing; 1997.

26. Barni M, Bartolini F. Data hiding for fighting piracy. *IEEE Mag Signal Process* 2004;21(2):28–39.

27. Takeda H, Matsumura Y, Kuwata S, Nakano H, Shanmai J, Qiyan Z, et al. An assessment of PKI and networked electronic patient record system: lessons learned from real patient data exchange at the platform of OCHIS. *Int J Med Inform* 2004;73(3):311–316.

28. Sandhu RS, Samarati P. Access control: principle and practice. *IEEE Mag Commun* 1994;32(9):40–48.

29. Blander J, Bergeron B. *Clinical management systems: a guide for deployment*, first edition. Chicago: Healthcare Information and Management Systems Society; 2004.

30. Ciccarese P, Caffi E, Quaglini S, Stefanelli M Architectures and tools for innovative health information systems: the guide project. *Int J Med Inform* 2005;74:553–562.

31. Muller H, Michoux N, Bandon D, Geissbuhler A. A review of content-based image retrieval systems in medical applications—clinical benefits and future directions. *Int J Med Inform* 2004;73:1–23.

32. Schabetsberger T, Gross E, Haux R, Lechleitner G, Pellizzari T, Schindelwig K, et al. Approaches towards a regional, shared electronic patient record for healthcare facilities of different healthcare organizations—IT strategy and first results. In: *Proceedings of 11th World Congress MEDINFO*; 2004, pp. 979–982.
33. Digital Imaging and Communications in Medicine (DICOM). Supplement 61: JPEG 2000 Transfer Syntaxes. DICOM Standards Committee, Working Group 4 Compression, September 2001.
34. Miles KA. Diagnostic imaging in undergraduate medical education: an expanding role. *Clin Radiol* 2005;60:742–745.
35. Ramnarayan P, Britto J. Pediatric clinical decision support systems. *Arch Dis Childhood* 2002;87:361–362.
36. Rossille D, Laurent JF, Burgun A. Modelling a decision-support system for oncology using rule-based and case-based reasoning methodologies. *Int J Med Inform* 2005;74:299–306.
37. Pedersen KV. A framework for a clinical reasoning knowledge warehouse. In: *Proceedings of IDEAS Workshop on Medical Information Systems: The Digital Hospital*, 2004; pp. 25–34.
38. Cauvin JM, Le Guillou C, Solaiman B, Robaszkiewicz M, Le Beux P, Roux C. Computer-assisted diagnosis system in digestive endoscopy. *IEEE Trans Info Technol Biomed* 2003;7(4):256–262.
39. Bemmel JH, Mulligen EM, Mons B, Wijk M, Kors JA, Lei J. Databases for knowledge discovery: examples from biomedicine and healthcare. *Int J Med Inform* 2006;75 (3–4):257–267.
40. Cios KJ, editor. *Medical data mining and knowledge discovery*, first edition. Heidelberg: Physica-Verlag; 2001.
41. Chen H, Fuller S, Friedman C, Hersh W. Knowledge management, data mining, and text mining in medical informatics. In: Chen H, Fuller S, Friedman C, Hersh W, editors, *Medical informatics: knowledge management and data mining in biomedicine*. New York: Springer-Verlag; 2005, pp. 3–33.
42. Tan KC, Yu Q, Heng CM, et al. Evolutionary computing for knowledge discovery in medical diagnosis. *Art Intell Med* 2003;27:2129–2154.
43. Kaplan B. Evaluating informatics applications—clinical decision support systems literature review. *Int J Med Inform* 2001;64(1):15–37.
44. Pluye P, Grad RM, Dunikowski LG, Stephenson R Impact of clinical information-retrieval technology on physicians: a literature review of quantitative, qualitative and mixed methods studies. *Int J Med Inform* 2005;74:745–768.

Section III
Healthcare Knowledge Management Implementations: Evidence from Practice

13
Knowledge Management and the National Health Service in England

Caroline De Brún

Abstract

The aim of this chapter is to discuss the application of knowledge management (KM) in healthcare, with a particular focus on the National Health Service in England. Key issues surrounding the implementation of knowledge management in healthcare and examples of good practice will be identified. Although the term KM is not widely accepted in health services, there are a number of examples where KM initiatives are being successfully applied to support clinical decision making and improve patient safety.

13.1 Introduction

There is much debate in healthcare over the use of the phrase "knowledge management" (KM), particularly when applied to healthcare operations. It is generally viewed as a term associated with business and industry, a buzzword representing a commercial environment where the preferred outcome is financial gain and, therefore, of no relevance to health. Within healthcare, the outcome of a patient's stay is the key measure of success, with the preferred outcome being patient satisfaction and improved wellbeing.

However, despite the resistance to the terminology, there is a place for KM activities in healthcare organizations, and there are several initiatives which are currently being embedded into the organizational culture of the National Health Service (NHS) in England.

13.2 Knowledge Management

A popular definition of KM is provided by Royal Dutch/Shell:

The capabilities by which communities within an organisation capture the knowledge that is critical to them, constantly improve it and make it available in the most effective manner

179

to those people who need it, so that they can exploit it creatively to add value as a normal part of their work. (Royal Dutch/Shell as reported by British Standards Institute 2001 [1])

Within healthcare this could translate to:

The way in which multidisciplinary teams, working in healthcare, harvest the personal expertise that is essential to patient safety, learn from it, adapt it to local situations and individual patients, and distribute it via reliable networks to the people caring for the patients, so that they can use it to improve the quality of care delivered.

In healthcare, KM should be about:

• coordinating experts in a particular specialism;
• giving them resources to collaborate;
• enabling clinicians to discuss the best treatment methods and reach a consensus, based on explicit knowledge and personal experience;
• disseminating it in a validated, robust format, such as a guideline.

But this is only part of the formula. For fully-informed patient care decisions, the complete knowledge package should comprise of all of the following, thus enabling the local knowledge to work with the localised evidence-base:

• individual wisdom (also known as personal expertise, clinician knowledge, tacit knowledge)
• evidence based practice (expertise backed up by high quality research)
• patient preference (based on choice and values)

Knowledge management can only improve healthcare when knowledge has been successfully integrated with evidence-based practice [2].

13.3   Intellectual Capital

With many definitions of KM available, it is generally agreed that people are the driving component. Arthur Anderson, one of the largest accounting/consulting firms in the US, came up with the following equation:

$$K = (P + I)^S$$

where *Knowledge* = *People* connected by technology to allow the *Sharing* of *Information* [3].

This model illustrates the use of technology in bridging the gaps across geographical distances to facilitate knowledge sharing. As in many countries, the state health system is spread nationwide; therefore, it is imperative that employees understand the importance of sharing their knowledge with other employees across the organization. Technology, such as e-mail, online communities, and intranets, can facilitate this process.

The knowledge that needs to be managed is the intellectual capital, the individual knowledge people possess, gained through experience and contact with like-minded experts, the tacit knowledge that is stored in people's minds and memories, and which is often carelessly lost by the organization when people move on, through resignation, redeployment, or retirement.

13.4 Importance of Knowledge Management in Healthcare

Particularly in healthcare, time, energy, and resources are wasted because different teams, be they operating in the community, on the ward, or in the operating theatre, often repeat the same practices and develop new methods over and over again, rather than sharing what they know via reliable national networks so that they can learn from each other.

KM should be an extension of evidence-based medicine, which draws on the documented evidence of treatment effectiveness to calculate the best care for the patient. Patients are individuals and may react to treatments in different ways. Only health professionals at the front line are aware of these adverse incidents, and they need to make sure that this tacit knowledge, which is locally specific (but may be applicable to other localities), is documented, backed up by research, and passed on via robust systems to other clinicians facing similar situations.

13.5 Benefits of Knowledge Management in Healthcare

Sharing knowledge of lessons learned offers staff, patients, and the healthcare organization numerous benefits, including:

- improved patient care, patient safety, and ultimately patient satisfaction;
- increased motivation, with the fact that everyone is working together and better results are being achieved;
- team-building, across the nation and across the globe;
- opportunities for research and innovation, supported by the new networks being built across the specialties;
- increased learning opportunities, via new contacts within other organizations;
- efficient healthcare systems, both in terms of effectiveness of treatments and cost effectiveness, because healthcare staff are working out the most effective way of treating patients and carrying out routine tasks, learning from other departments and thus creating a reduction in duplication;
- better communication with computer systems in place to allow health professionals to effectively communicate electronically;
- more informed decision making by learning from others and building on individual experiences.

13.6 Barriers to Knowledge Management in Healthcare

There are a number of issues hindering the adoption of KM into healthcare, the four main issues being:

13.6.1 Terminology

As stated previously, the term KM is associated with business, power, and profit. However, when broken down into what it actually is, i.e. sharing and building on what is known to improve a service, the outcome can mean anything that will benefit all involved, be they patients, carers, health professionals, or health organizations.

It would be difficult to change the terminology, as it is firmly established in other industry sectors, but translations could be made available to put KM into a clinical context. For example, ward rounds are a community of practice. They enable health professionals with different expertise, but with a common goal, to meet with the patient and collaborate to identify the most effective treatment. Care pathways are templates detailing the local procedures a patient with a particular condition will follow during the course of treatment. Because these documents do not contain confidential information, they can be shared between healthcare organizations, avoiding duplication of effort, enabling staff to learn from each other, and ensuring that a uniform service is being offered throughout the health service.

A consequence of the lack of appropriate terminology is that one of the most challenging issues is finding research, about in health environments, on healthcare databases. Evidence is necessary to support the implementation of KM initiatives, but the term does not exist in the indexes of most of the databases relating to health.

A list of 15 key articles on KM in healthcare was compiled for a Department of Health project in 2004, and a search strategy designed to find these articles was developed. The publication date of the articles ranged from 1986 to 2002. Only three of the articles were found using the search strategy. On examining the key words for each reference, it was found that they were all indexed with different terms, and there was no specific term identifying them as articles about KM in a clinical setting. This is because the term "knowledge management" is relatively new to healthcare. The term "knowledge" was added as an index term (also known as MeSH, Medical Subject Headings, thesaurus, descriptors, keywords) to Medline and the Cochrane Library in 1997, but it is too broad. PsycInfo (a database containing psychological abstracts) has used "knowledge level" as an index term since 1978, and this term would seem more appropriate to KM. CINAHL (Cumulative Index of Nursing and Allied Health Literature) added the index term "knowledge management" to its thesaurus in 2002. The lack of a common term for research about knowledge management in health is one of the difficulties facing health professionals when looking for research examples of KM applied to clinical settings. A new search strategy was compiled and is currently 100 steps long, but it needs frequent updating to reflect the changing terminology of KM in healthcare.

Once the terminology is translated into the language of the health service, it will be easier to find examples and apply KM concepts, because staff will have a clearer understanding of what is expected. They will also discover that KM is already embedded in some of their activities, albeit under a different name.

13.6.2   Trust

Trust is integral to the success of KM in health, particularly if mistakes have been made and lessons need to be learned. Errors do occur and need to be investigated; but, more often than not, it is the design of the system at fault, rather than the individual involved. Furthermore, if it is system failure then the system could fail elsewhere in the UK, and this is why the incident should be reported and acted upon, with the information being disseminated throughout the country. Systems are being put into place to ensure this happens; but, for this work to continue and develop, health professionals must feel reassured that they will not be blamed for mistakes if it was due to a general failure in the system, and they must not be used as scapegoats. If it is a general systems failure, then the organization must take responsibility and show how improvements will be made. In 2000, the Department of Health published the document "An Organisation with a Memory," [4] which will help with this process, although it will take time to build the level of trust required. People are beginning to talk more when mistakes occur, but putting them in writing requires a greater level of trust and support.

Trust is also important for cooperative behavior, as people will be more willing to share what they know in an open, trusting environment.

13.6.3   Technology

Technological advances mean that health professionals' roles are becoming more information technology (IT)-based, which for people who have not grown up with technology can be quite daunting. Currently, in healthcare, IT-based KM initiatives include:

• Decision support systems, to help clinicians make informed decisions.
• Intranets, to enable secure sharing of patient data.
• Blogs, to encourage collaboration.
• Online communities, to support networking and sharing of expertise.

These are all used in healthcare and should be promoted and developed further to help improve patient care.

In the NHS, the infrastructure for a robust computer system countrywide is making progress. It is a monumental project, which needs input from all involved, and cannot be achieved overnight. But the structure is in place; and in the not too distant future, patient information and tacit and explicit knowledge will all be safely shared across the country via secure networks, meaning that all health professionals will have the same access to the best information needed to treat patients.

13.6.4   Time

Time is always an important issue, particularly when change is involved. However, as demonstrated earlier, KM concepts are already being applied in healthcare settings, albeit in disguise. These concepts are increasing knowledge levels and saving health professionals time and effort, because they no longer have to "re-invent the wheel." They can adapt existing systems that have already proved successful. For example, why write a new procedure when one already exists that can be adapted to suit local situations. Initially, adopting a new technique, already applied elsewhere in a similar environment, will require an investment of time, but in the long term the benefits will be worth it in terms of improved patient care, reduction in workload for healthcare staff, and more efficient use of resources.

13.7   Overcoming Barriers to Knowledge Management in Healthcare

These barriers can be overcome, but successful KM does require the commitment of all staff within the organization, from cleaners to catering staff, to administration, to allied health, to clinicians. Everyone within the organization plays an essential role in the delivery of healthcare, and for that reason everyone needs to know that their knowledge contribution is valuable to the improved care of patients.

Some of the key steps to overcoming barriers include:

- Finding someone with influence within the organization who believes in, and practices, KM and supports them in making KM part of the organization's culture.
- Educating by example, using stories to demonstrate successful and achievable implementation of KM in healthcare.
- Providing opportunities and time for people to meet and share good practice.
- Developing a secure and simple computer system, such as an intranet, so that experiences can be easily shared.
- Rewarding good practice and innovation with recognition.
- Encouraging a trusting environment. This is possibly the most difficult step to achieve, but trust is the foundation stone of KM.

In terms of the NHS in England, barriers are being overcome. KM is being implemented, and this will be discussed further in Section 13.8.

13.8   Background to the National Health Service in England

The National Health Service in England operates in accordance with policies developed by the Department of Health. These policies are implemented by 10 Strategic Health Authorities (SHAs), which commission the services of the Primary Care Trusts (PCTs) and Acute Trusts. The Primary Care Trusts are responsible for commissioning local community health services, (such as general practice staff, community nurses, and allied health professionals), and the Acute Trusts provide emergency and hospital care.

The NHS has undergone several reorganisations over recent years, thereby strengthening the case for knowledge management in the NHS, as employees move within the organisation or leave as a consequence of change, taking their knowledge with them. The document, "Creating a Patient-Led NHS" [5], is set to further influence changes in the way services are commissioned, by halving the number of PCTs in England. This reflects patient choice and preferences, and will simplify management and administration processes, enabling staff to concentrate on health improvement.

A snapshot of the current situation shows one SHA, the South Central NHS, serving a population of 3,922,301, with health services provided by 10 Acute Trusts, 47 community hospitals, and 516 GP practices.

This is an example of just one Strategic Health Authority. In September 2005, the NHS employed 1.3 million staff across the whole country, in a range of settings, including emergency care, mental health, ambulance services, rehabilitation, general practice, and policy and administration.

From this, we can see the NHS contains an abundance of relatively uncontrolled knowledge, which needs to be coordinated, harvested, and appropriately distributed throughout the health service, with the aim of improving patient care. Furthermore, with the many recent changes to the organisation, which have lead to promotion, redeployment, redundancy, resignation and retirement, departments within the NHS are losing large quantities of expertise, because systems are not in place to harvest tacit knowledge. While working for the NHS, employees gather vast amounts of knowledge from their experiences, and without careful management, this valuable knowledge could be lost and the opportunity to learn from others may be missed.

The NHS does deliver an excellent service; but the more it delivers, the more is expected and demanded. Resources often cannot be implemented quickly enough to meet the increasing expectations, and mistakes do occur [4], which, although rare, do cause devastation to patients, their families, and also NHS staff, whose main priority is patient well-being. The findings of "An Organisation with a Memory" [4], chaired by the UK Chief Medical Officer, showed that human errors were often caused by systems failures rather than carelessness or incompetence [6]. The report suggested that, to improve patient safety, better reporting systems should be introduced, together with a more open culture, within the NHS, allowing people to learn from mistakes.

Prior to that publication, the Information for Health: An Information Strategy for the Modern NHS [7] was published, highlighting three explicit needs of clinicians:

1. Fast, reliable and accurate information about patients in their care.
2. Access to knowledge to inform clinical practice.
3. Access to information to underpin evaluation of clinical practice, planning and research, clinical governance, and continuing professional development [8].

The strategy recommended that a National Electronic Library for Health (National Library for Health, as of November 2004), (NeLH) be developed, whose aim it would be "to provide easy access to best current knowledge to improve health and healthcare, patient choice, and clinical practice" [9]. The justification for this digital library was that decision makers, unless they have access to good knowledge, would face barriers in providing high-quality healthcare.

To support the lessons learned and other KM initiatives, the National Library for Health (http://www.library.nhs.uk) launched the prototype for the Knowledge Management Specialist Library (http://www.library.nhs.uk/knowledgemanagement), in 2003, as part of the range of specialist libraries offered by the NeLH. This project is being funded as part of the National Knowledge Service (NKS) Mobilisation work-strand.

13.9   Knowledge Management in the National Health Service

With an increasing realization that KM could help prevent some of the medical errors occurring, the NHS concentrated on developing KM activities via the NKS.

The aim of the NKS is to provide NHS employees with the best current knowledge and the resources to capture this knowledge and turn it into an appropriate format so that it can be disseminated throughout the NHS, with the ultimate aim of improving patient safety and standardizing practice. Within the NKS sit a number of projects, including the "Do Once and Share" (DOAS) project and the Knowledge Management Specialist Library, accessible via the National Library for Health.

DOAS focuses on the 50 major clinical topics, some examples being renal failure, child health, asthma, and oral health, and aims to minimize duplication of effort by developing a common management approach across the NHS. The project will develop national clinical communities of practice, to facilitate collaboration and joint working. The following paragraphs look at other examples of KM in the NHS.

Lesson cards and Eurekas were developed by the NHS Modernisation Agency. They are functional and concise documents containing lessons learned from experience and examples of innovation in the NHS. The NHS Modernisation Agency and the NHS University have since evolved into the NHS Institute for Innovation and Improvement, (http://www.institute.nhs.uk), which will support the development of new ideas and work-based learning, use of technologies and build on good practice to improve services to patients, NHS employees and members of the public.

The NHS in England has developed a Protocols and Care Pathways database (available via the National Library for Health), containing step-by-step guides to procedures from NHS trusts around the country, which can be adapted to suit the local environment.

Map of Medicine is another KM tool available via the National Library for Health, connecting health professionals to the evidence base and local guidelines.

NHS Networks (http://www.networks.nhs.uk) enables health professionals to set up work-related networks, facilitating the communication process and supporting collaboration.

This demonstrates that, throughout the NHS, there are many innovative projects in place to gather and use professional expertise. The aim of the Department of Health and the NHS is to provide a gateway to these initiatives, encourage the development of new ideas, and to support a knowledge-sharing environment, and this is why the Knowledge Management Specialist Library is being developed.

Originally, the Knowledge Management Specialist Library was an introduction to KM, containing articles describing KM, book references, and information on a range of KM tools and techniques, such as exit interviews, white papers, communities of practice, etc.

More recently, the content of the site has been updated and migrated to a new resource management system. The aim of this portal is to direct health professionals to practical examples of KM applied to health, backed up by evidence, with the opportunity to join a community of practice to share experiences. The updated site was designed to provide the following:

- access to quality research on KM in healthcare;
- information on tools to implement KM in healthcare;
- networks to discuss and share ideas;
- glossary to make KM more understandable;
- diary dates, so that health professionals can attend relevant events;
- good practice examples, in the form of case studies, strategies, and lessons learned.

Content now includes links to full-text research articles or summaries demonstrating the application of KM techniques in health settings, together with introductory articles defining different KM concepts. The site provides access to a community of practice, which has been set up by the Northumberland Tyne and Wear Strategic Health Authority (now part of the North East SHA), and is available to all KM practitioners in the NHS. Communication currently takes place via a weblog called Talking KM, available at http://talkingkm.blogspot.com/

The adoption of RSS (Really Simple Syndication) feeds will ease the process of keeping up to date by allowing the website to send new content links to subscribers.

The updated Knowledge Management Specialist Library was launched in September 2005, but the site is not complete and it cannot be while knowledge management is being actively developed in the NHS, as it relies on user participation. This resource is being promoted via a monthly newsletter called Knowledge Flow, which highlights key resources on a different KM topic each month.

13.10   Conclusions

Communication, trust, and understanding are the keys to successful KM in healthcare.

There is still a lot of work that needs to be done to build a knowledge-sharing culture in healthcare. Without robust communication channels, whether newly developed or built on existing networks, people will not be able to share their expertise. With regards to the NHS, communities of practice need to be more flexible, and allow for networking, information sharing, collaboration, etc.

For healthcare to embrace KM successfully into the heart of their industry, there needs to be a greater understanding of the concept. Another important step for improving KM in the NHS, and healthcare generally, is to overcome the terminology barrier, and this can be done by demonstrating to NHS employees that KM is being practiced in the NHS, in the form of communities of practice (ward rounds), lessons learned from experience and good practice, decision-support systems, and intranets.

Time is also an important factor in the success of KM. People need to be encouraged to write up their experiences. Developing templates, enabling staff to can fill in the gaps with their experiences, can facilitate this process, and these documents should then be uploaded onto a centrally accessible resource, such as an Intranet. Naturally, if this document is directly concerned with patient safety or a change in procedure, then a process for quality evaluation needs to be in place, and then it should be circulated nationally, in case it can benefit other NHS organisations.

As KM becomes increasingly understood in the NHS, more content will be created by NHS staff, which will be added to the Knowledge Management Specialist Library and disseminated via the growing communities of practice. This continuing development will support the ultimate aim of improving patient care and reducing inefficiency, by enabling staff to learn from each other and build on innovative practice, which can be shared locally, nationally, and perhaps even globally.

References

1. British Standards Institute. *PAS 2001: Knowledge management: a guide to good practice.* London (UK): British Standards Institute; 2001.
2. Sackett David et al. *Evidence Based Medicine: How to Practice and Teach EBM.* Edinburgh (UK): Churchill Livingstone; 2000.
3. Probst G, Romhardt K, Raub S. *Managing knowledge: building blocks for success.* Chichester: Wiley; 2000.
4. Department of Health. *An organisation with a memory: report of an expert group on learning from adverse events in the NHS.* London: The Stationery Office; 2000. Available from: http://www.dh.gov.uk/assetRoot/04/06/50/86/04065086.pdf.
5. Department of Health. Creating a patientled NHS: delivering the NHS improvement plan. London (UK): The Stationery Office; 2005. Available from http://www.dh.gov.uk/assetRoot/04/10/65/07/04106507.pdf
6. Leape LL. Reporting of medical errors: time for a reality check. *Qual Health Care* 2000;9(3):144–145. Available from: http://qhc.bmjjournals.com/cgi/content/full/9/3/144.
7. NHS Executive. *Information for Health: An Information Strategy for the Modern NHS 1998–2005.* Wetherby: Department of Health; 1998. Available from http://www.dh.gov.uk/assetRoot/04/01/44/69/04014469.pdf
8. Sensky T. Knowledge management. *Adv Psychiatr Treat* 2002;8(5):387–396. Available from: http://apt.rcpsych.org/cgi/content/full/8/5/387.
9. Gray JAM, de Lusignan S. National Electronic Library for Health (NeLH). *Br Med J* 1999;319(7223):1476–1479. Available from: http://bmj.com/cgi/content/full/319/7223/1476

14
Knowledge Management and the National Health Service in Scotland

OLIVER HARDING AND ANN WALES

14.1 Introduction

This chapter aims to consider the National Health Service (NHS) in Scotland (NHSiS) from a knowledge management (KM) perspective and describe some of the issues, advances, and successes. It begins with some background information on the NHSiS. There follows a discussion on the advances made in terms of developing the NHSiS as a knowledge-based organization, based on some models from the KM literature. Finally, there is a case study: the National Pathways Project, giving an example of KM in practice.

14.2 Background

The NHSiS was established in July 1948 as a result of the National Health Service (Scotland) Act 1947. Since that time there have been some organizational changes; but, in general, the NHSiS has consisted of "operational units," some form of management system, and governance arrangements through a board structure.

Currently, the NHSiS can be described as comprising the following:

- front-line staff
- service units
- organizational units
- local NHS boards
- NHS national organizations.

The government department managing the NHSiS is the Scottish Executive Health Department (SEHD), which includes within it the Centre for Change and Innovation (CCI).

Although this is the basic, traditional structure, there are an increasing number of strategic and operational configurations that cross the traditional boundaries of organization and sector, e.g. community health partnerships, managed clinical networks, regional planning partnerships. The cross-boundary nature of these models has major implications for KM.

14.2.1 Frontline Staff

Doctors, nurses, allied health professionals, and other healthcare professionals deliver healthcare activity to their patients or clients. Such activity may consist of assessment (through interview, physical testing, or more technical tests) and intervention (carrying out procedures or prescribing medication or some other device or treatment). The healthcare professions tend to have their own professional bodies, such as the various Royal Colleges, which are involved in teaching, education, and maintaining standards of practice by their members.

14.2.2 Service Units

The organization of front-line staff usually forms a relatively small unit to start with, e.g. the hospital ward, outpatient departments, or the general practice (which is, in fact, contracted to the NHS rather than being a part of the organization). There may be organization of these units into larger departments.

14.2.3 Organizational Units

The next major level of organization is that around which most planning can be carried out. Hospitals may be organized into acute operating divisions; primary care is currently organized around community health partnerships (which are strategic bodies working across sectoral boundaries, and includes organizations other than those within the NHS, such as local authorities and voluntary organizations).

14.2.4 Local National Health Service Boards

The next level of organization is the local NHS board. This covers a defined geographic area, and encompasses all operating divisions within what is known as a single system. They have a degree of autonomy and a decision-making system based on a board consisting of executive and nonexecutive members. Since the move to "single system working," NHS boards form the single employing organization for the NHSiS at the local level.

14.2.5 National Health Service National Organizations

There are other NHS boards which have a remit across Scotland. These boards have a range of functions.

National Services Scotland. This covers a number of national roles, such as a central legal function, communicable diseases and environmental health, managing data from the NHSiS on a national basis, national screening programs, blood transfusion services, some other national services, and administrative functions.

NHS Health Scotland. This is described as a national resource for improving Scotland's health.

NHS for Education Scotland (NES). This has a remit for supporting best practice in education, training, and lifelong learning for NHSiS staff.

NHS Quality Improvement Scotland. This aims to improve the effectiveness and efficiency of the NHSiS.

NHS24. This a telephone health advice and information service available across Scotland (equivalent to NHS Direct in England).

SEHD. The SEHD has responsibility for the NHSiS, and for the development and implementation of health and community care policy, the accountability for which is to the Scottish Parliament. It communicates with the NHS through Health Department Letters and other means. It includes within it mechanisms to performance manage and support the NHSiS, such as the CCI, which supports service modernization and redesign.

14.2.6   Summary

The ultimate aim of the NHSiS is to deliver appropriate assessment and intervention to patients/clients (including that relating to the public health and health improvement function). It can reasonably be assumed that knowledge is crucial to the process of achieving this aim through the resources available to the NHSiS, and that this applies across all the parts of the NHSiS described above.

Until recently the main knowledge focus has been the practitioner. Library services aimed to provide knowledge from research literature and other sources to practitioners in order to allow them to gain personal knowledge and skills, which would translate into high-quality patient care. Now, however, a broader concept of knowledge means that the remit extends beyond library services. There is a recognition that the interrelationship between people, hardware, and systems forms the basis for knowledge generation and use.

It is on this basis that NES, the lead organization for KM in the NHSiS, is taking forward the NHSiS strategy in KM. In "From Knowing to Doing: Transforming Knowledge into Practice in NHS Scotland" [1] the context described above is redefined from a KM perspective as the "Scottish Health Information Environment." This has the patient at the center, with practitioners and others forming a local environment, with supporting knowledge/information processes on the outside.

14.3   Knowledge Management in the National Health Service in Scotland

In this section we describe some of the general theories and models used in KM, and relate these to the NHSiS.

TABLE 14.1. Applying KM methods to NHSiS.

KM element	NHSiS
People	• Practitioners, support staff, managers, policy makers within NHSiS • Patients or clients themselves • Partners, e.g. individuals in other public-sector organizations
Processes	The range of possible processes is large, some more formalized than others, but includes: • Professional qualification and accreditation • Quality assurance processes • Clinical workflow processes
Activities	• Interacting with patients or clients • Interacting with colleagues • Communication in general: reading, dialogue, writing • Searching for material/literature • Thinking, reflecting, assimilating • Group work
Technology	• Information technology (IT): pen and paper, computer • "Soft" technologies, e.g. interpersonal skills
Environment	• Time management • Culture

14.3.1   Attributes of Knowledge Management Systems

Lehaney et al. [2] suggest that there is no single unifying definition or approach to KM, but there is some consistency in the underlying principles and content. KM involves:

- people,
- processes,
- activities,
- technology, and
- the broader environment,

the purpose being to enable the identification, creation, communication or sharing, and use of organizational and individual knowledge. How this applies to the NHSiS is presented in Table 14.1.

Lehaney et al. [2] go on to describe a model based around staff, structures, and technologies, applied to the NHSiS as highlighted below.

14.3.1.1   People/staff

Although staff are key to any organization, other people within the NHSiS are important too. The latest KM strategies for NHSiS put the patient firmly at the center; and this is appropriate, as the ultimate organizational goals are around patients and their health. For this reason also, patients are seen as key participants in the activity of the health services, with their own information and knowledge needs that can have a significant influence on outcome. Patients, and the public at large, are seen as key stakeholders at a number of levels, and one of the main themes of the KM strategy for the NHSiS is around patient focus and public involvement.

Within the NHSiS, staff development takes place through a number of mechanisms, such as:

- Professional development. This is often encouraged by specific professional bodies, or there may be formal requirements for continuous professional development in place.
- Local NHS board staff-development programs.
- Local programs for research, development, and audit.
- Local clinical governance arrangements.
- Contracts of employment. When reviewed, may take account of staff attributes, e.g. the knowledge and skills framework within "Agenda for change" [3].

Often the development of "know-how," "know-when," etc. occurs as experience is gained, and there are informal means of gaining individual knowledge, through working with colleagues for instance.

As well as developing staff in relation to these attributes, local departments of human resources and/or organizational development have a role in developing the broader skills to enable gains in individual knowledge, e.g. in developing critical thinking and emotional intelligence.

"Building a knowledge competent workforce" is seen as key to the success of the implementation of the KM strategy.

14.3.1.2 Structures

Structures may relate to the environment, activities, and processes. Within the KM strategy for the NHSiS a lot of emphasis has been placed on the development of "managed knowledge networks" (MKNs), which aim to support extended virtual communities, such as managed clinical networks. At present, MKN members are connected largely by technology via the NHSiS e-Library portals and knowledge exchanges, and are supported principally by explicit knowledge sources in the form of published primary and secondary literature; but, in the future, they should also involve more social interaction among participants.

14.3.1.3 Technologies

A lot of emphasis is placed on the use of IT in the KM strategy for the NHSiS. Much of this is based on obtaining explicit knowledge through the searching of databases, with an emphasis on the interoperability of databases. The human–IT interface is seen as important too, with a recognized need to develop individually flexible, relevant systems that can be used (almost) instantaneously with clinical activity.

14.3.2   The Balance Between Attributes of the Knowledge Management System

It is likely to be the interrelationships among the parts of the system described above which will determine the overall strengths of the system. If this is the case, then it is likely to be the least sufficiently developed attributes which will determine the overall strength of the system. Edwards et al. [4] carried out a survey of people involved in KM, comparing the perceived and desired levels of importance placed on different KM factors. They found that, for technology, the perceived importance was greater than the desired importance. In other words, too great an emphasis is placed on IT solutions to KM. The same survey found that insufficient importance is placed on culture and people. To some extent this is the situation within the NHSiS, where advances in technologies seem very much further ahead than changes in culture and other aspects of the environment.

Often, a practitioner's work plans focus mainly on activity, with insufficient emphasis on reflection and acquiring knowledge. Time management, with sufficient allocation to knowledge-based attributes, is required. More importantly, there needs to be the development of a culture which values knowledge and encourages continued learning. This is emphasized by Anderson [5], who describes certain attributes of culture in the NHSiS which may form barriers to creativity in KM and knowledge sharing.

With the changes in employment policy and practice comes, perhaps, the opportunity to address this, e.g. through the knowledge and skills framework of "Agenda for change" [3]. These sorts of changes in human resource management may provide an opportunity for a more flexible system of rewards and incentives, as suggested by Anderson [5].

14.3.3   Further Exploration of Processes

It is the interrelationship among staff, structures, and technology which allow and facilitate the basic KM processes [2] of:

- identification, or creation
- acquisition
- retention
- utilization
- sharing
- measurement.

Within the NHSiS there are three main domains of functioning: clinical practice (i.e. focused on the activities of assessment and intervention), management (i.e. organizing people, processes, and materials and equipment, etc., to allow activity to take place), and policy development and planning (i.e. developing plans and strategies for the future direction of the service). For each domain there are examples for each KM process (Table 14.2).

TABLE 14.2. KM process examples for each domain.

	Clinical practice	Management	Policy and planning
Identification or creation	Identification of existing national clinical guidelines or development of local guidelines	Setting up an employee database	Identification of data and information on a population health need
Acquisition	Order from the library	Populating database from other data/employees themselves	Obtaining this from sources, e.g. ISD, NHSHS, eLib
Retention	Keep nearby	Store on local computer server	Store on local computer server
Utilization	Refer to when seeing a patient (or before or after)	Refer to when carrying out reviews	Production of a report
Sharing	Telling others in the team	Summarizing data for executives	Present to the NHS board
Measurement	Audit on the use of guidelines	Identification of completeness/external audit	Evaluation of report, outcome, decision making

Table 14.2 gives a few examples only; the range and depth of KM processes across the three domains is huge. Within the KM strategy for Scotland [1], most focus seems to be on the "clinical practice" domain, and the management domain is considered also. Of the KM processes, acquisition, utilization, and sharing are considered, but there is scope to develop measurement further. Such approaches as knowledge audit, mapping, and gap analysis may be useful. Although the main focus has quite rightly been on practice, KM is also equally important in parts of the NHS which do not involve direct patient activity (e.g. policy and planning).

14.3.4   The SECI Model of Knowledge Management in the National Health Service in Scotland

Nonaka and Toyama [6] have proposed the SECI model of KM building on the concepts of tacit and explicit knowledge:

- Socialization—tacit to tacit transformation. This involves the interaction between individuals within an environment, and includes sharing and creating tacit knowledge through direct experience.
- Externalization—tacit to explicit transformation. This is described as articulating tacit knowledge through dialogue and reflection. It is about "translating" tacit knowledge. It may involve local codification of knowledge.

TABLE 14.3. General examples of applying SECI model to the NHSiS.

	General example
Socialization	Sharing of tacit knowledge within clinical teams—in the process of caring
Externalization	More formal exchange of tacit knowledge within clinical teams, which may involve some codification. For example, writing a local policy or procedure
Combination	A literature review where knowledge from a range of sources is gathered and interpreted
Internalization	Reading and using a new guideline or protocol

- Combination—explicit to explicit transformation. This is described as systemizing and applying explicit knowledge and information, characterized by gathering and integrating explicit knowledge and information, transferring and diffusing explicit knowledge, and editing explicit knowledge
- Internalization—explicit to tacit transformation. This is defined as learning and acquiring new tacit knowledge in practice, characterized by embodying explicit knowledge through action and practice, using simulation and experiments.

To apply the SECI model, the NHSiS gives the general examples shown in Table 14.3; there are many more.

In terms of the Scottish Health Information Environment described in "From knowing to doing" [1] the model seems to be one largely based on local tacit knowledge, and sharing of this, with the support functions being targeted on the management of explicit knowledge. Further work is required in looking at how local externalization can be developed and used to inform the development of the overall information environment. This again relates to culture in some ways, as there is a better understanding and acceptance of explicit knowledge as a central, remote form of knowledge than as a form of local knowledge.

14.4   Case Study: The National Patient Pathways Project

The purpose of National Patient Pathways project [7] was to provide evidence-based best-practice recommendations for the appropriate referral of patients from general practice to specialist outpatient care and appropriate follow-up care. The National Patient Pathways have been developed by the NHSiS with the assistance of the Scottish Intercollegiate Guidelines Network (SIGN) and the CCI.

A number of steps have been outlined in the pathway development process:

- recruit multidisciplinary and geographically representative topic-specific group;
- hold first group meeting to agree remit;
- conduct literature searches and identify existing material;
- assess quality of the literature;
- complete evidence tables;
- draft pathways;
- consult;

- pilot;
- finalize pathways;
- support implementation.

Each step can be seen as demonstrating attributes of the SECI model:

- The recruitment to the group and meeting of the group may be described as socialization. The exchange of information is largely tacit-to-tacit exchange. There may be some externalization through the writing of minutes and the development of planning documents.
- Literature searches and assessment of the quality of literature are about internalization and combination, within the individual reviewer.
- The evidence tables and draft pathways produced involve the generation of explicit knowledge from tacit knowledge, i.e. externalization. Consultation involves some internalization and combination. Piloting involves socialization.
- The finalization of pathways involves feedback from piloting and consulting, the tacit knowledge of which needs ultimately to modify the explicit knowledge held within the pathways.

Ultimately what is produced (the pathway) constitutes explicit knowledge, and a distillation of the explicit and related tacit knowledge that has gone into its development. The final stage is described as "support implementation." This implementation phase will require a whole range of SECI processes to put the pathway into practice.

The completed development of a set of pathways represents a success. Implementation, however, is an issue, and is often recognized as the most difficult aspect of guideline development.

The implementation phase includes the following stages (which can be considered in terms of the KM literature, especially the SECI model):

1. Linking with other CCI projects (connecting processes).
2. Working with local healthcare professionals (engaging with people who are intended to use the pathway, which, as a minimum, will include internalization by this group).
3. Linking with electronic communication tools (technological aspects of KM).
4. Implementation through referral information/management services (again linking to existing systems).
5. Access educational and training support (means for facilitating internalization).
6. Form a support network and spread good practice (socialization).

Overall the approach to implementation has been fairly pragmatic and realistic, with consideration and resource allocation to this phase built in from the beginning. Also, the implementation process has been based on the best available evidence for this from the literature—a further example of a KM processes.

It is expected that local areas will adapt and adopt these pathways. In effect, it is recognized that SECI processes will be required within each implementation area. One of the main ways of beginning the implementation process is through raising awareness. It is recognized that much of the transfer of knowledge will be tacit–tacit, socialization, through existing structures: redesign projects, existing referral management initiatives, managed clinical networks, and clinical governance structures. However, it is also recognized that a multifaceted approach to awareness raising is likely to be beneficial, e.g. using a range of media and methods, each with SECI elements within.

An alternative approach for exploring implementation in local areas is to consider what is needed in terms of models from the KM literature, namely people, structure, and technologies:

- People. Staff with an awareness of the pathway and appropriate skills and attitudes; patients who are likely to have a positive attitude to pathways, and a willingness to comply.
- Structure. An appropriate environment and culture for the implementation of the pathway, and sufficient general systems in place to allow it to work.
- Technologies. For example, software which will allow tracking against a pathway, and/ or automatically generate letters, etc.

In particular, the specific processes are likely to be important:

- Identification or creation. Identification, i.e. people at the local level will have to be aware of the pathway, its contents, and supporting evidence.
- Acquisition. People will need to know how to obtain the material (i.e. download from the CCI Website), but also where to go for support, etc.
- Retention. Presumably there will be a need for some form of retention locally. This may vary from printing out the material and sticking on the wall or keeping nearby, to creating electronic files or even patient databases.
- Utilization. This will require all the above to be in place, but also the motivation of staff to use the pathway, based on feedback on patient care or other aspects, or some other reward structure.
- Sharing. Aspects of the utilization of the pathway itself require the sharing of information. More importantly, the experiences of staff using the pathway need to be shared locally and more widely in order to build up knowledge on the utilization of the pathway.
- Measurement. Some form of local measurement needs to be built in, in order to provide feedback on the use of the pathway, and improvements in patient outcomes, locally and more widely.

14.4.1   Reflection on the National Patient Pathways from a Knowledge Management Perspective

Much of the process detailed relates well to the KM theory, especially the SECI model. Most of the explicit–implicit transformations are clear. However, the links between the consultation and piloting phases and the finalization of the pathway were indistinct in the National Patient Pathways process, and could be explored further, i.e. by what process exactly is this internalization, combination, externalization process actually carried out? Overall, to be explicit about the relevant SECI stages/processes within future projects is likely to be useful.

Ideally, the learning from this project will be collected and shared, for it has produced knowledge in itself. A further issue relating to this is research: a means of generating knowledge. Ideally, this project would have included a related research program.

Local implementation of the pathways is a KM issue in itself, and likely to vary between local areas depending on circumstances.

Evaluation is a further issue. The original SIGN methodology [8] that the pathway development process is based on has a further stage of audit and review. This needs to be considered, and it may be taken forward through local areas. Audit and review would provide evidence regarding the success of the project beyond simply providing a pathway, to see whether they had ultimately been used, and whether this had made a difference to the patient/client. Ultimately, KM initiatives need to have an impact on organizational goals that is demonstrable.

14.5   Conclusions

In this chapter we have provided some insight into the NHSiS from a KM perspective. We believe that significant advances have been made in terms of introducing KM as a concept to the NHSiS, building on library services to give a broader view of knowledge and its use. We have reviewed our KM strategy against some of the existing theories of KM, and given an example of KM in action, in the form of a case study on patient pathways.

Some of the issues that have been identified for future work are:

- Addressing 'softer' issues of culture in the context of technological advancement.
- Considering nonclinical domains of the NHS which also need a KM perspective.
- The links between national development projects, and local implementation, and the potential for the use of KM frameworks in this.

References

1. Knowledge Services Group NHS Education for Scotland. From knowing to doing: transforming knowledge into practice in NHS Scotland implementation plan 2005–2008; in draft, 2006.
2. Lehaney B, Jack G, Clarke S, Coakes E. *Beyond knowledge management.* Idea Group USA; 2003
3. Agenda for change: modernising the NHS pay system. HSC 1999/227. Department of Health; 1999.
4. Edwards JS, Handzic M, Carlsson S, Nissen M. Knowledge management research & practice: visions and directions. *Knowl Manage Res Pract* 2003;1:49–60.

5. Anderson JM. Strategic knowledge management paper for MBA, 2004–2005.
6. Nonaka I, Toyama R. The knowledge-creating theory revisited: knowledge creation as a synthesizing process. *Knowl Manag Res Pract* 2003;1:2–10.
7. Frigola-Capell E, Watson F. National Pathways Project, Centre for Change and Innovation, personal communication.
8. Scottish Intercollegiate Guideline Network. SIGN 50: a guideline developers' handbook,, February 2001, last updated May 2004.

15
Knowledge Management for Primary Healthcare Services

ALAN EARDLEY AND ALEX CZERWINSKI

Abstract

This chapter looks at some of the issues of knowledge management in the UK's National Health Service and in healthcare in general. An examination of some of the concepts of knowledge and of knowledge management is carried out, including knowledge management tools, systems, and strategies. The characteristics of healthcare organizations are examined and it is concluded that the National Health Service relies on knowledge and would benefit from the effective application of knowledge management. A number of knowledge management initiatives (i.e. the National Electronic Library for Health and the Map of Medicine™) are examined. The current approach to knowledge management in the National Health Service is reviewed and recommendations are made for promoting "best practice" in the organization.

15.1 Introduction

The UK's National Health Service (NHS) employs over 1.2 million people, working in 28 strategic health authorities (SHAs), which in turn manage 276 hospital trusts and 302 primary care trusts. As one of the largest identifiable government-funded bodies in the UK, it is not surprising that the NHS has taken on board wide-scale application of computer-based information systems in virtually every aspect of its service provision. Until 7 years ago, however, there was little evidence of an overall strategic element to its policy. More recently, public and government pressure to improve services has led to critical examination of health service information standards (DOH CMO, 1998). This led to the establishment of the National Heath Service Information Authority (NHSIA) in 1999. The remit of this body is to deliver a set of national information technology (IT) services for the health service and its patients. A national program is now under way with the aim of revolutionizing the way health service information is handled.

The National Programme for IT (NPIT), which is being delivered by the new Department of Health (DoH) agency "NHS Connecting for Health" (NHSCH), is charged with "bringing modern computer systems into the NHS which will improve patient care and services" [1]. Over the next 10 years, the NPIT is intended to connect over 30,000 "first-line" general practitioners (GPs) in the UK to almost 300 hospitals employing over 100,000 doctors, 380,000 nurses and 50,000 assorted healthcare professionals. In doing so, it will benefit more than 50 million patients, transforming NHS business processes as well as structures.

This strategy is based on the foundation of a standardized IT infrastructure allowing common healthcare applications to be "rolled out" as an integrated national project. NHSCH aims to overcome long-standing problems, including "lost medical records, inconvenient appointments, and repeated journeys to hospital" [1]. The IT infrastructure is intended to link a number of disparate "islands of automation," including the following important healthcare IT applications:

- the NHS patient care records spine (NHS CRS);
- the electronic transmission of prescriptions (ETP) system;
- a newly established national broadband network for IT in the NHS (N3)
- picture archiving and communication systems (PACS);
- an on-line appointment booking service "Choose and Book."

In addition, a number of management and administrational applications (e.g. Quality Management and Analysis System (QMAS)) are integrated into the program. It can be argued that this is characteristic of the "problem-centric" approaches to IT system and infrastructure design that may have typified large government-backed IT projects in the UK. The concentration appears to be on data and information in the form of facts (e.g. patient care histories), events (e.g. clinical episodes and appointments) and transactions (e.g. IT-supported GP payments). For more information on the NHS project, the reader can refer to NHS strategic plan [NHSIA 2002]. The background to the first NHS prototypes can be seen within the context of the Electronic Records Development and Implementation Programme (ERDIP) work, which looked at performing an initial evaluation of the role of IT within the health service. Primary healthcare [47].

It is understandable that the NPIT intends to solve immediate patient problems such as "missing files, scans and x-rays" and needs to "reduce form filling" so that "basic information will not have to be repeatedly recorded every time a patient enters the NHS system" [1]. It cannot be doubted that solving these immediate problems and providing these advantages will make the NHS administration more efficient, and patient care more effective through online "customer facing" systems such as "Choose and Book." There are, therefore, four main strands or themes to the services being delivered to these professions by the organization as the "National Service Delivery" to support knowledge work. These strands are as follows:

- The "information infrastructure" strand, which will provide connectivity and support all of the common applications.
- The electronic patient record and electronic health record provision, which will manage and maintain the data on which many administration and healthcare applications can be based.

- The "key service stream" establishing "health informatics" as a recognized profession within the NHS to encourage both IT and non-IT staff at various levels in NHS trusts to promote the use of computing and IT in all parts of the NHS.
- The "information, knowledge and management services" provision, which can be seen in some ways as a "late addition" to the NPIT, but which is being promoted as a way of improving clinical practice within the NHS. This "fourth strand," therefore, is of particular importance to the NHS as a "knowledge organization," and providing support to the front-line healthcare professionals (rather than just the supporting administrators) should, therefore, be a high priority with the NPIT.

It is contended in this chapter that, because of the characteristics of the NHS, it is important for NPIT to develop IT applications that are useful and supportive of healthcare in the wider sense. It is possible that the IT applications that were originally being promoted by the NPIT may have focused too much on administration and support activities, rather than on the "core businesses" of healthcare, which is usually the province of the nursing and medical professions. There is a growing body of evidence that the importance of knowledge management (KM) in the NHS is recognized by an important and influential "community of practice" [2].

15.2   The Case for Knowledge Management

KM in the NHS has a considerable pedigree. The UK Government started the Knowledge Network as a pilot project in the DoH in 1997 when a briefing system was developed to bring together information into a common repository. Given this early date (KM was not a well-developed discipline at the time), it is perhaps not surprising that the IT tools were not originally intended for application in KM, but would today be considered as "content management" tools. A project manager within the KM events team points out that [3]:

To be honest, in the beginning we did not think of the system as a knowledge management system but rather as a tool that helped us to do our jobs better. It was only after the event that someone pointed out that we actually had a model KM system.

This approach implies an approach to KM that is less than strategic, perhaps containing elements of *bricolage* or "development by experiment" that seems to have characterized the early days of strategic IT applications in business [4].

The NHS is a classic example of a "knowledge organization" that contains specialist and general "communities of practice" [2] in which "knowledge workers" carry out their professional activities. Communities of practice (CoPs) are "groups of people who interact on an ongoing basis to discuss a shared, specific interest" or who "share a concern, a set of problems, or a passion about a topic and who deepen their knowledge and expertise on an ongoing basis" [5]. This clearly describes healthcare practitioners at a number of levels and is very relevant to both the development and the dissemination of knowledge in a wide range of healthcare domains. This topic will, therefore, be explored in more depth later in the chapter. The topic of knowledge work and the knowledge worker are also of great relevance to healthcare. To understand the role of the knowledge workers is to understand many of the issues that have developed around professions in the NHS, even though the term may have originated in a business context. "The term 'knowledge worker' was coined by Peter Drucker . . . to describe someone who adds value by processing existing information to create new information which could be used to define and solve problems" [3].

15.3   Knowledge Management as a Concept

Knowledge is classically defined as, "A fluid mix of framed experience, values, contextual information and expert insight that provides a framework for evaluating and incorporating new experiences and information" [6]. This implies that knowledge can develop and expand in relation to experience, have value in relation to the context in which it is used, and be flexible in its application. It is contended that healthcare knowledge is typical of this definition. The NHS is a knowledge-rich, knowledge-dependent organization. Further, there are several types of knowledge that are relevant to the medical domain.

First, there can be tacit knowledge [7], which is equivalent to "know-how," is related to the use of experience to take action in a particular context, and is often difficult to communicate, but can be learned. Second, there can be explicit knowledge, which is equivalent to "knowing what" and is capable of being represented in a codified form (e.g. a practice manual) and can be communicated, taught, and shared with others. There are also levels of knowledge, as knowledge can be embodied in individuals (e.g. medical specialists), in groups (e.g. CoPs), and in organizations (e.g. hospitals). Knowledge at the various levels is related through a fluid process that transforms knowledge from one type to another as it moves between levels. Also, each CoP will have its own specialist vocabulary of knowledge that will enable knowledge transfer within the group, but which can inhibit communication across group boundaries [5].

These are generally regarded as the attributes of a "body of knowledge," in this case applied to professions in an organization. These professions contain specialists who have one thing in common, i.e. they all undertake "knowledge work" and, therefore, are involved in the domain of KM. The healthcare professions tend to exhibit features such as:

• *An ontology.* Gruber [9] calls this a "specification of a conceptualisation or description of the concepts and relationships that exist for an agent or a community of agents" (e.g. doctors or nurses) or "a shared and common understanding of some domain that can be communicated across people and computers" [10] for the purpose of enabling knowledge sharing and reuse. This equates with the shared concepts and definitions that allow and enable the communication of knowledge to take place both within and between CoPs.

- An epistemology. Practically, this translates into the issues of scientific methodology that inform a knowledge domain. In medicine and healthcare it equates to the "process of knowing" [11] by which knowledge is acquired, organized, refined, and distributed to the benefit of the knowledge users and recipients [10]. This clearly equates with the extensive education and training that such professions undergo and the continued professional development.

There is broad agreement in the literature as to the definition of the KM process. According to one of the most frequently cited sources, the KM process is, "The systematic process of identifying, capturing and transferring information and knowledge (that) people can use to create, compete and improve" [12]. Alternatively, the KM process is defined as, "The systematic and organizationally specified process for acquiring, organizing and communicating (the) knowledge of employees so that other employees may make use of it to be more effective in their work" [13]. Both definitions stress the systematic nature of the phenomenon and agree on the essential nature of the process. The main difference in these definitions is that the former stresses the differential or competitive benefits of the use of KM, while the latter emphasizes the benefits of effectiveness. It would seem that the second definition (i.e. KM for work effectiveness) has more to offer for healthcare in the NHS, so this definition will be used in this work.

15.4 Knowledge Management Systems

It has been pointed out that, "Knowledge management is not a product in itself, or a solution that organizations can buy off the shelf or assemble from various components" [14]. Also, the KM process cannot be established instantaneously, but for most purposes must be built up over time. Further, it is linked to personal relationships and informal communications and processes as much as it is to formal organizational structures and technologies [6]. Four stages or phases can be identified in the KM process [14]:

- *Knowledge gathering*. The knowledge artifact is identified acquired and collected, possibly involving procedural or technical support (e.g. a learning or teaching process or the use of a search engine or online information source).
- *Knowledge organization and structuring*. The knowledge artifacts are codified and structured to enable them to be managed and to improve the effectiveness of the other stages or phases.
- *Knowledge refinement*. The knowledge artifacts are corrected and improved, updated, and deleted.
- *Knowledge dissemination*. The knowledge is represented in an appropriate form and distributed to the knowledge users in an appropriate and useful form.

To achieve its optimum efficiency, the KM process in a typical organization will be supported by an appropriate KM system, which will be based on processes and technology. It is possible to distinguish between two broad types of KM system:

horizontal and vertical. Horizontal KM systems provide generalized or infrastructural support across organizational and process boundaries and can be applied to a variety of knowledge applications. A variety of "horizontal" IT applications are available in industry, including BackWeb, Wincite, and KnowledgeX [15], and there are a variety of knowledge portals. By contrast, vertical KM systems are intended to be applied to one domain of knowledge and are specific to one type of situation.

This type of KM system is often developed "in house" from existing information applications and is generally highly effective in the area in which it is applied (e.g. a particular CoP), but it may contain features that make it difficult to apply to other areas of knowledge and, therefore, may restrict its ability to provide "engagement" with other specialist areas or CoPs [8]. To ensure that the healthcare organization gains maximum benefit from its knowledge network system or systems, therefore, it is important that it follows a KM strategy.

15.5   Knowledge Management Strategies

To be effective, the organizational unit needs to have a KM strategy in place. KM strategies can be divided into two broad categories: "personalized" and "codified" [16]. A personalized KM strategy relates to the tacit type of knowledge and it is recognized that the KM process will tend to be based on direct, informal, and interpersonal communication. A codified strategy applies to the explicit type of knowledge and assumes that knowledge can be represented as artifacts that can be processed formally (e.g. stored in databases and represented in documents). This view of KM strategy may be oversimplistic compared with the complexity of the concept of knowledge, as the total knowledge base of a CoP or organization will almost certainly be represented by both types of knowledge, making it impossible to concentrate on one class of strategy. An alternative view is that the choice of KM strategy depends on the sum of a specific range of problems based on the uncertainty, ambiguity, or complexity of the CoP's or the organization's KM process [17].

15.6   Knowledge Management in the National Health Service

Perhaps the original vision for KM in the NHS came in 1997 with the publication of the report "The new NHS—modern, dependable" that promoted various information services for patients and staff that would use the then-new Internet-based technology. These include NHS Direct, NHSnet and Book and Choose, as well as the use of the World-Wide Web "to provide knowledge about health, illness and best treatment practice to the general public" [18]. This was followed by several initiatives that sought to raise the profile of information services and IT in support of healthcare, resulting in the 1998 reports "Our information age" [19] and

"Information for health" [20], which together contained the outline NHS information strategy outlining a program of modernization based on better access, storage, and distribution of information. Although not directly related to KM, it can be argued that these developments were necessary precursors to the KM initiatives that were to follow. The first of these was probably the proposal contained in "A first class service: quality in the new NHS" in 1998, which suggested a framework for quality in clinical governance based on the support of KM systems [21]. The first reports containing concrete proposals for KM systems were published 2 years later. These were "R&D for a first class service" [22] and "An organisation with a memory" [23], which proposed the development of new KM systems that would enable clinicians to access scientific advancements and research findings and made the case for KM systems to disseminate tacit knowledge and the results of experience. These initiatives were followed by "Working together, learning together" in 2001, which proposed a framework of learning strategies to maximize the use of knowledge assets in a variety of healthcare applications, and proposed the establishment of the NHS University.

The suggestions and proposals that were put forward in these reports and "white papers" led to a range of important knowledge initiatives, including NHS UK, NHS Direct Online, the National Electronic Library for Health (NeLH), and the Connections database developed by the NHS Modernisation Agency. These initiatives were later brought under the control of the National Knowledge Service (NKS), which was formed to combine and coordinate the growing number of national agencies and providers of information and knowledge to provide "... a common core of evidence-based health knowledge delivered by a single integrated knowledge service ... by fully integrating the development of NHS knowledge systems" [24]. The NKS project, which is funded by the DoH, includes the following:

• An analysis and definition of the knowledge needs of clinicians and patients in a variety of health services.
• The creation of knowledge resources and knowledge artifacts, which are either created "in-house" or outsourced to specification.
• The implementation or delivery of those knowledge resources and knowledge artifacts using approved technologies to agreed standards.
• The development of knowledge skills and practices at an organizational level to use those resources effectively.
• The active promotion of the NKS to foster and spread good practice and encourage the development of local KM strategies [24].

It was recognized that the sheer size of the NHS is likely to create problems in promoting KM. Initiatives tend to be successful on a local rather than global scale, and the implementation of the KM strategy is "... in pockets rather than across the board" [24]. Clearly, the challenge is to adopt a KM strategy that "... avoids a postcode lottery in terms of good knowledge management practice ... to strike a balance between national coherence and local creativity" [24]. The danger of focusing on vertical (i.e. narrowly based) KM systems that focus on clinical and evidence-based medicine is also recognized by the need to keep in view other domains of knowledge and develop horizontal (i.e. generic) KM systems. This is important in recognizing the importance of the "customer service" aspect of healthcare, which is an important part of the NHS modernization program: "the biggest healthcare project in the world" [24].

15.7   Responsibility for Knowledge Management Strategy

The responsibility for the overall direction of the KM strategy in NHS trusts is being devolved to local organizations, in theory to allow ". . . local choice consistent with a nationally integrated service" [24], as was first proposed in 2001 in "Shifting the balance of power" [25]. This important document in effect served to consolidate the previous initiatives by placing the DoH in a position where it provides national leadership, sets national guidelines, and undertakes some central procurement (i.e. "the strategy"), while the implementation of KM initiatives and projects is carried out at local level, overseen by SHAs (i.e. "the policies"). The DoH is a member of the UK Government's Knowledge Network, which is overseen directly by the office of the e-Envoy. The DoH has a KM strategy founded on three components, i.e. people, processes, and technology, with four key components: people and change, leadership and accountability, content and processes, and information and technical infrastructure. This strategy is based on two basic precepts, expressed in a singularly informal manner:

• Recognizing the ways in which you/we/they are doing it (knowledge management) already, e.g. through the use of e-mail, shared document drives, desktop access to information and knowledge bases, the departmental intranet, online staff directories meetings, seminars, informal chats at the coffee machine, etc.
• Building on this by doing it better, e.g. by improving access to information and "joining up" information assets, providing training and guidance, piloting new ways to capture and share knowledge, etc. [24].

Two of the most important "national initiatives" in support of the KM strategy that are in various stages of development in the UK are described in Section 15.8 (namely the NeLH) and Section 15.9 (namely the Map of Medicine^{TM}).

15.8   The National Electronic Library for Health

The NeLH was founded in 1998 by Sir Muir Grey, who received recognition for his commitment to knowledge management and his input to the NPIT in the Queen's Birthday Honours List in 2005. Reference [26] states that ". . . knowledge is the enemy of disease and it is only through the work we are doing (at NHS Connecting for Health) that we can turn knowledge into action." Sir Muir went on to become the Director of NeLH and Programme Director of the National Screening Committee.

This view, coming from such an eminent clinician, is unequivocal in its support for KM within the NPIT. Further, at a meeting of the NPIT National Clinical Advisory Board (NCAB) in January 2004, a presentation was given on "Knowledge—the enemy of disease" [11], in which the importance of KM and the differences between knowledge support and decision support were discussed. An appeal was made for representatives from each of the organizations represented on NCAB who are "interested in knowledge and decision support" to examine potential applications of decision support in a KM context [11, p. 3]. From initiatives such as these and the influence of medical practitioners within the NHS on the NPIT, some interesting and important KM applications have been developed and are already in use.

Writing in 2003, Anne Brice, the Specialist Libraries Development Co-ordinator for the NeLH, points out that "The application of the knowledge we already possess has greater potential to improve the health of patients than any drug or technology likely to be developed in the next decade" [27]. Sir Muir Gray identified that knowledge resources were not being used effectively, and such medical knowledge that was available outside its immediate domain was often not made available nationally where it was needed. The types of knowledge that are needed by clinicians and patients are knowledge from research, knowledge from data, and knowledge from experience [27]. The NeLH gives specific advice to NHS professionals, describing the KM process as ". . . the activities or initiatives you put into place to enable and facilitate the creation, sharing and use of knowledge for the benefit of your organisation" [28]. The NeLH was aimed to contribute to health and healthcare in the UK by providing users with the opportunity to become actively involved in the development and integration of systems enabling them to access to high-quality information to support local decision making [29]. The NeLH was seen as being critical to the successful delivery of the modernization agenda and was envisaged as having an important role in the "patient' empowerment" agenda of the NKS, which sought to develop an integrated approach to quality management which sought to address specific problems related to pediatric surgery [30].

The NeLH project soon recognized that research and knowledge needed to be "mobilized and localized" to cross the divide between the existence of knowledge and its practical use, and that time (to be spent in research) was the most critical constraint in making this happen. The balance between the need for information (and, therefore, knowledge) and the ability of the practitioners to access such information was very unequal. A study showed that practitioners in a "traditional" clinical setting needed to obtain important (i.e. non-routine) medical information about various patients up to 60 times in the average week (on average, twice for every two patients examined) and that the use of the knowledge gained from this information could have a significant effect on eight medical decisions every day. The research shows that the necessary information was obtained successfully in approximately 30% of cases, and that much of the information is from informal sources (e.g. colleagues' opinions), obsolete (e.g. out-of-date textbooks), or unqualified (e.g. biased or inaccurate primary research sources) [31]. An interesting comparison is made in a later study (but still in a similar environment) with the amount of time that clinicians had to obtain the necessary information [32].

In fact, there seemed to be an inverse relationship between the level of importance of the medical decision and the access to information that was required to support it. Medical students (who, it may be assumed, need comparatively basic medical knowledge) might spend 60 min per week reading medical journals, while house officers did not spend any time at all acquiring/accessing such knowledge sources. Time was not the only constraint highlighted in the study on the practitioner's ability to acquire useful knowledge. The indiscriminate proliferation of information that is offered to healthcare professionals may have restricted their ability to use it effectively [33], as practitioners during 1998 were sent an average of almost 23 kg of medical guidelines, and more than eight sources of medical advice from the DoH and NHS. Other studies show that some practitioners spent more time in a typical week driving than reading [34]. The other major restriction on the acquisition of knowledge was poor IT literacy, which was identified in research carried out at approximately the same time involving community nurses, in which 60% had experienced a specific need for clinical information during the 6-month period of the study, but only 6% had succeeded in obtaining the necessary information from a specialist nursing database [34].

"Information for health" [20] specified that the design, development, and implementation of the NeLH should be undertaken by a partnership of healthcare professionals and IT and library professionals—in effect a CoP [2]. The construction of the NeLH was based on a process that first requires the creation of specialist libraries (SLs; originally termed virtual branch libraries), each of which services a CoP with specialist knowledge, each based on one of three types of specialism: demographic grouping (e.g. pediatric or geriatric medicine), healthcare activity (e.g. primary care or public health), and disease grouping (based on the MeSH system) [27]. Each SL is a dedicated repository with the primary task of organizing a common knowledge core. It is managed by leading healthcare professionals (both the producers and consumers of knowledge) and is maintained by accredited NHS IT specialists. This knowledge is integrated into databases of care pathways, a "search engine" for medical guidelines, and "information zones to support key NHS priorities" [27]. The SL management teams identify ways in which information needs can be met, identify gaps in the knowledge, and develop new knowledge resources according to recognized quality standards. The SLs integrate the following types of knowledge:

• Research knowledge containing refereed and systematically updated reviews of the effectiveness of treatments, drawn from sources such as Clinical Evidence, the Cochrane Library, and the National Institute for Clinical Excellence.
• Experiential knowledge derived from good practice and service improvement guides and communications from the NHS Modernisation Agency.
• Empirical intelligence of practice and treatment effectiveness, such as that provided by the Public Health Observatory.

The effectiveness of the IT component of the NeLH program in supporting CoPs was evaluated in a study undertaken in 2002 by the University of Aberystwyth, which sought to place NHS CoPs according to four development stages:

- *Potential* for connecting specialists into a CoP. Activities at this stage include engaging SL stakeholders, establishing reference groups, and liaising with other CoPs and the NeLH core team.
- *Building* the CoP based on sharing experiences, developing stories, and case studies, establishing a common vocabulary and identifying resources in the domain that may be added to the SL.
- *Engaged* in access to knowledge and learning by CoP members. At this stage the accent will be on "outreach," offering support to CoP members and involving stakeholders in contributing to the SL.
- *Active* in operating and maintaining the CoP and the SL for "real-world" applications, such as treatment planning and benchmarking.

The characteristics of each of the above stages were compared with the objectives that were specified in the SL development plans and the CoP was placed in one of the stages according to its characteristics. The report found that few of the CoP SL "teams" had reached the "active" stage (i.e. were fully functional), a significant number were at the "engaged" stage. Many more were at the "building" stage and all had passed the "potential" stage [27]. The study identified some key result areas that should be considered if CoPs are to develop and remain viable in supporting SLs. These include the following:

- Promoting stakeholder involvement through the involvement of a variety of collaborative frameworks and models of sponsorship and extended partnership. The development of collaborative procedures to unite stakeholder organizations is a core competence of SL teams [35].
- Establishing a "community of networks" by linking individual centers of excellence and expertise (i.e. other SLs and CoPs) as a basis for building further cooperation between specialists.
- Developing a support program for training and development in the technical aspects of KM (e.g. research methods, IT and communication, and knowledge elicitation and representation) to maximize the quality and utility of the knowledge base [35].
- Building a flexible technical platform (it may be implied that this is a form of portal) [36] that presents information from different sources (internal and external to the SL) in a way that is transparent to the user (or "knowledge worker").
- Ensuring rapid and "on demand" presentation of information in "24/7" mode (i.e. continuous service) that "reflects the rhythm of the workplace" [27] and presents information at an appropriate level of detail for its clinical purpose.
- Arriving at an appropriate combination of the type of knowledge (e.g. knowledge from experience and knowledge from research) and the balance of quality and timeliness of knowledge (i.e. "best current knowledge") derived from the SL.

It is not stated, but it may be implied that clinical KM systems are more broadly effective when the contents are shared with patients. The NeLH is completely open to patients and the public, working closely with NHS Direct Online in involving both these groups in CoPs [37].

15.9   The Map of Medicine™

The Map of Medicine™ is described by its creators as "a fast intuitive, easy-to-use support tool that is reflective of the way clinicians think" and "a visual representation of specialist knowledge enabling clinicians to use the exact information required to help patients along their journey within the NHS" (www.mapofmedicine.co.uk). In other words, it is a decision-support system based on "clinical processes" or items of medical information that are hyperlinked in a way that can be used to represent knowledge in support of the decision-making process. The interface is designed to allow clinicians to navigate through over 300 possible "patient journeys" to find the relevant information that will advise them on patient treatment. The map includes patient journeys in areas such as accident and emergency, internal medicine, obstetrics, gynecology, and oncology. Examples of journeys or pathways are shown with a demonstration on the NHS Library for Health Website [38]. It is noticeable that the map was developed as a result of a medical initiative by Dr Owen Epstein and more than 300 doctors and nurses in the Royal Free Hospital and University College Medical Schools, the Royal Free Hampstead NHS Trust and the NHS National Library for Health. The software is the intellectual property of Medic-to-Medic, a subsidiary company of UCL BioMedica PLC, a wholly owned investment fund of University College London, which signed its first (local) contract with Fujitsu Services, one of the NPITs local service providers (LSPs) in 2004 [12].

According to its originator, the stimulus to the development of the map was the need to distribute existing knowledge more widely among practitioners and to unite disparate knowledge elements within a standard framework [39]:

Imagine if every NHS clinician knew what all (the other) NHS clinicians know—the Map is the electronic glue to bring local specialist knowledge together acting as a virtual "desktop consultant" for healthcare professionals to use when the patient's journey leads them into unfamiliar territory.

Trials conducted by the Royal Free Hospital into 13 general practices and its own Accident and Emergency Department show positive results, demonstrating [39]

that doctors (i.e. GPs) use the Map to support their decision-making, often after morning surgery. Two thirds of them now use the Map on a regular basis and work in A&E shows that the Map is improving decision making on admissions to hospital.

At the moment the map is being used in a localized area where it was developed, but Medic-to-Medic are in discussions with other LSPs across the country with the aim of making the map available nationally and to integrate it into the NPIT. Under this program, Fujitsu will initially deploy the map across the south of England in parallel with an upgrade of local NHS IT systems as part of the NPIT. According to its Medical Director, Dr. Michael Stein, there are plans to introduce the Map into the Canadian Health Service [48].

15.10   The Current National Health Service Approach to Knowledge Management

The NeLH recognizes that early approaches to KM had a strong focus on the technology and on vendor-driven "knowledge management solutions" based on IT. The role of IT as "a solution" (rather than an enabler) led to the abandonment of some early KM projects or a lack of utility in their deliverables, leading to the so-called "knowledge management graveyard" [40]. More recently, the approach to the use of IT has been to recognize that KM is about the interaction of "people, processes, and technology" and the use of IT to support KM in two ways:

- Organizing, storing, and accessing *explicit* knowledge in electronic libraries and "best practice" databases.
- Connecting individuals and CoPs so that they can share *tacit* knowledge in a way that overcomes time and location barriers through the use of forums, groupware, and video-conferencing systems.

It is worth remarking that, until relatively recently, the characteristics of the technology were more suited to explicit knowledge, i.e. to the storage and processing of *facts* in the form of data and information relating to knowledge. This seems to be at odds with opinions that up to 80% of an organization's knowledge (and this possibly applies more to the NHS than most organizations) is in tacit form. Appropriately, more recent developments in technology (such as those which support NeLH and the Map of Medicine^{TM}) are tending to focus more on communication and collaboration processes than on storage and display [41]. Further, the importance of aligning the KM technology closely with individual preferences in terms of work practices and with organizational forms is generally recognized [42]. The same source sets out a "rule of thumb" that the proportion of the organizational investment in technology in terms of cost and effort should be less than 50% of the investment in the total KM effort.

This is intended to show the importance of people, processes, and structure in the KM effort, but also serves to focus the mind of nontechnical managers on the importance of making the correct choices and decisions when using IT as a part of the KM infrastructure in ensuring that it "adds value" by reducing "the cost, time and effort needed for people to share knowledge and information" [40]. Without going into specific detail about the individual proprietary IT packages, applications, and techniques, the NHS strategic plan has identified and recommend the generic tools, technologies, and techniques [40] on which the NHS KM infrastructure may be based:

- *Personal knowledge tools.* These are technologies or techniques that are intended primarily for use by individuals in developing, augmenting, and storing their personal "knowledge base." In other words, they support the generic mental processes in which knowledge workers are involved. Such tools can include: decision support tools, which may be graphical (e.g. decision trees and

Ishikawa diagrams); statistical (e.g. quantitative analysis) or technological tools (e.g. decision-support systems, intelligent knowledge-based systems, data mining tools, and intelligent agents); and electronic learning (e-learning) tools. Online dictionaries and thesauri and search engines (e.g. Google or Yahoo) and portals (which may be customized versions of search engines or specially design Internet applications) also fit into this category;

- *Connecting tools.* These are processes or technologies that seek to promote the objectives of "connecting people with people" or "providing a one-stop knowledge shop." Factors which need to be borne in mind when selecting connecting tools include the "time factor" (i.e. whether the connection needs to take place "in real time"), place (i.e. the location of the people to be connected), and the importance of "social presence" (i.e. the importance of the personal presence of those taking part in the communication). Tools in this category will be based on the principles of universal access to information and ease of access and use. They can involve synchronous or asynchronous communication modes. Such tools could include something so basic as electronic mail systems (e.g. Microsoft Outlook), video-conferencing meetings (either from specialized studios or from the workstation), special-interest discussion boards or forums, and intranets and extranets (i.e. Internet technology restricted to a given interest group or part of the organization);

- *Collaborative tools.* These allow people to work together in teams and enable the sharing of tacit knowledge among those teams and beyond. They imply tangible advantages (e.g. the saving of traveling time and subsistence costs) or intangible advantages (e.g. enabling people to share tacit knowledge and access the knowledge of remote experts and allowing people to work together in teams irrespective of location or time factors). Such tools include groupware (e.g. proprietary packages such as Lotus Notes and Microsoft Exchange), workflow and project-support tools (which enable the modeling of joint work processes and the sharing of documents), and virtual working tools (which can be used to perform remote processes). This latter category is potentially important, as it can involve tools that enable manual as well as intellectual tasks to be carried out remotely (e.g. doctors in the US have performed surgical operations on patients in Europe [40] by controlling robot arms over the Internet).

15.11   Recommendations for Best Practice

Clearly, there is considerable potential for the use of such tools and technologies in support of KM in NHS healthcare in general, and it is clear that the NeLH managers are aware of that potential. There are, however, a number of specific problems in implementing such systems and adopting such tools in an organization so large and so wide in scope as the NHS. It is important that certain factors need to be in place if their implementation, "roll out," and use is to be effective in practice. Ensuring that a healthcare organization is able to deploy these tools in support of a KM strategy requires a complex interrelationship between processes and structures. It is recommended that the following organizational and KM processes and structures are considered and addressed.

15.11.1   *Organizational Processes*

This factor relates to the way people carry out their work and how they interact with other actors in the "knowledge chain." The organization should consider the extent to which there is scope of individuals to be innovative or creative in obtaining access to knowledge, the degree to which the processes of an organization are based on rules or routine and the amount of time and opportunity that people have to access and share knowledge in both formal and informal ways. Formal processes of favor the promulgation of explicit knowledge, while informal processes are often matched with tacit knowledge. It should be noted that he formalization of processes is often a characteristic of healthcare organizations, whereas much of the knowledge that is used in healthcare is of the tacit variety.

15.11.2   *Organizational Structure*

The organizational processes will be supported by an appropriate organizational structure. This can include factors that typify an organization that is long established or has been created by amalgamating organization units into large conglomerations. This would certainly include SHAs and NHS trusts. The organization should examine the location and temporal factors that may promote or inhibit KM processes. For instance, the relationship between the different departments or CoPs should be noted. This relationship may favor competition rather than collaboration where the departments are expected to compete for resources (e.g. for IT projects), and some departments may be competing in terms of a professional status based on expertise. In such situations it can be difficult to promote the sharing of knowledge.

A similar situation can apply where the organization has a very "traditional" or a hierarchical structure. If there are many layers of line management and administrational staff (i.e. a long "chain of command"), then it can be more difficult to implement KM principles than with flatter, more "functional" structures which place expertise near the point at which knowledge is used.

15.11.3   *Knowledge Management Processes*

There is a clear relationship between the organizational processes and the organizational infrastructure. Both of these factors will need to be appropriate to support the KM processes that will be needed in the organization. KM processes are those that form the KM lifecycle, in other words the creation or acquisition of new knowledge, the organization and storage of knowledge which is in the organization, and the sharing and usage of organizational knowledge for specific purposes. In order to support KM processes, a number of factors have been identified by NeLH [40]:

- There should be a KM strategy in place at the strategic business unit level. This is are being encouraged throughout the NHS, at SHA and hospital trust level [43].
- Organizations should conduct knowledge audits to identify knowledge needs and knowledge resources and existing applications of and needs for knowledge. Methods such as MaKE [44] have been suggested for this application.
- Specific attention should be given to establishing processes and events for creating and acquiring "new" knowledge (i.e. new to the organization) through training initiatives and collaborations.
- There should be encouragement for "connecting people to people" through workshops, focus groups, and the establishment of CoPs.
- Formal KM processes should be supported by the use of KM tools (e.g. "best-practice databases, content management tools, and knowledge portals). The use of these tools should be encouraged through the use of mentoring and peer assistance programs.
- Workers should be encouraged to think and work in a way that recognizes KM practices in their day-to-day work, such as the use of log books, self-evaluation, and "story-telling" sessions [45].

It is worth pointing out that some of these recommendations constitute existing practices or "common sense." In fact, they are often examples of good practice in organizational processes that are being applied to KM. They are simply being considered from a new perspective and with a focus on knowledge. This can make them more acceptable to workers who are suspicious of radical new concepts such as KM. Unfortunately, recommendations for applying these KM processes cannot be prescriptive: the "KM toolkit" [40] will depend on the organization processes and structure relating to each healthcare unit.

15.11.4   Knowledge Management Infrastructure

The KM processes will need to be supported by an appropriate KM infrastructure in the same way as the organizational processes use the organizational infrastructure. Again, a set of principles or recommendations can be offered for consideration to ensure that this match is effective. Some of these are as follows:

- Serious steps should be taken to ensure management "buy-in" and support for KM processes. In principle, support for KM at a senior level is needed, but it may not be enough on its own. The support of a wide range of managers across the organization will be needed to ensure the effective identification and implementation of KM processes. Therefore, as well as a "mission statement," steering groups involving representatives from different functions will be needed to ensure that people feel recognized and are involved in the communication chain;
- The ownership or "place" of KM in the organization should be defined. Issues such as responsibility for promoting and organizing KM initiatives and the relationship between KM and other organizational issues and priorities need to be considered. It has been observed in the NHS [40] that there may be too much

emphasis on the technology at the expense of organizational or personnel factors if KM is "placed" within IT. Conversely, if responsibility for KM is lodged within a research faculty, then the development of new knowledge may take priority over the reuse of existing knowledge.

- There should be a "core team" of KM managers, facilitators, and champions which is aligned with the organizational structure. This KM function will be responsible for initiating, coordinating, and monitoring the effectiveness of KM initiatives throughout the organization. As with a number of the other factors in the KM field, the structure (i.e. the number of "levels") and use of the core team (i.e. its responsibilities) will vary greatly between healthcare organizations, according to their size and structure. It is worth pointing out that, as KM is by definition a "functional" (rather than a line management) issue, the "management overhead" for KM should be kept to the minimum to be effective. Most sizeable organizations will need have a KM Director and a network of Knowledge Managers.

- The organization should encourage experts to engage in the KM process, by creating a network of KM knowledge "brokers," "facilitators," or "champions." These are people who are in a position to aid the KM processes and to interact efficiently with the organizational processes and structure. It may be possible to identify people who are already undertaking this role (e.g. researchers, librarians, Web-masters) even though they may not consider themselves to be involved in KM. If an effective network of such people is not already in place, then it will be necessary to recruit or train them.

- External contacts should be established and maintained. Such "networking" initiatives are important, as healthcare knowledge is frequently more readily available outside the organization than within it and because KM is a rapidly evolving discipline. In this respect, the membership of professional bodies, attendance at conferences, and subscription to academic journals can be important. Also, external consultants are often instrumental in implementing KM initiatives, particularly where IT tools are involved. Clearly, this involves expense (as well as effort) on the part of the organization. The healthcare organization must consider its own individual characteristics and "tailor" a system to suit its specific needs.

It is worth pointing out that the distinction between the various structures and processes will become less distinct as KM becomes more integrated into the organization.

15.12   Summary

The NHS is a large and diverse organization which has a complex range of disciplines and practices and a variety of infrastructures and technologies. It is also "knowledge rich" and takes part in many of the practices that are associated with KM and has a noticeable emphasis on the existence of "bodies of knowledge and

"CoPs." The NHS can, therefore, benefit from the latest KM practices and processes and from the tools and technologies that are being developed to support them. There is clear evidence that the importance of KM is recognized within the NHS, as many initiatives are in place and initiatives are being followed (e.g. the Map of Medicine™). There is a wide range of guidance available to managers in the form of Websites and portals and through the NeLH. Many of the organizations and trusts that make up the NHS have implemented KM strategies and have put into place organizational structures that are intended to promote KM.

There is evidence that this approach is proving to be effective, but KM is a rapidly evolving discipline, and organizations must be careful to keep up with changes in the field. It is possible to identify key factors that can improve the effectiveness of KM in the NHS in four areas: organizational processes, organizational structure, KM processes, and KM infrastructure. Recommendations for ensuring effectiveness in these areas include organizational and personnel factors, as well as the use of technological tools.

References

1. National Programme for IT in Health. 'Connecting for health'. Available from: http://www.connectingforhealth.nhs.uk/ [20 October 2005].
2. Brown JS, Duguid P. Organisational learning and communities of practice: towards a unified view of learning and innovation. *Organ Sci* 1991;2(1):40–57.
3. Bran J. The 60 second interview—inside knowledge. *Knowl Manage Mag* 2002;5(6). Available from: http://www.kmmagazine.com/xq/asp. [10 November 2005].
4. Ciborra C. The Limits Of Strategic Information Systems. *Int J Inf Resource Manage* 1991;2(3):11–17.
5. Endsley S, Kirkegaaard M, Linares A. Working together: communities of practice in family medicine; 2005. Available from: http://www.aafp.org/fpm/20050100/28work.html [10 October 2005].
6. Nonaka I. A dynamic theory of organisational knowledge creation. *Organ Sci* 1994;5(1): 14–37.
7. Polanyi M. *The tacit dimension.* New York: Doubleday; 1967.
8. Endsley S, Kirkegaard M, Linares A. Working together—communities of practice in family medicine. *Fam Pract Manage* 2005;12(1):28–33.
9. Gruber TR. A translation approach to portable ontologies. *Knowl Acquis* 1993;5(2): 199–220.
10. Benjamins VR, Fensel D, Gomez Perez A. Knowledge management through ontologies. In: Reimer U, editor, *Proceedings of the 2nd International Conference on Practical Aspects of Knowledge Management (PAKM98)*, Basel, Switzerland, 29–30 October 1998.
11. National Programme for Information Technology minutes of the National Clinical Advisory Board meeting held on the 15 January 2004. Available at http://www.connectingforhealth.nhs.uk/publications/ncab_minutes_jan04.pdf [20 October 2005].
12. The Map of Medicine: 13 Million People to Benefit from Improved Clinical Practice Thanks to the Map of Medicine[TM]. Website of the Country Doctor's Association. Available at http://www.countrydoctor.co.uk/precis%20–%20Map%20of%20Medicine.htm. Accessed 1st July 2006.

13. Alavi M, Leidner DE. Knowledge management systems: issues, challenges and benefits. *Commun AIS* 1999;1(7).
14. Benjamins VR, Fensel D, Gomez Perez A. Knowledge management through ontologies. In: Reimer U, editor, *Proceedings of the 2nd International Conference on Practical Aspects of Knowledge Management (PAKM98)*, Basel, Switzerland, 29–30 October 1998.
15. Angus J, Patel J, Harty J. Knowledge management: great concept, but what is it? *Inf Week*. 1998;(June).
16. Hahn J, Subramani MR. A framework of knowledge management systems: issues and challenges for theory and practice. In: *Proceedings of the International Conference on Information Systems, ICIS*, 13–15 December 2000, Brisbane, Australia.
17. Zack MH. Developing a knowledge strategy. *Calif Manage Rev* 1999;41(3):125–145.
18. Department of Health. *The new NHS—modern, dependable*; 1997.
19. *Our information age*. London: HMSO; 1998.
20. Department of Health. *Information for health*; 1998.
21. Department of Health. *A first class service: quality in the new NHS*; 1998.
22. Department of Health. *R&D for a first class service*; 2000.
23. Department of Health. *An organisation with a memory*; 2000.
24. *Knowledge management in the NHS*; 2003. Available from: http://www.nelh.nhs.uk/knowledge_management/km1/nhs.asp [3 November 2005].
25. Department of Health. *Shifting the balance of power*; 2001.
26. *Knighthood for NHS connecting for Health Director*. Available from: http://www.connectingforhealth.nhs.uk/publications/ncab_minutes_jan04.pdf [10 October 2005].
27. Brice A, Gray M. Knowledge is the enemy of disease. *Update Mag* 2003;(March). Available from: http://www.cilip.org.uk/publications/updatemagazine/archive/archive2003/march/update03 [10 November 2005].
28. NeLH Specialist Library. *Entry "Knowledge management."* Available from: http://libraries.nelh.nhs.uk/knowledgemanagement/viewResource.asp? [20 November 2005].
29. Turner A. A first-class knowledge service: developing the National Electronic Library for Health. *Health Inf J* 2002;(19):133–145.
30. T.S.O. Learning from Bristol: the Department of Health's response to the report of the public enquiry into children's heart surgery at the Bristol Royal Infirmary 1984–1995. Cm 5363; 2002.
31. Covell DG, Uman GC, Manning PR. Information needs in office practice, are they being met? *Ann Intern Med* 1985;(103):596–599.
32. Sackett DL, Richardson WS, Rosenberg WMC, Haynes RB. Surveys of self-reported reading times of consultants in Oxford, Birmingham, Milton Keynes, Leicester and Glasgow. In: Rosenberg WMC, et al., editors, *Evidence-based medicine*. Churchill Livingstone; 1997.
33. De Lusignan S, Chan T, Pritchard K, Wells S. Can the implementation of a KM strategy in primary healthcare provide an antidote for information overload? *Curr Persp Healthcare Comput Year* 2003;151–158.
34. Farmer J. Improving access to information for nursing staff in remote areas: the potential of the Internet and other networked information sources. Unpublished Working Paper. Robert Gordon University; 1997.
35. Guah MW, Currie WL. Factors affecting IT-based knowledge management strategy in the UK healthcare system. *J Inf Knowl Manage* 2004;3(4):279–290.

36. Skyrme DJ. Portals—panacea or pig? *I³ Update—Entovation Int News* 2000;(44) (October). Available from: http://www.skyrme.com/updates/u44_f2.htm.

37. Neves A. Achieving a health KM assessment: how a knowledge-audit exercise recently carried out at the NHS Modernisation Agency has helped to gauge the success of the KM strategy already in place. *Knowl Manage* 2004;7(10):29–31.

38. NHS Library for Health. *Map of Medicine*. Available from: http://www.mtmsolutions. com/sample/index.html [1 December 2005].

39. Press release: 13 million people to benefit from improved clinical practice thanks to the Map of Medicine™. Available from: http://213.130.38.90/pressrelease.pdf [20 October 2005].

40. NHS Library for Health. *Knowledge management technology*. Available from: http://www.nelh.nhs.uk/knowledge_management/km2/technology.asp [21 December 2005].

41. Coyne C. On the Web: a sense of place. *Knowl Manage* 2003;6(5)(January). Available from: http://www.KMmagazine.com.

42. Davenport TH, Prusak L. *Working knowledge: how organisations manage what they know.* Harvard Business School Press; 2000.

43. NHS Information Authority Strategic Plan Version 2.4. January 2002. NHSIA.

44. Sharp PJ. MaKE—a knowledge management method. Unpublished PhD thesis, Staffordshire University, UK; 2003.

45. Snowden D. Complex acts of knowledge: paradox and descriptive Self-awareness. *J Knowl Manage* 2002;6(2):1–13.

46. Davenport TH, Prusak L. *Working knowledge: how organisations manage what they know.* Harvard Business School Press; 1997.

47. Electronic Health Records: from Concept to Patient-held Reality. Freer D. and Crouch P. Proceedings of the 3rd Annual Southern Institute for Health Informatics 2000 Conference, September 2000, University of Portsmouth. Available at http://www.disco.port.ac.uk/hcc/sihi/sihi2000/proceedings/Freer/sld001.htm. Accessed 1st July 2006.

48. Zeidenberg J. Map of Medicine provides 'best practices' support to clinicians via web. Website of Canadian Healthcare Technology. Available at http://www.canhealth.com/jul05.html#05junstory3. Accessed 1st July 2006.

16
We Haven't Got a Plan, so What Can Go Wrong? Where is the NHS Coming from?

ANNETTE COPPER

Abstract

There is no getting away from the fact that the UK's National Health Service (NHS) needs managing. However, it seems there is no word that sits more uncomfortably than this one when it comes to the necessary business of administering the NHS. There are a hundred-and-one ways to interpret the form and function of the NHS, but one thing is for sure: it is an unsettled environment. There is a direct correlation between its perceived public health efficacy and the "reforms" instituted and administered down the years, both nationally and locally; and for those who are the administrators of the system, both front line and managerially, these reforms come so thick and fast that it seems there is never an opportunity to consolidate change.

At the apex of all this change are the political taskmasters devolving politics straight into the NHS via the NHS strategic health authorities (SHAs). The SHAs offer their vision for the future in their strategic frameworks, offering glimpses of the future via policy interpretation.

However, more is needed beyond strategic frameworks and the increased use of targeted performance measures to address the ills of the NHS.

There is one thing that will never change, whatever the future holds: people make the NHS function. No matter how these relationships are as dictated in the future, no matter how systemically the NHS changes, it will always need people to make it function. The current political climate dictates that reform is a collection point that beleaguered clinicians and managers need to gather around. The time for clinicians and managers to argue whether they are playing on the same team is over. The story is no longer the polemic of individual patient care versus resources and productivity, but one of joint leadership and mutual dependence between clinicians and managers. Taking a systems approach to handling this relationship step change can help overcome the culturally habituated behaviors that have held back the development of satisfying working relationships so far. Modeling these relationships is easy, and they are the focus of this chapter; embedding them in the belief that they are the only way to protect the dispensing of services in a locally sensitive way is another story.

16.1   Introduction

There are a hundred-and-one ways to interpret the form and function of the UK's National Health Service (NHS), but one thing is for sure: it is an unsettled environment. The current temperature of the NHS is running high. Constantly in a state of "reform" incorporating the changes that are to be administered nationally and locally, it can never settle down into a system of good practice comprehensively understood across the service. It runs so hot all the time trying to incorporate change that there is never a cooling-off period to consolidate change.

At the apex of all this change are the political taskmasters devolving politics straight into the NHS via the NHS strategic health authorities (SHAs). The SHAs offer their vision for the future in their strategic frameworks, offering glimpses of the future via policy interpretation. A common example of this, and I use it because it is atypical of the vision many SHAs have, is the Trent Strategic Health Authority Strategic Framework 2005–10 [1]. The whole system approach based on learning, innovation, and devolution is intended to be responsive to the needs of staff to create a world-class workforce, to reduce inequality and to enable patients to be treated according to need. Their focus is:

- improving *equity*
- putting the *customer first*
- expanding *choice*
- improving *standards*
- strengthening *accountability*.

Strategic frameworks are all well and good on paper; however, for so many working in the NHS they just read like so much rhetoric. The problem is that detailed system change is often modeled on pilot site results that cannot translate directly into local service delivery, as detailed replication is unpredictable in a local setting. What really works has to be discovered through trying different interventions that can be evaluated. Novel approaches need defining and working out on a small scale initially, but how responsive are staff to experimenting with patient delivery? Truthfully, many feel fixed to the spot dealing with policy change delivering the NHS Improvement Plan and creating a patient-led NHS. What emerges is a gap between what is outlined in policy documents, plans, and frameworks and how they work out [2]. Redesign in healthcare then becomes a battlefield. The change may be described in terms of whole-system solutions, but the reality becomes a focus on line management and individual performances: redesign becomes short-term milestones, and encouraging entrepreneurship and innovative becomes "don't fail".

If this undercurrent is familiar to you, is there comfort to be found anywhere? Is there a more objective means of determining effectiveness and efficiency across the service? The NHS star rating system has offered the public a comparison between hospitals and primary care trusts (PCTs) using a standard evaluation process. They are also viewed as a benchmark for internal processes. The biggest question has to be whether the star rating system ultimately is an effective means of enhancing patients' experience of the NHS. Although the star rating system is not the only process used to measure performance, its results are published through the media for public scrutiny. The Centre for Health Economics, University of York, recently researched the impact of the star rating system in English acute hospitals [3]. There were many positive hospital responses to the star ratings, including the alignment of "internal performance management and reporting systems with key national targets" [3, p. 21]. The negative responses included "evidence of tunnel vision and a distortion of clinical priorities," reduced staff morale and public trust, and "bullying and intimidation" [3, p. 20]. Although this report does not cover all healthcare settings, there was one part of the report that could well describe the experiences of all. Not surprisingly, the critical feedback was that star ratings fail to take into consideration "local contingencies" and specific "mitigating factors that might help explain variations in the measure performance of hospitals." Many of these unique conditions are beyond the hospital's control; therefore, it is viewed as unfair that this would not be taken into consideration when the rating is calculated.

16.2   Targets and Management

The point is that the increased use of targeted performance measures to monitor the impact of health service reforms is by no means the only panacea to the NHS ills. It does, however, form an important component of the inevitable bundle of responses needed to bring the NHS into line with levels of efficiency and effectiveness that are acceptable to objective formulae and critical observers. Currently, the Economic and Social Research Council are conducting research examining the effectiveness of targets currently used in the NHS to develop and analyze a number of alternative performance measures. The project "Metrics, targets and performance: the case of NHS Trusts" [4], ran from April 2005 to March 2006:

...the NHS as a whole has not yet been reformed. There are still important problems to be solved and there is as yet no firm evidence to show that Labour's reforms have produced a marked difference in health outcomes. While much of the improvement in the NHS ... has been achieved through central fiat and targets, it is too early to predict whether the more recently introduced tools to lever up performance—greater use of market incentives and regulation—will achieve the desired outcome.

There is no getting away from the fact that the NHS needs managing. It seems there is no word that sits more uncomfortably than this one when it comes to the necessary business of administering the NHS. In terms of political involvement and administering the future NHS, the government's idea of a more cohesive management approach is [5]:

- To devolve more responsibilities to the NHS itself to take corporate decisions and actions, e.g. through the SHAs working together to manage the NHS Bank or through the NHS Confederation taking on a new role as an employers' organization.

- To move away from a system of departmental monitoring and regulation of organizations, to one where responsibility sits with new inspectorates and the new Office of the Independent Regulator for NHS Foundation Trusts, and developing a system where incentives start to have an impact.
- To strengthen commissioning of services by PCTs to create a system of alternative service providers within which patients can exercise individual choices and where they have more control over their care.
- To develop new relationships between the Department of Health, the NHS, local authorities and the new bodies—the Healthcare Commission, the Office of the Independent Regulator for NHS Foundation Trusts, the Commission for Social Care Inspection and National Institute for Clinical Excellence, and the Social Care Institute for Excellence—which between them manage and shape the whole system within which health and social care are delivered.

The key words here seem to be restructuring, devolution, incentives, and commissioning. Cleary, the changes to the NHS are going to continue apace. Having consolidated centrally to produce national standards, the government is now moving into phase two. The future, as seen through the eyes of the politicians, has an increasing emphasis on devolving decision making through partnership between commissioners, service providers, and patients so that the point of delivery has had all the necessary good-practice filters to ensure optimum care for the patient. "The objective is to create a dynamic system where responsibilities and roles increasingly gravitate to those best able to deliver them" [5].

16.3   The Clinician–Manager Relationship

There is a large publication list of literature addressing the current state and projected future of the NHS, and there may be any number of policy, strategy, and succession plans to be applied on a local level now and in the future. One thing that will never change, whatever the future holds, is that people are needed to make the NHS function; and no matter how these relationships are dictated in the future, no matter how systemically the NHS changes, it will always need people to make it function.

This reality is both the strength and the weakness of the NHS. The investment and reform that is the signature of the NHS Plan requires people to make it work. It sets an agenda addressing national standards, accountability and the diversification of service providers and patient choice. These drivers seem to be the source for a trend that has developed over time: the dysfunction between clinicians and managers. Healthcare delivery cannot function without them, so this discord cannot be swept under the carpet. Organizational and structural issues can be prescribed through policy and healthcare administration, but behavioral dynamics have to be uncovered to be addressed. This is not to say that all clinician and manager relationships are somewhere on the bipolar continuum between strained politeness and outright relationship breakdown, but a culture seems to have evolved around this relationship that has generated enough negative reporting to be a cause for concern for the delivery of quality patient care [6].

The tensions are not beyond understanding. The occupational lives of managers and clinicians can seem polarized, with managers focused on cost and efficiency and clinicians on treatment efficacy and pushing back the boundaries of healthcare. It can seem as though, year in year out, different managers are paraded in front of the same clinicians as if on a conveyer belt, as they advocate the latest management solution they want to effect which, much to the chagrin of clinicians, cannot be completely ignored. The central government health agenda is currently the ball game. One of the pitches in the ball game is patient-centered care. It is intended that "the NHS will shape its services around the needs and preferences of individual patients, their families, and their carers" [7], and maybe this is the pitch over which managers and clinicians can agree. Even here, though, there is a creeping anxiety among clinicians that managers are poaching on their territory, threatening their clinical autonomy when it comes to control over diagnosis and treatment, evaluation of care, nature, and volume of medical tasks and contractual independence [8].

Another frequently cited reason for this tension is public changes in attitudes to clinical autonomy and increased calls for accountability. Clinicians are always going to argue the need to exercise judgment when applying the reflective practice model of patient care, wanting to perform unfettered by any structural constraints that would impinge on their practice. The tension here is that their clinical delivery of care, expanding clinical knowledge, and the use of their individual discretion could be subsumed into a scientific–bureaucratic model that would undermine their individual discretion. Having said that, the government and the public have become increasingly demanding in the way they hold healthcare providers to account. And high-profile medical malpractice, e.g. the Harold Shipman and Bristol Hospital inquiries, has prompted the government to exercise a more regulatory approach and increased the pressure for the activity of clinicians to come under greater scrutiny. In addition, the growing costs of healthcare and its growing demands on the economy have meant that the decisions of doctors have come under examination and there are increasing attempts to control them.

Five new regulatory bodies were created in the NHS between 1998 and 2002. These bodies, some of which are now defunct, are, or were, all concerned primarily with the clinical quality of healthcare. Past regulation often focused on more peripheral administrative and managerial matters, not on clinical practice. Historically, regulation had assumed that clinical practice was fundamentally sound and impeccable in its intentions. The current approach, however, implicitly assumes that the NHS needs watching, perhaps as not all its motives serve the public good [9].

This has brought about a diminishing of trust and increased suspicion of professional influence, power, and autonomy. Clinical reflective practice derived from individual expertise and professional consensus, and based on expert opinion, is being replaced by critical appraisal and a benchmarking bureaucratic model.

Having sketched the changing status of clinicians, that of the managers in the NHS also needs addressing. The introduction of a quasi-internal market in 1991 significantly impacted on the NHS, and the managerial agenda shifted to the dictates of central government agendas. This increased government involvement was partly prompted by the need to get public expenditure under control. As this political focus narrowed in on public services generally, and the management of these services specifically, the previously held relationship between doctors and managers began shifting. At first, clinicians held their ground and employed their clinical status to underscore their authority. Managers at that time usually were administrators and did no more than offer administrative support without challenging the clinical view. However, the arrival of general management, internal market forces, and the introduction of clinical governance shifted this bias radically and placed more authority in the hands of managers, fueling the tension between themselves and clinicians.

However, this newly acquired power deposited on managers has not gone so well. Managers have to respond to the spending provisos of their funding organizations and there is an unrealizable expectation to improve and extend the service within the existing resources. By 2002, the Commission for Health Improvement concluded that very few NHS organizations were examples of good management and that more than 80% of NHS organizations tend to be reactive rather than proactive, they lack organization-wide policies and often have differing policies in multiple departments, and they communicate ineffectively and lack communication between managers and service providers and between doctors and nurses [10].

What is the cause of this poor performance? Arguably, the answer is less likely to be found in the abilities of NHS managers than in the system they have to work in. The NHS has a culture of compliance, where managers are accountable upwards, rather than outwards to patients, and they lack the freedom that general management needs and on which successful public service delivery depends.

Nigel Edwards of the NHS Confederation's Policy Director, is backing the King's Fund findings [11], saying:

Government health reforms such as Patient Choice, the new financial system Payment by Results and increased use of private sector providers are making NHS finances more volatile and less predictable. They are contributing to a projected NHS deficit of £620 million for 2005/06 which the Health Secretary announced last week so sending in 'turnaround teams' to achieve rapid reductions in deficits, as announced by Patricia Hewitt last week, may only provide a short-term solution. Blaming NHS managers for deficits is a diversion from the fact that the introduction of market mechanisms into the health service requires a more flexible financial regime [12].

So, if the clinicians are not really to blame and the managers are not really to blame, then who is? Politics always seems a good place to start. It has been argued that "the government's desperation to find ways of engaging with the public on issues close to its heart has led to a feverish obsession with healthcare" [13]. With healthcare policy having become increasingly prescriptive since the 1990s, it seems that riding the back of this obsession are management healthcare initiatives like so much frantic activity, swirling above the heads of NHS staff. It could be argued that anyone trying to ignore changes is not doing so as an act of sabotage, but more from conscientious objection. So, here we are, in the middle of things, or rather in the middle of 1.3 million staff wondering what to do.

16.4   The Way Forward for Clinicians and Managers

The current climate dictates that this relationship is one that needs resolving, and the political storm advancing itself as reform is the only collection point that these two beleaguered groups can gather around. It is not the intention here to minimize the historical and cultural differences between managers and clinicians, but these differences are now being superseded by political reform that could undermine the NHS to the point that it transforms into something no longer recognizable as a national health service. The truth is that managers are more than bean counters and can provide an overview of the systemic needs of the whole service they administer and target resources to optimize this administration, whilst clinicians are more than delivery points for healthcare and can be a reality check for managers concerning clinical realities and the apportioning of resources. Basically, whether they like it or not, they need each other (Table 16.1).

TABLE 16.1. Doctors and managers: who needs whom [14]?.

Doctors need managers	Managers need doctors
To resolve complexity of the working environment, which needs managing	Doctors are the vehicle of the "health delivery product"
To help them with unrealistic expectations	To ground them in the human and clinical reality of patient care
To mediate with the state	To translate government policy into clinical reality
To set boundaries of care	To recognize where boundaries are ineffective, unrealistic, or inhumane
To act as repositories of negative comments from patients and to deal with complaints against the omnipotence of doctors	To contain their anxiety in certain situations
To have an overview of the needs of the whole service and not be influenced by parochial needs or those of the most powerful and influential	To inform them about the clinical realities in order to decide on apportionment of resources
To get the resources that are required to deliver the service	To use resources effectively and efficiently
To help them understand networking and committee skills	To communicate evidence-based clinical practice based on sound scientific principles

Managers and doctors have more than one obvious thing in common, i.e. working for the same employer; more importantly, they share professional characteristics. Both are often following a career pathway, both are committed to working long and hard, in both professions there are specialists, and both have the need for effective communication to overcome their use of language exclusive to their professions. Despite these common factors, their different cultures and pressures can cause considerable difficulties in their relationships with each other.

Of course, an important aspect determining whether mutual interdependence is taken seriously is whether both partners are equal. Doctors can manage, although arguably not to the same level of expertise, but without a doubt managers cannot doctor. Managers will say that in order to manage effectively they need the support of doctors, but doctors rarely think that they need management support in order to practice effectively. Management skills are, however, essential for doctors heading a unit or clinical team.

It would seem that what really gets clinicians and managers agitated is the fact that resources are finite and in this way both are caught in the same fiscal trap. Conflict between the two almost always flares up around financial considerations; and in this current climate of accountability, management also now monitors risk and handles complaints against clinical staff, suspensions, internal inquiries, and external consultations.

The point is that they can either continue to be at loggerheads with one another or they can cooperate to maximize the likelihood of their managing their local services in a way that satisfies both adequately. The facts are that, currently, one-third of hospitals are going to have to cut services, funding agreements revisions are turning on a dime, freezing clinical recruitment and redundancies are becoming real possibilities, and the government is having a major case of denial [15].

The time for managers and clinicians to argue whether they are playing on the same team is over. The government is promising private healthcare providers with volumes of work to embed a more market-based system for healthcare. Payment by results [16] means that patient choice may create an unacceptable level of volatility. The Audit Commission says that this new funding method, where money follows the patient, is destabilizing the NHS and exacerbating the current financial crisis. Instead of increasing choice it could have the opposite effect, with services going to the wall unless the payment system is radically reformed, says the commission. It also cautions that critical services essential to support emergency admissions could close down in some hospitals because of the failure to attract patient referrals [17]. The NHS is continuing to morph into something else; and if the opportunity is not taken to redefine relationships now, then market forces will define them later.

The days when managers and clinicians scapegoated one another is no longer an exercise that can be indulged in at will. They need to work together to mitigate the systemic vulnerabilities in the NHS that they are going to be exposed to. The story is no longer the polemic of individual patient care versus resources and productivity, but of joint leadership and mutual dependence between managers and clinicians [18].

TABLE 16.2. Strategies for improvement [14].

Relationships
- Respect for differences between managers and doctors
- Ability to develop goals and strategies that are aligned with the clinicians involved
- Education: managers to learn about medicine and doctors about management techniques and how to navigate bureaucracies
- Staff stability to enable working relationships to develop

Reflective practice
- The capacity to stand back when there are conflicts in order to analyze the problem
- Consult a disinterested party

Educational
- For both doctors and managers to be educated on the impact of psychological processes at the organizational level
- Develop an academic basis for management and medical management/clinical leadership
- Foster early interdisciplinary education. Managers attending ward rounds and doctors attending management programs
- Better management research to redesign care processes based on best practice

Taking a systems approach to handling this relationship step change can help overcome the culturally habituated behaviors that have held back the development of satisfying working relationships. The point is that clinicians and managers alike make mistakes, and these are to be expected. If your organization has successfully set up risk management around both clinical and general management risk, then the foundation work has been done to allow systems of support and strategies to be developed that can mitigate risk. This can be very helpful in analyzing and finding solutions to perceived clinical and managerial failures. However, not all change can be handled indiscriminately by an individual; it requires input and representation from across all managers and clinicians to create a shared understanding of this organizational task and to legitimize the outcome.

The pressure is on in the NHS. It always has been, but it now seems to be at a tipping point that is genuinely causing deep anxiety, with the main contributory factor being the financial concerns wracking it. It is at times like these that falling into predictable patterns of behavior for clinicians and mangers can offer some comfort; retreating into a "them and us" position to apportion blame for real or perceived mishandling of healthcare administration is one way of avoiding seeing the bigger picture, which is the real issue, and which inevitably includes all those involved in delivering healthcare. Personal and group agendas resurface on meeting-room tables in a bid for self-preservation, and old neuroses play out rather than open dialogue in a search for joint and realistic resolutions. Unless logic and accord, rather than fear and worn-out expectations based on old grievances, become the standard, then the gap between clinicians and managers will remain. A variety of approaches can be used to address this relationship, but what must come first is the intent on the part of managers and clinicians to tackle whatever is coming at them over the next few weeks and months with an agreed understanding that they will be responsive rather than reactive to the vagaries of policy windshift and financial constraints. Some suggested headlines that each healthcare setting needs to consider to flesh out into a plan that will move this understanding are given in Table 16.2.

For each local healthcare setting, it is time to get a plan if they do not want their roles and responsibilities defined for them by forces beyond their control. There is a need to synthesize performance information and clinical reality for systemic healthcare improvement. This synthesis needs to become naturalized into managerial and clinical ways of working. Better solutions require a community of ambition. From being reactive to being proactive, from blaming to better problem solving, from command and control to shared leadership; and if you work in the NHS and you don't think that this is your job, then you definitely don't have a plan.

References

1. Trent Strategic Health Authority. *Planning with a purpose.* Available from: http://www.tsha.nhs.uk/strategic-framework/planning-for-the-future/planning-with-a-purpose [19 October 2005].
2. Leading Edge 2. *Aligning what we say and how we behave.* The NHS Confederation; 2001.
3. Davies H, Marshall M, Mannion R. *Impact of star performance ratings in English acute hospital trusts*; 2005. Available from: http://www.rsm.ac.uk/new/pdfs/art_stars05.pdf [19 October 2005].
4. *An independent audit of the NHS under Labour (1997–2005)*; April 2005. Available from: http://www.kingsfund.org.uk/resources/publications/an_independent.html [7 December 2005].
5. Department of Health. *Empowering local communities*; 2005. Available from: http://www.dh.gov.uk/PublicationsAndStatistics/Publications/PublicationsPolicyAnd Guidance/PublicationsPAmpGBrowsableDocument/fs/en?CONTENT_ID=4097241 &MULTIPAGE_ID=4914654&chk=0DNFbU [7 December 2005].
6. Edwards N. Doctors and managers: poor relationships may be damaging patients—what can be done? *Qual Saf Health Care* 2003;12:i21 (free full text).
7. NHS Core Principles. Available from: http://www.nhs.uk/England/AboutTheNhs/Core Principles.cmsx [7 December2005].
8. Davies HTO, Harrison S. Trends in doctor–manager relationships. *Br Med J* 2003;326: 646–649 (free full text).
9. Walshe K. The rise of regulation in the NHS. *Br Med J* 2002;324:967–970. Available from: http://bmj.bmjjournals.com/cgi/content/full/324/7343/967 (free text) [10 December 2005].
10. Haldenby A. *NHS management—part of the problem or part of the solution?* 2004. Available from: http://www.reform.co.uk/website/pressroom/articles.aspx?o=9 [10 December 2005].
11. Palmer K. *How should we deal with hospital failure? Facing the challenges of the new NHS market.* Available from: http://www.kingsfund.org.uk/resources/publications/ (free to download from the King's Fund Website) [10 December 2005].
12. Press release for NHS Confederation. *NHS Confederation response to King's Fund report. How should we deal with hospital failure? Facing the challenges of the new NHS*

market. Available from: http://www.nhsconfed.org/press/releases/nhs_confederation_response_to_kings_fund_report_how_should_we_deal_with_hospital_failur.asp [10 December 2005].

13. *Power to the patients?* Available from: http://www.spiked-online.com/Articles/0000000CA5CD.htm [7 December 2005].

14. Garelick A, Fagin L. The doctor–manager relationship. *Adv Psychiatr Treat* 2005;11: 241–250.

15. One in three NHS trusts plan to reduce services, BMA survey reveals, UK http://www.medicalnewstoday.com/medicalnews.php?newsid=31119 (accessed 5 December 2005)

16. Audit Commission. *Early lessons from payments by results*. Available from: http://www.audit-commission.gov.uk/reports/NATIONAL-REPORT.asp?CategoryID=ENGLISH^574&ProdID=B502F0FC-E007-4925-AD24-529C4889AD02&SectionID=sect66# [11 December 2005].

17. Times Online. *Patient choice is damaging hospitals says NHS watchdog*; 11 October 2005. Available from: http://www.timesonline.co.uk/article/0,,2-1820311,00.html [5 December 2005].

18. Crosson F. Kaiser Permanente: a propensity for partnership. *Br Med J* 2003;326:654 (free full text).

17
Healthcare Knowledge Management: Knowledge Management in the Perinatal Care Environment

MONIQUE FRIZE, ROBIN C. WALKER AND CHRISTINA CATLEY

Abstract

The chapter presents four key steps in the knowledge management process: access to quality clinical data; knowledge discovery; knowledge translation; and knowledge integration and sharing. Examples are provided for each of these steps for the perinatal care clinical environment and a number of artificial intelligence tools and analyses results are described. The usefulness of this approach for clinical decision support is discussed and the chapter concludes with suggestions on knowledge integration and sharing using Web services.

17.1   Introduction

17.1.1   Integrating Knowledge Management into Clinical Care

When a patient needs medical attention, the physician interacts with the patient through the constructs of the medical model, an ancient ethical and intellectual code for the physician which provides structured interview and examination techniques directed towards establishing a diagnosis and a management plan. The diagnosis is usually stated as a pathophysiologic condition due to an anatomic abnormality. Until a definitive diagnosis is established about the presenting problem, the physician deals with a working diagnosis, which implies the concepts of a differential diagnosis, investigative plan, and treatment plan. The differential diagnosis is a list of the other likely pathologic entities which may explain the patient's condition. The investigative plan deals with the uncertainty in the differential diagnosis by invoking testing strategies to "rule out" or "rule in" the conditions listed in the differential diagnosis. With the treatment plan, the patient's need for comfort is attended to and an attempt is made, using a variety of interventions, to return the pathologic state to as normal a physiologic state as possible.

The modern interaction between the physician and the patient is generally supplemented, especially in hospital practice, by testing systems (e.g. body fluid analysis, imaging, electrical signal analysis). Testing systems are used to increase or decrease the likelihood of a disease process and to monitor treatment. If the patient is healthy or the diagnosis and prognosis are known, then no testing need be done. Even if a definitive diagnosis is established, then the natural history (i.e. how the illness unfolds over time) is often uncertain for any one patient. The testing systems help to deal with the uncertainty in the diagnosis and management of patients [1].

17.1.2   The Healthcare Knowledge Management Process

The clinical databases, data-mining techniques, clinical decision-support (CDS) tools, and integration technologies discussed in this chapter, in relation to the perinatal care environment, are linked together in a four-step circular knowledge management (KM) process for perinatal care. Figure 17.1 shows a diagram of the four steps described in the KM process; an overview of the four steps of KM in perinatal care follows.

17.1.2.1   Step 1: Access to Clinical Data

The first step in the KM process is the collection, storage, and retrieval of data. The current developments of electronic patient records (EPRs), hospital information

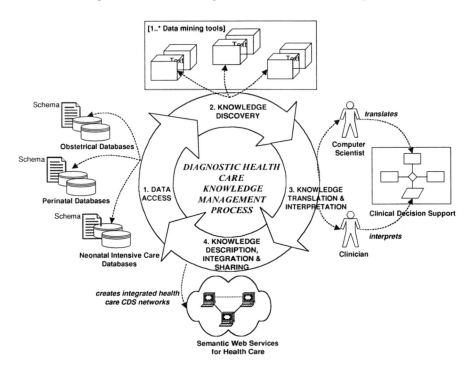

FIGURE 17.1. Diagnostic healthcare KM process.

systems, patient archiving and communication system (PACS), and the quick tempo of illness in critically ill patients has spawned numerous monitoring technologies which are evolving rapidly and generate large volumes of information. However, these monitors and hospital information systems are often unconnected, uncoordinated, and can generate confusing outputs. This highlights the importance of developing healthcare KM processes to deal with the huge amount of data in today's healthcare facility.

One essential ingredient is data quality, which is critical for meaningful analyses and use of the data; training of hospital personnel involved in data collection and performing regular data audits to ensure high concordance with the caseroom logbook and maintain data integrity. Examples of databases used for studies reported in this chapter are found in Appendix A. Obtaining access to data is a key ingredient in the KM process. This requires the development of strong partnerships between caregivers and artificial intelligence (AI) specialists. It is important to note that, prior to obtaining clinical data, the partners must apply to the appropriate ethics review board to obtain clearance for the work proposed. Involving the clinical personnel at all stages of the research and development work is essential for its ultimate success, as experience has shown that healthcare practitioners are more likely to incorporate information technology (IT) tools into daily practice if they are involved in the conception and development of the tools.

17.1.2.2   Step 2: Knowledge Discovery

In this phase of the KM process, a variety of data-mining tools are used to extract important features, observe trends, and develop prediction models for future patient cases. This step transforms data into knowledge. Some of the tools that show promising results are statistical techniques, artificial neural networks (ANNs), case-based reasoning (CBR), and fuzzy-logic sets (FLSs). A more detailed discussion of these tools is found later in the chapter.

17.1.2.3   Step 3: Knowledge Translation

In this step, the output of the knowledge discovery (KD) tools is transformed into information useful for the clinician. In this phase, graphical user interfaces (GUIs) are integrated to make the tools intuitive and user friendly. Examples of useful features that can be included are providing the probability attached to predictions, and initiating alerts for caregivers when the outcomes estimated present a clinical situation that urgently needs attention. Knowledge translation (KT) includes the development of CDS tools, which are becoming increasingly part of the IT applications in the delivery of healthcare.

17.1.2.4   Step 4: Knowledge Integration and Sharing

Results from KT will eventually be shared with all practitioners involved in a patient's care, possibly integrated into clinical repositories, such as the patient's

EPR, and possibly processed by other CDS tools. A promising technology to achieve this integration and sharing is the use of Web services (intranet or Internet) to provide caregivers easy and quick access to data, tools, data analyses, clinical alerts, etc. Access should be provided at the point of care and in remote locations, such as a caregiver's office or home, and enable utilization of tools in all steps of the KM process, at will.

An important aspect to ensure success of any of the steps and tools used in the KM process is to position them to work within the traditional medical model. For example, Case-based reasoner (CBR) that finds the 10 closest matching patient cases to the new patient arrival simulates a physician thinking: "I have seen patients like this . . . and this is what happened to them." Similarly, an Artificial neural network (ANN) which predicts a clinical outcome, e.g. whether the patient is expected to live or die, simulates a physician thinking: "And for this patient, this is what I think will happen." System development for CDS must never attempt to replace physicians and caregivers and must remain as close as possible to the way in which physicians perform their diagnosis and patient management. ITs applied to KM should be intuitive, easy to use, and provide information quickly and effectively.

17.2   The Perinatal Environment

Perinatal care includes the period before birth (obstetric care of a fetus), and the care given to newborns after delivery. Thus, the period encompasses the 28th week of gestation through to the 7th day after delivery [2]. Data collection during these different stages of development of the fetus, and later of the infant, especially when things go wrong, is intense. The type of data collected depends on the medical environment, clinical or research plans for data utilization, and prediction models expected to be derived from or used on the data. Integrating data that comes from so many sources, in an intelligent manner, provides knowledge that should help caregivers in making a diagnosis or in selecting a course of therapy. Caregivers also need to estimate outcomes or whether severe complications are likely to arise. In a neonatal intensive care unit (NICU), for example, accurate outcome prediction has the potential to facilitate patient management, parental counseling, and resource allocation.

To date, most prediction models are made up of scores based on a combination of demographic, therapeutic, and physiologic variables. The Score for Neonatal Acute Physiology (SNAP) [3] is based on the adult intensive care unit prediction model, the Acute Physiology and Chronic Health Evaluation (APACHE) [4]. APACHE assigned a weight ranging from 0 to 4 to each of 34 possible physiological measurements to indicate a deviation from normality; the total score, therefore, reflected the patient's severity of illness. The SNAP weights ranged from 0 to 5 and had 37 possible measurements whose choice was based on clinical expertise. SNAP-II was developed by logistic regression analysis using the SNAP variables and data from the 17 NICUs comprising the membership of the Canadian

Neonatal Network (CNN); this database includes slightly more than 20,000 babies [5]. SNAP-II achieves similar performance to SNAP, but it requires only six of the 37 variables (lowest blood pressure, lowest serum, pH, lowest temperature, lowest pO_2/FiO_2 ratio, seizures, and urine output—all variables being collected in the first 12 h from admission to the NICU). These scoring systems (APACHE, SNAP, SNAP-II) classify patients according to their severity of illness, which is closely correlated with mortality. Death is a rare outcome in the NICU, given that the overall mortality rate in the CNN database is less than 4% [6].

However, accurate outcome prediction for single patients in the NICU could facilitate clinical and ethical decision making, patient management, provision of accurate parental information, and appropriate resource allocation planning. Although illness severity and therapeutic intensity scores have been useful as research tools, they also have important limitations. For example, at its highest score, the predictive power of SNAP is about 50% [7].

Scoring systems are not easily updated to reflect new practices, nor are they designed to be specific to the practice in a particular unit or region. None has been shown to be of sufficient accuracy in predicting the outcome of individual patients for use in supporting clinical or ethical decisions. Moreover, all scores have limitations in the outcomes that they predict and they do not appear to have any utility in improving diagnostic accuracy or reducing medical errors. Richardson and Tarnow-Mordi [8] reviewed 30 neonatal scoring systems and found that few had been validated on large, concurrent samples of newborns. Scoring systems have been compared [9,10] to help choose such tools, but it is reported that many clinicians remain skeptical about using scoring models in actual patient care [11,12]. Indeed, scoring systems appear to be little better than clinical judgment alone in predicting probability of death where the probability approaches 50%. Therefore, an automatic system to predict important outcomes with adequate sensitivity and specificity, based on a unit- or region-specific database, may have greater utility as a decision aid in the NICU.

17.3   Estimating Clinical Outcomes in the Perinatal Environment

From conception to birth, a vast quantity of patient information relating to an infant and the mother is accumulated and stored in medical databases. Infant-related data are stored in obstetrical, perinatal, and neonatal intensive care (for very sick infants) databases that are frequently distributed temporally and geographically. When developing systems for outcome estimation, it is essential to find ways to reduce the number of variables used to estimate outcomes, i.e. define a minimum dataset (MDS) for each of the models of outcome estimation to be created. Moreover, there is a need to obtain faster test results and to predict the onset of significant and life-threatening changes [13]. This need, coupled with the limitation of current illness severity indices, has been a motivating force behind research and development efforts to create CDS tools .

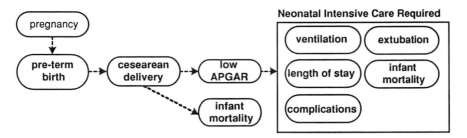

FIGURE 17.2. Perinatal clinical outcomes of interest.

Figure 17.2 shows the outcomes that can be estimated at various stages of perinatal care, both during the pre- and post-natal periods. These outcomes are felt to be highly relevant for obstetricians, neonatologists, and pediatricians, and they are discussed in more detail below.

17.3.1   Estimating Pre-Natal Outcomes

17.3.1.1   Pre-Term Births

Defined as birth before 37 completed weeks' gestation, pre-term birth (PTB) is the leading cause of mortality occurring before 28 days of age, accounting for 85% of all neonatal deaths not due to lethal congenital malformations [14]. Owing to its direct correlation with infant mortality and increased risk of long-term health problems, reducing the burden of PTB has become the number one neonatal health priority. Many studies have attempted to predict women at risk of PTB; so far, no scoring system has proven itself superior to clinical judgment. One of the major obstacles is that most women who deliver prematurely have no obvious risk factors, and over half of all PTBs occur in low-risk pregnancies [15,16]. Owing to a lack of complete obstetric data, it is often difficult to perform risk estimation based on sophisticated medical markers and extensive medical histories, as published in large clinical trials [17]. We used ANNs to predict PTBs by classifying each new patient case using an obstetrical CDS tool that identifies mothers at high risk of delivering premature infants [18].

17.3.1.2   Delivery Type

This outcome variable predicts whether the delivery of the baby will be by cesarean section or a vaginal delivery. Successfully predicting the delivery type can help to prepare for the care of mothers during delivery. The cesarean birth rate has been increasing slowly every year in Ontario (Canada), from 19.9% in 1999, to 20.9% in 2000, to 22.8% in 2001. The increase occurred in both teaching hospitals and large community hospitals. The debate continues on whether the present cesarean birth rate is too high. Six years ago, the cesarean birth rate in the Ottawa area hospitals was 16%. A recent study reported the development of a prediction model for delivery type. The study used two different AI approaches to estimate this outcome: ANNs and fuzzy-logic neural networks. Both resulted in high performance measured by the sensitivity, specificity, and area under the receiver operating characteristic (ROC) curve [19].

17.3.1.3   Apgar Score

This test is done 1 min and 5 min after delivery of the newborn to evaluate its condition immediately after delivery. The Apgar tests five attributes: appearance (color); pulse (heartbeat); grimace (reflex); activity (muscle tone); and respiration (breathing). A score is determined by awarding zero, one or two points in each category. Scores of seven and higher indicate that the baby is in good clinical condition. The Apgar score was developed in 1952 by the late pediatrician Dr Virginia Apgar [20]. Again, a prediction model was developed for this rarely studied outcome, with encouraging results [19].

17.3.2   Estimating Neonatal Intensive Care Outcomes

17.3.2.1   Newborns Requiring Intensive Care

Development of neonatal technology and practices have resulted in sophisticated care, capable of sustaining life for infants as small as 500 g and as premature as 23 weeks' gestation. There has been a substantial reduction of mortality in premature infants, and the rate of handicap or significant morbidity appears to have remained steady or declined in survivors of NICUs of nearly all gestational ages and weights. Despite these positive results, current neonatal care decisions are frequently based on uncertain conditions, and the use of aggressive treatments is increasingly being questioned. A serious concern for healthcare providers and for parents is: To whom should this intensive care be administered and in what circumstances should it be withdrawn? Are there factors with respect to these babies' health status to guide physicians and parents in whether to administer treatment or not, or to end it if it has been started? In the NICU, ethical dilemmas and decision conflicts are unavoidable. The challenge is to provide guidance that is practical and specific, but not prescriptive [21–23]. There are suggestions that appropriate technologies can improve the decision-making process [24,25]. However, physicians often perceive current outcome estimates as unreliable and are seeking better-performing algorithms for predictions. If estimates can be provided with acceptable accuracy, then the potential exists to enhance significantly the evidence on which critical decision making is based in NICUs.

17.3.2.2   Mortality

Neonatal mortality is defined by the World Health Organization as death occurring before 28 days of age [26]. In the CNN database, only deaths to discharge were recorded, because there was no follow up after discharge from the hospital. Moribund babies were excluded from the database, since they only receive comfort measures rather than aggressive therapy [27]. Initial studies using SNAP showed that moribund infants were assigned a zero SNAP because no tests were performed or monitoring values were not recorded; this inaccurately estimates their risk of death, because a lower score should indicate a lower risk of mortality.

All current methods, including illness severity scores, have difficulty in accurately predicting mortality of very low birth weight (VLBW) and extremely low birth weight (ELBW) infants. Regression analysis on a tertiary center database did not outperform neural networks in prediction of ELBW neonatal mortality [28] and the positive predictive values (PPVs) were similar to those reported for illness severity scores. However, in a study using ANNs, the PPV of 62.7% in <1000 g infants in one experiment was better than previous reports of other methods and suggests the possibility that further performance improvement may be possible with this approach. Furthermore, the ANN system consistently demonstrated high specificity and negative predictive value (NPV), suggesting that it was relatively accurate in predicting survival. This is an important finding for clinical utility. More caution must be exercised in predicting death, as this might lead to inappropriate counseling of parents and subsequent inappropriate ethical and therapeutic decision making.

Given that caregivers predict death quite well early in the course of an NICU patient's stay [7], but predict survival less well, the ANN might be an excellent complement to clinical judgment, since it predicts survival much more accurately than caregivers. Nonetheless, improving sensitivity and PPV for the outcome of mortality is an important aspect to improve the potential utility of these systems for use in evidence-based ethical decision making [29].

17.3.2.3 Other Neonatal Intensive Care Unit Outcomes

Other outcomes studied in the NICU are: estimating the duration of artificial ventilation, i.e. whether the ventilator will be used for 12 h, 24 h, 48 h, 7 days, 14 days, or longer [30–32]; another study estimating whether an extubation will succeed or fail [33]; length of stay (LOS) [34]; mortality [28,35]. Potential clinical complications of neonates in the intensive care unit are currently being studied with encouraging results; examples are major neuro-imaging abnormality, chronic lung disease (bronchopulmonary dysplasia), necrotizing enterocolitis, and retinopathy of prematurity.

17.3.3 Databases to Estimate Perinatal Outcomes

Two principal databases were used for the studies mentioned above. The CNN data were collected across Canada from 1996 to 1997 (17 centers, about 20,000 infants and 1000 deaths). A second database was obtained from the Perinatal Partnership Program of Eastern Ontario (PPPESO) program in Ontario, Canada. In 2001, 17,406 women gave birth in hospitals in the Eastern and Southeastern Regions; the information on these women and babies born was collected in the

2001 Niday Enhanced Perinatal Database. The databases used are described more fully in Appendix A.

17.4 Knowledge Discovery

Research efforts have focused on the application of IT and AI, particularly data integration and tools such as CBR, ANN, and FLSs to provide easy access to information and KM at the point of care. The literature on adult uses of ANNs in outcome prediction is now large and rapidly growing: a Medline search using only the single MeSH term "Neural Networks (Computer)" recorded approximately 2000 "hits" in March 2003, but 9636 hits as of November 2005. There are, however, only a few studies using ANNs in prediction of outcomes for pre-term newborns. A number of studies compared ANNs with regression models, and in each study the ANN approach outperformed the statistical method, but usually by only a small margin, suggesting that these approaches may be complementary [28,36,37].

A review of evidence of health benefit from ANNs in medical intervention has recently been published [38]. This surveyed randomized and nonrandomized clinical trials of ANNs in the domains of oncology, critical care, and cardiovascular medicine, including four studies in perinatal or neonatal care. The review notes the potential for extensive benefit, but criticizes poor methodology and exaggerated claims in many studies. The design blueprint for decision-support research contained in Lisboa's review has the following components: *Clarify the purpose of the study*; *Model design* (particularly to control for overfitting); *Network regularization* (e.g. using a Bayesian regularization framework); *Variable selection* (number of observations should be 5–10 times the number of available covariates); *Validation: support for learned intermediaries* (ensure experts accept integrity of the model); *Benchmarking against a suitable alternative* (e.g. against logistic regression-derived scores); *Robustness in performance evaluation* (e.g. effect of prevalence of different conditions); *Comparative trials* [38]. Following these suggestions will help to inject credibility in CDS tool developments.

17.4.1 Artificial Neural Networks

ANNs are widely used and are effective in a broad range of applications for analysis (e.g. voice recognition), control (industrial applications), and forecasting (e.g. market and weather forecasts). An ANN uses a process analogous to information processing by the human brain, acquiring knowledge through a learning process and storing it using inter-neuron connection strengths (synaptic weights). The ANN thus develops a set of outputs based on a system of input conditions. In this respect the ANN serves a similar function to common statistical techniques. The main advantage of neural networks over statistical techniques is that the model does not have to be explicitly defined before beginning the experiments. ANNs can recognize the relevant data and patterns, whereas a statistical model requires prior knowledge of the relationships between the factors under investigation [39].

Also, with statistics, it is difficult to integrate data of different formats (i.e. working simultaneously with continuous, binary, ordinal, and nominal data), but this can easily be achieved using ANNs.

17.4.1.1   Improving the Performance of Artificial Neural Networks in Analyzing Medical Data

The versatility of available software such as MATLAB [40] makes ANNs accessible to newcomers to this field of work, yet seasoned users can also modify the basic networks using more complex functions to achieve even better classification performance. We have experimented with a variety of structures over the past decade and have chosen the backpropagation feedforward neural network with the weight-elimination cost function and the hyperbolic tangent transfer function [32]. Originally, the training sets typically contained two-thirds of the data randomly selected, with the remaining used for a test set. More recent experiments tend to use one-third of the data set for each of: training, testing, and validation.

Two and three layer networks were used with the weight-elimination cost function to prune the network and the logarithmic-sensitivity index as a stopping criterion, which optimizes for both sensitivity and specificity [41]. Multiple trials were executed using different random-number generator seeds. A serious limitation can occur when one outcome class contains less than 85% of patients [42]. This was overcome by increasing the smallest class through multiple random sampling of patients in this class until their presence reached 20% of cases [43]. Tedious manual tweaking of nine ANN parameters to obtain optimal performance for each set of experiments was overcome by developing a fully automated ANN that runs day and night with little user supervision, saving weeks and months of work for each analysis. An automated calculation of ROC curves was added [44]. A verification program allows a previously defined ANN estimation model to be applied to a new database to ensure that the ANN was generalizing, rather than overfitting to the training data. The verification tool runs only one epoch, using the weights and biases obtained from the best results from the training runs.

17.4.1.2   Input Variable Reduction: Finding a Minimum Dataset

Medical databases are generally large, containing more variables than are needed to predict the desired outcome. After the database has been cleaned (removal of outliers and ambiguous data), the first step is to pare down the database to a workable size by removing unimportant input variables. The difficulty lies in knowing which variables to remove. When only the most important variables remain, the MDS has been reached. The MDS not only defines the most important input variables for a prediction model, but also defines a list of indicators and their relative importance. When a database is mined, sometimes the ability to predict case-by-case results is not the goal.

In these instances, often a set of indicators is desired in order to make overall declarations about the factors that lead to certain results. The variables of the MDS with the largest relative weights are these factors or indicators. A number of methods exist for input variable elimination with ANNs. Complex, mathematically-intensive examples will not be explored, which includes examples such as independent component analysis and higher order cross-statistics, p-value test reduction, and complex dimensionality reduction. Several methods have been proposed to identify the weights of the inputs and hidden nodes in order to establish the importance of each variable with respect to the outcome. One approach is to reduce the input variables one by one and observe when the performance deteriorates [45–47]. The remaining variables then form an MDS to estimate a particular outcome.

Another method to extract weights for (with a hidden layer) was proposed by Garson [48], and was later simplified by Goh [49]. One problem with Goh's technique is that it is presented as an approach for extracting weights in nonlinear ANNs (with hidden layers), but the algorithm in its current form tackles linear networks and does not allow one to compute weights in the hidden layer when applied to the problems described here [50].

17.4.2   Case-Based Reasoning

A CBR system is an expert system that derives solutions to problems based on cases. Functionally speaking, CBR-based medical systems provide "analogy-based" solutions/diagnosis to clinical problems by manipulating knowledge derived from similar previously experienced situations, called *cases* [51].

A basic premise in CBR is that many problems that decision makers encounter are not unique; rather, they are variations of a problem type. Thus, it is more efficient to solve a problem by analogy and starting with the solution to a previous similar problem than it is to generate the entire solution again from first principles [52]. A problem can be solved in a cycle of four steps, referred to as the *CBR R^4 Cycle*: *Retrieve*, *Reuse*, *Revise* and *Retain*. In solving a current problem, the CBR retrieves a similar past case and its solution. It then adapts the successful solution of the retrieved case to adjust for any differences between the current case and the retrieved case. Finally, the CBR stores the solution to the current case along with feedback about the outcome so that it can be used in solving future problems [53].

A CBR has been used to match entire cases for inspection by physicians in an adult intensive care unit and to generate warnings if any of the 10 closest matched case patients had died [54]. It was suggested that a database could be extended using the imputation process, so that it could be successfully merged with another database that contained different input variables. A CBR was used by Ennett in conjunction with an ANN to impute missing input values into medical databases [55]. The weights at the input nodes of an ANN, after optimal performance is attained, and used in the CBR as match weights. Ten closest patient cases are found, and then missing values in the variables of these 10 patients are imputed by the mean of the value of each variable for this set of patients. There are other methods to impute missing values, such as replacing them with normal values. However, the approach described above was found to perform as well or better than others described in the literature.

17.5   Results

17.5.1   Estimations of Pre-Natal Outcomes

17.5.1.1   Pre-Term Birth

All experiments were performed on three PPPESO databases, using years 1999, 2000, and 2001. Based on physician input, eight obstetrical variables were selected as being nonconfounding for predicting PTB: maternal age, number of babies this pregnancy, number of previous term babies, number of previous PTBs, parity (total number of previous children), baby's gender, whether mother has intention to breast-feed, and maternal smoking after 20 weeks' gestation. The outcome assessed was whether birth occurred at less than 37 weeks' gestation.

Table 17.1 summarizes the database distributions; notice that the PTB rate is similar for all three years. The ANN architecture was a three layer architecture (input-hidden-output) layers feedforward network based on the backpropagation training algorithm with the hyperbolic tangent transfer function. All experiments used weight elimination added to the error function. Two categorized datasets were created: the first combined all PTB cases from each of the three PPPESO years of data collected, and the second contained all term delivery cases for a specific year (2001). Each categorized dataset was randomly separated into training and test sets (two-thirds and one-third respectively). The 2/3-term training set and the 2/3-pre-term training set were combined, yielding an approximate 80:20 distribution (term to preterm respectively). Finally, the 1/3-term test set and 1/3-pre-term test set were combined, randomly deleting pre-term cases until an approximate 90:10 "real" distribution was obtained.

The study assessed whether changing the PTB rate distribution of the training datasets increased the performance of the ANNs. Given the current lack of success in predicting with high sensitivity PTB in nonsymptomatic populations, sensitivity was chosen as the key measure of performance. Additionally, the ANN performance was measured using specificity, correct classification rate (CCR), and the area under the ROC curve, i.e. the C-index. The performance was also compared with the CCR of a constant predictor (CP), a statistical benchmark that classifies all test set cases as belonging to the outcome class with the highest a

TABLE 17.1. PPPESO PTB statistics by year.

	1999	2000	2001
PTB cases (%)	8.7	9.2	8.4
Prevalence in PTB cases (%)			
Smoking	17.45	17.32	17.13
Breast-feeding	71.45	75.42	79.78
Previous PTB	10.28	11.33	12.19
Previous term	42.14	42.70	43.29
# Babies = 1	75.79	80.55	77.62
Gender = Male	55.24	52.43	51.23

TABLE 17.2. Network settings of the best-performing networks
for predicting PTB (PPPESO).

Experiment	Train PTBR = 8.59% Test PTBR = 8.67%	Train PTBR = 23% Test PTBR = 10%
Number of hidden layers	2	2
Hidden nodes	3	3
Learning rate	0.0004	0.0004
Learning rate increment	1.7685	1.2865
Learning rate decrement	0.5	0.9092
Weight decay constant	0.501	0.501
Momentum	0.95	0.85
Error ratio	1	1
Lambda increment	1.01	1.01
Lambda decrement	0.99	0.99

priori probability of the training set. Table 17.2 summarizes the optimized network
parameters for both the original and artificial datasets.

It can be argued that the ANNs trained on the artificial datasets were of more
value to physicians because a greater number of mothers at risk of PTB were
correctly classified. In general, at-risk patients are more difficult to classify using
risk stratification models; therefore, preference should be given to a model that is
better able to classify these individuals. The three-layer ANN optimized to predict
PTB using the 2001 artificial training dataset outperformed the original dataset for
predicting PTB: sensitivity increased by 13%, peaking at 33.4%; CCR was slightly
higher than CP, and the area under the ROC curve, which assesses the ability of
the model to discriminate between outcomes, increased to 0.71.

The ANN identified four variables as having the highest connection weights;
listed in order of significance, these are: the number of babies this pregnancy;
number of previous term babies; total number of previous children; and maternal
smoking after 20 weeks' gestation. These results are encouraging in terms of
validating the applicability of the ANN to clinical PTB prediction, as each of the
four variables is commonly believed to be a risk factor associated with an increased
frequency of PTB [56].

Using only a very limited eight-variable obstetrical input set, a maximum sensitivity of 36.64% was achieved with an artificial distribution of PTB cases of just
over 20%. These initial results are encouraging, because if women at risk of PTB
could be accurately identified using basic obstetrical and socio-demographic information, then this would reduce the need for invasive and costly predictive tests.

17.5.1.2 Delivery Type

As described earlier, two approaches were used to estimate this outcome and the
next one (Apgar5): a neural network with the weight-elimination cost function
and hyperbolic tangent transfer function; and fuzzy K-nearest-neighbor (KNN)

algorithm. The maximum CCR of the ANN test set was 86.8% for a two-layer network and 85.7% for a three-layer network with seven nodes in the hidden layer. The corresponding sensitivity was 80.6 for the two-layer network and 84.0 for the three-layer networks. The specificity was 88.5 and 86.2 in the two- and three-layer networks respectively. With the FLC the CCR was 89.2, the sensitivity 71.3, and the specificity 94.3% [19]. These results show a very good performance of both AI approaches in estimating delivery type.

17.5.1.3   Apgar5

With the ANN, the specificity was very high (99.7%), but the sensitivity was lower (31.4%). The CCR was also very high (98.2%). This particular outcome does not appear to have been studied to date by AI tools. This first attempt is encouraging, and the ANN will be optimized by a variety of approaches to obtain a higher specificity in the future. With the FLC the CCR was 97.6%, the sensitivity was 19.5%, and the specificity was 99.3% [19].

17.5.2   Estimations of Neonatal Intensive Care Outcomes

17.5.2.1   Very Low Birth Weight Mortality

The CNN database contains a large number of variables, which are more fully described in Appendix A. For this outcome, nine were selected for analysis; these variables also comprise the components of the SNAPPE-II illness severity score, which is the SNAP-II and three perinatal variables (hence "perinatal extension" or PE), namely Apgar score, birth weight and "small for gestational age" (newborns whose birth weight is below the third percentile for gestational age). These were studied for infants <1500 g birth weight (VLBW) and <1000 g (ELBW).

The total number of cases of all birth weights in the database was 20,008. After exclusion of cases with missing values there were 2079 cases with <1500 g birth weight and 1050 cases with <1000 g birth weight in the database (admission data). Several separate experiments were performed with three to eight hidden nodes in a single hidden layer of the ANN. The CP, CCR, PPV, NPV, likelihood ratio (LR) and negative LR (NLR) were measured for all experiments.

The CP (in this study the proportion of infants in each set *not* dying before discharge home) was 79.3% for infants <1000 g and 86.7% for those <1500 g; the latter high proportion might be expected to be difficult for an ANN to improve upon. Nonetheless, the ANN always performed better than the CP. After training, CCRs on the test set at best performance were 83.8% for infants <1000 g and 88.4–88.8% for those <1500 g. Sensitivity for the outcome in this experiment was about 50%; best was 50.6% for <1000 g, 47.4% for <1500 g, but specificity was uniformly high at 93.2–97.5%. Area under the ROC curve (0.7937–0.8021 for <1000 g, 0.82–0.8401 for <1500 g) was generally at least as good as or better than for SNAP-II or SNAPPE-II.

17.5.2.2 Scoring Systems

At best performance, the PPV for these data was 47.2–48.5% for all datasets except for the <1000 g test set using the eight-node hidden layer network, where PPV was 62.1%. NPV was 77.3–79.7% for all test sets except in this case for the <1500 g test set using the eight-node hidden layer network, where it was 85.5%. This provides some evidence that the eight-node hidden layer provided a small, but important, improvement in performance. LR similarly was slightly higher for the eight-node hidden layer network. LR with three nodes was 2.3 (both <1000 g and <1500 g); with eight nodes in the hidden layer, the values were 3.5 (<1000 g) and 3.3 (<1500 g).

NLR was similar for both systems: 1.6 (three nodes <1000 g), 1.3 (three nodes <1500 g), 1.7 (eight nodes <1000 g), and 1.6 (eight nodes <1500 g). While these results are not yet good enough for application in the clinical setting, they again show that ANN predictions are as good as or better than currently available scoring systems, and they provide encouragement for further work to optimize performance.

17.5.2.3 Contribution of Variables to Mortality in Neonatal Intensive Care Unit Patients

For this experiment there were 5102 infants in the CNN database after exclusion for missing values (infants of all birth weights were included in this analysis.) When adjusted so that the variable with the highest contribution had a value of 100, the relative contributions of the variables in the SNAP-II and SNAPPE-II were estimated (Table 17.3). CCR, sensitivity, specificity, PPV, NPV, LR, NLR and area under the ROC curve were measured to evaluate this system's performance. Performance measures for the test set were: CCR = 90.2%; sensitivity 24.5%; specificity 97.7%; PPV = 82.5%; NPV = 74.5%; LR = 10.7; NLR = 1.3; area

TABLE 17.3. Relative contributions of SNAP-II and SNAPPE-II variables to NICU mortality[a].

SNAP-II & SNAPPE-II Variable	SNAP-II Relative Weight	SNAPPE-II Relative Weight
Lowest pO_2/FiO_2 ratio	100	100
Urine cc/kg in 24 h	71	66
Apgar @ 5 min	N/a	43
Lowest temperature	51	42
Small for gestation	N/a	32
Lowest serum pH	42	28
Birth weight	N/a	19
Lowest blood pressure	37	19
Seizures	25	19

[a] Performance measures for the test set (infants of all birth weights): Sensitivity = 24.5%, Specificity = 97.7%, LR =10.7, NLR = 1.3, PPV= 82.5%, NPV = 74.5%, CCR = 90.2%, Area under ROC curve = 0.8253.

under the ROC curve was 0.8253. Thus, system performance was very good for prediction of mortality versus survival when using infants of all birth weights in this database.

17.5.2.4 Duration of Ventilation

The total cases in the database were 20,008 for admission data (day 1). After exclusion of cases with missing values for one or more SNAPPE-II variables, there were 1841 cases remaining. The estimations of probability of ventilation >12 h, >24 h and >36 h were studied with this dataset. System performance was evaluated by measuring CCR versus CP, sensitivity and specificity, area under the ROC curve, PPV and NPV, and LR and NLR. The correct classification rate of the ANN without replacement of missing values was generally high, ranging from a low of 78.4% for prediction of ventilation duration <12 h to 86.7% for <36 h. CCR was always higher than the CP (in this experiment the proportion *not* ventilated for the duration under study), which ranged from 60.0% for ventilation <12 h to 85.3% for <36 h. Specificity was 78.3% for <12 h, 85.3% for <24 h, and 93.4% for <36 h. Area under the ROC curve was 0.8217 for <12 h up to 0.8692 for <24 h. However, whereas specificity and ROC tended to be better for longer durations of ventilation, sensitivity was poorer for prediction of duration of ventilation <36 h (47.9%) than for <12 h or <24 h (74.3–79.4%).

The PPV for these data similarly became poorer for prediction of longer periods of ventilation: 70.6% for ventilation duration <12 h, 62.7% for <24 h and 51.9% <36 h. NPV, however, changed relatively little with differing periods of ventilation: 84.6% <12 h, 93.0% <24 h, and 83.8% <36 h. LR was similar for all predictions: 3.6 for ventilation duration <12 h, 5.4 for <24 h and 3.4 <36 h. NLR, however, was better for predictions of shorter ventilation periods: 3.7 for <12 h, 4.1 for <24 h, and 1.6 for <36 h.

Duration of ventilation is an important predictor of resource utilization in the NICU, with ventilated infants requiring much higher commitments of nursing, respiratory therapy, and other personnel, as well as elevated utilization of laboratory, medical imaging, pharmacy, and other investigational and therapeutic resources. These results suggest that further research to refine estimation of utilization indicators may have considerable future utility.

17.5.2.5 Extubation Success

Mueller et al. [33] compared the performance of an ANN with a multiple logistic regression (MLR) model in predicting extubation outcome in newborns weighing 900–1500 g. Mueller et al. used ANNs to estimate outcomes for a "new" patient, based on the experience acquired with a large database of a similar population of previous patients. They also compared both systems with clinical predictions of extubation failure or success from four neonatologists who were provided with the same datasets used to develop the mathematical models. In that study there was little difference in the ability to predict extubation success (although the ANN had marginally the best performance: 86% ANN versus 84% MLR and

clinicians), but for prediction of extubation failure the ANN significantly outperformed both the MLR model (86 versus 56%) and the clinicians (86 vs 41%).
There was some evidence that clinical predictions were more accurate from more
experienced clinicians [33].

17.5.2.6   Major Neuro-Imaging Problems

We have studied the estimation of probability of major neuro-imaging abnormality. Preterm newborns, particularly those <28 weeks' gestation or <1000 g birth
weight, have a high incidence of intraventricular hemorrhage (IVH), where bleed-
ing occurs from the fragile blood vessels around the ventricles (fluid spaces) in the
brain. Low degrees of such hemorrhage (classified as grades 1 and 2 according to
a system developed by Papile et al. [57]) are not associated with a significant increase in risk of adverse long-term neurodevelopmental outcome. Higher degrees
of IVH (grades 3 and 4, the latter also being known as intra-parenchymal hemorrhage (IPE)) carry increasing risk of poor outcomes such as cerebral palsy (CP)
and developmental delay. A separate, but often associated, abnormality of the brain
tissue itself, known as periventricular leukomalacia (PVL), is highly predictive of
CP. Grade 3 IVH, IPE (or grade 4 IVH) and PVL were combined into a single
outcome, which we titled "major neuro-imaging abnormality"; this included any
infant with any one or more of these findings on any brain ultrasound during the
infant's NICU stay.

The patient database was again the CNN database. Missing variables were imputed using a hybrid CBR–ANN system [55], thus producing 18,306 complete
matching cases. For this experiment, the input variables used were the nine variables from the full SNAP list that were found to be most predictive of mortality
in earlier ANN studies plus the six SNAP-II variables. Various experiments used
various ANN architectures, with no or one hidden layer and with varying numbers
of hidden nodes in the hidden layer. The best results using a three-layer ANN with
six hidden nodes in the hidden layer gave a very encouraging 70.10% sensitivity
and 90.13% specificity for this important NICU outcome.

While successful methods to prevent these adverse outcomes are not presently
known, the ability to predict the highest risk infants may have important implications for the neonatologist counseling an infant's parents on possible long-term
outcomes.

17.5.2.7   Necrotizing Enterocolitis

A second area already studied by us is probability of necrotizing enterocolitis
(NEC). NEC is a relatively common problem (~5% NICU admissions) that is most
often seen in pre-term newborns. Various risk factors are known or suspected, such
as episodes of low oxygen or circulation, rapid feeding advances, and infection.
The condition causes inflammation and necrosis of the bowel wall and may lead
to septic shock, gut perforation, and long-term bowel abnormalities. Mortality is
high, with about 15% of those affected dying. Our research team used the same
patient database from the CNN and the same variables as under the neuro-imaging

abnormality above. Among the ANNs used for this experiment, a three-layer ANN with five hidden nodes achieved the highest specificity and CCR, while a three-layer ANN with seven hidden nodes had the highest specificity (and only a very small difference in specificity from the ANN with five hidden nodes).

For the best balance of high sensitivity and specificity, therefore, the three-layer ANN with five hidden nodes appeared to be the best ANN architecture for this outcome; it achieved a test sensitivity of 42.5%, specificity of 90.79%, and a CCR of 89.95%. This performance is remarkable, since the prediction of NEC in the NICU setting is usually considered extremely difficult. This suggests that ANN prediction of babies at particularly high risk may be possible and might allow the use of early measures to prevent the onset of NEC related to hemodynamic stability, feeding, infection, etc.

17.5.2.8   Chronic Lung Disease and Retinopathy of Prematurity

These studies have commenced and results will be available and reported in due course.

17.6   Knowledge Translation and Interpretation

AI estimations need to be integrated into clinical social context to create value for healthcare decisions and provision. In sophisticated NICUs, decisions to continue or discontinue aggressive treatment are an integral part of clinical practice. High-quality evidence supports clinical decision making, and a decision-aid tool based on specific outcome information for individual NICU patients is expected to provide significant support for parents and caregivers in making difficult "ethical" treatment decisions.

17.6.1   Parent-Assist Decision Aid System

The concerns with neonatal intensive care treatment and decisions have led to some efforts at creating neonatal decision-support systems. Some examples are the NEONATE project (successor of the COGNATE project) [58], and the Baby CareLink® Tool [21]. The NEONATE project is an ongoing effort to develop a decision-support tool for clinical staff (doctors and nurses) in a neonatal intensive care environment. The focus is to help the NICU medical team deal with large amounts of (and many different types of) information in making clinical decisions. The development is in a preliminary phase where the neonatal practitioners' concepts and knowledge hierarchies are being identified and used to develop user interfaces. The researchers have taken a cognitive engineering approach in their design.

In the US, development efforts are under way on the Baby CareLink® system. This tool originated as a research project at the Harvard Medical School and is now a commercially supported product by Clinician Support Technology©.

The tool aims to provide a nurturing environment in which parents can, either locally or remotely, actively participate in NICU decisions for their baby. It is built on improved communication and customized education for parents so that they may be empowered to provide better care to their premature infant. The limitation of these two systems is that no AI is leveraged for supporting decision making. Moreover, the NEONATE system does not yet account for any parental involvement in the decision-making process, whereas the Baby Carelink® actively elicits parent participation but does not yet consider the input of physicians [21].

Yang and coworkers [59] developed a framework that integrates information on a newborn patient's likely outcomes with the physician's interpretation and incorporates the parents' perspectives into codified knowledge. Context-sensitive content adaptation delivers personalized and customized information to a variety of users, from physicians to parents. The system provides structuralized KT, interpretation, and exchange between all participants in the decision, facilitating collaborative decision making that involves parents at every stage on whether to initiate, continue, limit, or terminate intensive care for their infant. The major components of this system are as follows:

1. *Evidence-based estimation.* Provides intelligent outcome prediction based on an analysis of a set of diagnostic data input compared with past evidence of relationship between indicators and outcomes using an ANN and a CBR.
2. *Content management.* Captures, manages, and retrieves all data objects for decision making and data objects describing user context, and the content aggregation component including a local data repository for storing static and dynamic decision-support data.
3. *Communication management.* Allows public, protected, and private message delivery via simple message protocols.
4. *User interface.* Includes a content adaptation component, parent decision-support tool, and context-sensitive help.

These subsystems interact to provide services such as predictive analysis, document repository, customized delivery, and adaptive interfaces. By harnessing these functional blocks, the user-friendly system delivers improved outcome estimation and KM.

17.7   Knowledge Integration and Sharing Using Web Services

Integration is a pressing concern for the healthcare domain, which is defined by a "plethora of distributed data and knowledge, from which complex and timely high-value decisions must be made in a low-tolerance environment" [60]. The Semantic Web and Web services are two emerging and evolving technologies that IT experts predict will change the face of healthcare delivery [61,62], ultimately providing integrated healthcare data, knowledge, and computer-based applications.

Adding semantics to the Web is a necessary component towards realizing Web services' goal of application-to-application integration. To this end, the next generation Internet will be the Semantic Web. The vision of the Semantic Web is to associate meaning to all Web resources such that they can be discovered and consumed autonomously by applications [63], making the Semantic Web a meaningful indexed repository of documents and services [64].

Currently, interpretation of Web-based information requires human knowledge and intuition; humans and machines could interpret the Semantic Web. As decision-support-system environments are rapidly changing from centralized and closed to distributed and open, scalability and interoperability features are becoming more crucial to CDS development [65]. Combining the Semantic Web and Web services offers a solution, providing physicians with instant access to knowledge, not just data, in real-time decision-making environments.

To complete the KM cycle described in Figure 17.1, the data, knowledge, and services described in the previous sections must be accessible to all practitioners involved in perinatal care. We have employed Semantic Web services for healthcare [66] as the technological enabler to create an infrastructure for perinatal outcome estimation. Using the concepts of "Data as a Service" and "Software as a Service" [67], the infrastructure integrates both clinical data and CDS tools in a distributed healthcare environment, the objective being to compose Semantic Web services autonomously based on predefined physician service composition templates [68]. The composition templates model workflows for perinatal CDS; by formulating the physician's decision-making process, it is possible to alert physicians to potential adverse perinatal outcomes before they occur.

In the distributed field of perinatal care, developing models for outcome estimation (e.g. MDSs) involves integrating patient cases from obstetrical, perinatal, and neonatal care databases, such as those previously described. The term semantic in "Semantic Web services" implies meaning has been associated with the Web resources; this was accomplished by creating an ontology covering all relevant perinatal care and CDS terminology, essentially a predefined taxonomy for perinatal CDS. The perinatal CDSS ontology is a necessary prerequisite to integrating data from distributed databases, providing the standardization needed to rectify differences in terminology that occur when multiple databases represent the same information in different ways.

The AI tools described earlier, such as the ANN for outcome estimation and CBR–KNN system for matching an individual patient's condition to the most similar past cases, are key components of the "Software as a Service" element of the infrastructure. The IT tools used to achieve integration are based on the World Wide Web Consortium's (W3C) standards: specifically, XML to support standardized data and Web services to offer decentralized clinical decision support.

The infrastructure has three key concepts, shown by the three layers depicted in Figure 17.3. Layer 1 (*Knowledge Description*) encompasses all knowledge sources required by the higher layers: specifically, the clinical perinatal databases and practitioner's tacit domain knowledge. Each knowledge source must be formalized before being invoked by the Semantic Web services: a medical ontology

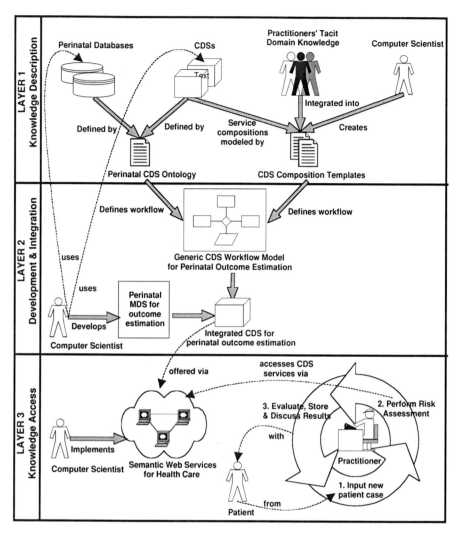

FIGURE 17.3. Knowledge description, integration, and sharing.

describes the database schemas, and composition templates model the manner in which core services are composed to perform complex service compositions. Layer 2 (*Integration*) involves developing MDSs for perinatal outcome prediction, as discussed. The MDSs are then integrated with the "Generic CDS Workflow model for Perinatal outcome estimation", which defines how the CDSSs are composed as Semantic Web services. Layer 3 (*Knowledge Sharing*) provides the Semantic Web services, which are the "glue" that integrates the inner layers and the means by which the practitioner accesses the perinatal outcome estimation tools.

When practitioners wish to interact with the system, they input new patient case data via a Web services user interface; data are obtained either directly from the patient or from a clinical repository. The practitioner can then perform outcome estimation and receive a real-time result. The result is evaluated, possibly discussed with the patient, and ideally stored in the patient's Electronic EPR. The three layers are interrelated, in that layer 2's objective cannot be met until layer 1's knowledge sources are described, and the trained outcome estimation tools developed in layer 2 cannot be ubiquitously invoked, shared, and evaluated until the Semantic Web services infrastructure described in layer 3 is designed and implemented.

17.8   Conclusion

Developments in the analysis and treatment of perinatal and neonatal intensive care data has progressed rapidly in the last decade and will continue to evolve as computers become more powerful and teams of engineers, computer scientists, and physicians work together to solve old problems with new approaches. With online acquisition of data now available (e.g. physiologic data from monitors, investigation data from laboratory, PACS, and other hospital systems) future ANN-based systems will be able to process data in "real time" so that outcome prediction will be immediate and continuously updated. Information, and even alerts, will be able to be sent to clinical staff immediately as the clinical situation requires.

The potential of these systems to support or even improve decision making by the healthcare team (or perhaps also by parents in pediatrics) is obvious and exciting. However, while the provision of better "evidence" to support clinical, "ethical," and resource decisions appears likely to be a valuable contribution to care and decision making, without clinical trials of such systems it cannot yet be said that this information will always lead to appropriate use or that knowledge gained through trials will lead to beneficial clinical application. Future work should assess not only the performance of the systems themselves, but also their use in and impact on clinical practice.

17.A   Appendix

17.A.1   Perinatal Data

17.A.1.1   Perinatal Partnership Program of Eastern Ontario Database

An excellent database was obtained by the author from the PPPESO program in Ontario (Canada) and is being used to predict PTB, delivery type (cesarean section or vaginal), Apgar score of the infant (at 5 min after birth), and mortality. The PPPESO works together with hospitals, health departments, community agencies, academic institutions, private practitioners, and consumers to effectively link perinatal care, education, and research. The PPPESO works with its partners to identify issues, develop and implement solutions, and produce results that will improve evidence-based regionalized perinatal care to child-bearing families in

Eastern and Southeastern Ontario. PPPESO's role is to provide support to this process among the partners by collecting and analyzing data, dissemination of information, communication, advice, facilitation, and education. In 2001, 17,406 women gave birth in hospitals in the Eastern and Southeastern Region, with an increase 16,957 than 2000. The information of these women and babies born was collected in the 2001 Niday Enhanced Perinatal Database (Niday 2001).

The list of variables collected were as follows. Input variables include: birth date, mother's age, postal code, inter-hospital transfer, number of previous term/pre-term babies, number of babies, baby's sex, baby's weight, presentation, monitoring methods used, maternal pain relief offered, antenatal steroids used, whether scalp or cord blood gases were performed, maternal intention to breast-feed, maternal smoking, and neonatal transfer. Outputs of interest include: number of weeks' gestation, labor type, Apgar score at 1 and 5 min, newborn resuscitation techniques, and neonatal death/stillbirth.

17.A.1.2   Canadian Neonatal Network Database

The CNN has provided data collected across Canada from 1996 to 1997 (17 centers, about 20,000 infants, and 1000 deaths.) The CNN database contains several subsets: admissions data; obstetric characteristics; illness severity information; discharge data elements; diagnoses and conditions; disposition. The database includes registration information (identifiers, demographic information, and obstetric characteristics verified from maternal records), illness severity data (SNAP, CRIB, NTISS, and SNAP-II data elements abstracted prospectively while the patient is in the NICU), specified diagnoses, complications, procedures and therapies, a discharge abstract completed after death or discharge of the patient from the last hospital to which the patient has been admitted, and summary data, collected two-weekly, such as staff/patient ratios and nursing acuity scores for all patients. Data collected annually include nursing wage rates, bed occupancy rates, patient turnover rates, adoption of new technologies in each unit, number of assisted reproduction births, total deliveries in the area, and NICU admission rate per 1000 deliveries. Outcome variables include: in-hospital death; major morbidities; resource utilization.

The current studies are: prediction of mortality in neonates of various gestations, duration of assisted ventilation and LOS, and complications such as bronchopulmonary dysplasia, IVH, NEC, and retinopathy of prematurity. The CNN variables are all recorded in raw numeric form, rather than categorical form, for ease of abstracting and analytic flexibility. The data are entered in a standardized format to study illness severity, practice variations, and resource consumption. Uniform conditions are established for all data collection by a comprehensive manual. The data are collected by a research assistant who visits NICUs daily and enters data from the patient record and other unit records directly into a laptop computer; the program permits error checking. Case numbers are assigned sequentially and can be cross-referenced with a code assigned by our local center to each patient. The system avoids paper and keyboard entry, duplicate assignment of study number, and filing/storage of data forms, while improving security and reliability. Obstetric information is verified from maternal records. The discharge abstract is completed after death or discharge of the patient from the last hospital to which the patient has been admitted, as many patients are retro-transferred to other hospitals. Summary data, collected every 2 weeks, include staff/patient ratios and nursing acuity scores for all patients.

Data collected annually include nursing wage rates, bed occupancy rates, patient turnover rates, adoption of new technologies in each unit (including certain ventilator technologies, pulmonary function monitoring, and magnetic resonance imaging), number of assisted reproduction births, total deliveries in the area, and NICU admission rate per 1000 deliveries. The abstractor is trained for the data collection study (EPIC). All data are cleaned on receipt at the coordinating center, e.g. by removing out-of-range entries. The CNN study includes re-abstraction of a random 5% of charts at each participating institution to check reliability; all centers have had excellent results.

References

1. Frize M, Solven FG, Stevenson M, Nickerson BG, Buskard R, Taylor K. Computer-assisted decision support systems for patient management in an intensive care unit. In: *Proceedings of Medinfo*, 23–27 July, Vancouver, British Columbia, IMIA 1995; pp. 1009–1012.
2. Medical Dictionary of Medical Terms. Available from: http://www.medicalglossary. org/patient_care_perinatal_care_definitions.html [31 October 2005].
3. Richardson DK, Gray JE, McCormick MC, Workmann K, Goldmann DA. Score for neonatal acute physiology: a physiologic severity index for neonatal intensive care. *Pediatrics* 1993;91:617–623.
4. Knaus WA, Zimmerman JE, Wagner DP, Draper EA, Lawrence DE. APACHE—acute physiology and chronic health evaluation: a physiologically based classification system. *Crit Care Med* 1981;9:591–597.
5. Richardson DK, Corcoran JD, Escobar GJ, Lee SK, Canadian NICU Network, Kaiser Permanente neonatal minimum data set area network, et al. SNAP-II and SNAPPE-II: simplified newborn illness severity and mortality risk scores. *J Pediatr* 2001;138:92–100.
6. Lee SK, McMillan DD, Ohlsson A, Pendray M, Synnes A, Whyte R, et al. Variations in practice and outcomes in the Canadian NICU network: 1996–1997. *Pediatrics* 2000;106:1070–1079.
7. Meadow W, Lantos J. Ethics at the limit of viability: a premie's progress. *NeoReviews* 2003;4(6):e157–e162 [serial online].
8. Richardson DK, Tarnow-Mordi WO. Measuring illness severity in newborn intensive care. *J Intensive Care Med* 1994;9:20–33.
9. Castella X, Artigas A, Bion J, Kari A. A comparison of severity of illness scoring systems for intensive care unit patients: results of a multicenter, multinational study. *Crit Care Med* 1995;23(8):1327–1335.
10. Fery-Lemonnier E, Landais P, Loirat P, Kleinknecht D, Brivet F. Evaluation of severity scoring systems in ICUs—translation, conversion and definition ambiguities as a source

of inter-observer variability in APACHE II, SAPS and OSF. *Int Care Med* 1995;21:356–360.

11. LeGall J, JR, Lemeshow S, Leleu G , Klar J, Huillard J, Rui M, et al. Customized probability models for early severe sepsis in adult intensive care patients. *J Am Med Assoc* 1995;273(8):644–650.

12. Hyzg RC. ICU scoring and clinical decision making. [Edit.] *Chest* 1995;107(2): 1482–1483.

13. Gardner RM, Shabot MM. Computerized ICU data management: pitfalls and promises. *Int J. Clin Monitor Comput* 1990;7:99–105.

14. Dawood Y. The obstetric view of premature labor. In: Smith GF, Vidyasagar D, editors, *Historical review and recent advances in neonatal and perinatal medicine.* Mead Johnson; 1980. Available from: http://www.neonatology.org/classics/mj1980/ch10.html [31 October 2005].

15. Iams JD, Goldenberg RL, Merber BM, Moawad AH, Meis PJ, Das AF, et al. The preterm prediction study: can low-risk women destined for spontaneous preterm birth be identified? *Gen Obstetr Gynecol* 2001;184(4):652–655.

16. Allan N, Aylward D, Berry E, Bowie J, Brooks F, Burgoyne W, et al. *Preterm birth: making a difference.* Toronto, Canada: Best Start Resource Centre; 2002.

17. Goldenberg RL, Iams JD, Mercer BM, Meis PJ, Moawad AH, Coper RL, et al. The preterm prediction study: the value of new vs. standard risk factors in predicting early and all spontaneous births. *Am J Public Health* 1998;88(2):233–238.

18. Catley C, Frize M, Petriu DC. Predicting preterm birth using artificial neural networks. In: *Proceedings of IEEE Computer-Based Medical Systems,* 22–24 June 2005, Dublin, Ireland. pp. 103–108.

19. Frize M, Ibrahim D, Seker H, Walker RC, Odetayo MO, Petrovic D, et al. Predicting clinical outcomes for newborns using two artificial intelligence approaches. In: *Proceedings of IEEE Engineering in Medicine and Biology Society Conference,* vol. 2, 1–5 September 2004, San Francisco ,CA; pp. 3202–3205.

20. Alexian Brother's Medical Center. Life with baby: pregnancy and beyond. Available from: http://www.alexian.org/progserv/babies/thirdtri/apgarscore.html [31 October 2005].

21. Wyatt JS. Neonatal care: withholding or withdrawal of treatment in the newborn infant. *Bailliére Clin Obstetr Gynaecol* 1999;13(4):503–501.

22. Carter BS. Ethical issues in neonatal care. *E-Medicine* [online journal] 2003. Available from: http://www.emedicine.com/ped/topic2767.htm [31 October 2005].

23. Tyson J. Evidence-based ethics and the care of premature infants. [Online] *The future of children.* The David and Lucile Packard Foundation; 2003. Available from: www.futureofchildren.org/information2826/information_show.htm?doc_id=79897[31 October 2005].

24. Larcher V, Hird MF. Withholding and withdrawing neonatal intensive care. *CurrPaediatr* 2002;12:470–475.

25. Dwivedi AN, Bali RK, Naguib RNG. Organization current knowledge design (OCKD): a knowledge management framework for healthcare institutions. In: *Proceedings of the 25th Annual International Conference of the IEEE Engineering in Medicine and Biology Society;* 17–21 September 2003, Cancun, Mexico; pp. 1236–1239.

26. Health Canada. *Perinatal health indicators for Canada: a resource manual.* Minister of Public Works and Government Services Canada, 2000. Available from: http://www.phac-aspc.gc.ca/rhs-ssg/phic-ispc/ [October 31 2005].

27. Chien LY, Whyte R, Thiessen P, Walker R, Brabyn D, Lee SK, and the Canadian Neonatal Network. SNAP-II predicts severe intraventricular hemorrhage and chronic lung disease in the neonatal intensive care unit. *J Perinatol* 2002 Jan;22(1): 26–30.
28. Ambalavanan N, Carlo WA. Comparison of the prediction of extremely low birth weight neonatal mortality by regression analysis and by neural networks. *Early Hum Dev* 2001;65:123–137.
29. Walker RC, Frize M. Are artificial neural networks "ready to use" for decision-making in the NICU? *J Paediatr Res* 2004;56:6–8.
30. Tong Y, Frize M, Walker R. Extending ventilation duration estimations approach from adult to neonatal intensive care patients using artificial neural networks. *Trans Inf Technol Biomed* 2002;6(2):188–191.
31. Walker CR, Frize M. Clinical decision-making in the NICU: a computerized system to assist diagnosis and therapy. *Paediatr Child Health* 2000;5:29A.
32. Frize M, Ennett CM, Stevenson M, Trigg HCE. Clinical decision-support systems for intensive care units using artificial neural networks. *Med Eng Phys* 2001;23(3):217–225.
33. Ennett CM, Frize M. Selective sampling to overcome skewed a priori probabilities with neural networks. In: *Proceedings of American Medical Informatics Association Annual Symposium*, 4–8 November 2000, Los Angeles, CA; pp. 225–229.
34. Zernikow B, Holtmannspotter K, Michel E, Hornschuh F, Groote K, Hennecke KH. Predicting length-of-stay in preterm infants. *Eur J Pediatr* 1999;158:59–62.
35. Walker CR, Ennett CM, Frize M. Use of an artificial neural network to estimate probability of mortality and duration of ventilation in neonatal intensive care patients. In: Patel V, Rogers R, Haux R, editors, *MedInfo 01*, 2–5 September, London. Amsterdam: IOS Press, 2001(CD-Rom).
36. Sargent DJ. Comparison of artificial neural networks with other statistical approaches—results from medical data sets. *Cancer* 2001;91(8 Suppl S):1636–1642.
37. Livingstone DH, Manallack DT, Tetko IV. Data modelling with neural networks: advantages and limitations. *J Comput-Aided Mol Des* 1997;11:135–142.
38. Lisboa PJG. A review of evidence of health benefit from artificial neural networks in medical intervention. *Neural Networks* 2002;15:11–39.
39. Blum A. *Neural networks in C++*. New York: John Wiley, 1992.
40. The Mathworks Inc. *Mathworks (2004)*. Retrieved from: http://www.mathworks.com [5 May 2003].
41. Ennett CM, Frize M, Scales N. Logarithmic-sensitivity index as a stopping criterion for neural networks. In: *Proceedings of 24th Annual Conference of the Engineering in Medicine and Biology and the Annual Fall Meeting of the Biomedical Engineering Society*, 23–26 October 2002, Houston, TX; pp. 74–75.
42. Frize M, Wang L, Ennett CM, Nickerson BG, Solven FG, Stevenson M. New advances and validation of knowledge management tools for critical care using classifier techniques. In: *Proceedings of American Medical Informatics Association Annual Symposium*, 7–11 November1998, Orlando, FL; pp. 553–558.
43. Frize M, Ennett CM, Charette E. Automated optimization of the performance of artificial neural networks to estimate medical outcomes. In: *Proceedings of the 3rd ITAB Conference (Information Technology Applications in Biomedicine) and ITIS (International Telemedical Information Society)*, 9–10 November 2000, Arlington VA, pp. 168–173.

44. Ennett CM, Frize M, Charette E. Automated optimisation of neural networks performance. *Med Eng Phys* 2004;26:321–328.
45. Zernikow B, Holtmannspoetter K, Michel E, Pielemeier W, Hornschuh F, Westermann A, et al. Artificial neural network for risk assessment in preterm neonates. *Arch Dis Child Fetal Neonatal* 1998;79:F129–F134.
46. Shi Y. Development of a model for prediction of repeat injuries in injured children using artificial neural networks. ISS Master's thesis, Systems and Computer Engineering, Carleton University, Ottawa, Canada; 2004.
47. Frize M, Ennett CM, Hebert P. Improving the efficiency and effectiveness of artificial neural networks as decision-support systems. In: Patel V, Rogers R, Haux R, editors, *Medinfo*, September, London. Amsterdam: IOS Press; 2001 (CD-Rom).
48. Garson GD. Interpreting neural-network connection weights. *AI Expert* 1991;6(4): 46–51.
49. Goh TC. Back-propagation neural networks for modeling complex systems. *Artificial Intell Eng* 1995;9(3):143–151.
50. Rybchynski D. Design of an artificial neural network framework to enhance the development of clinical prediction models. MScE thesis, School of Information Technology and Engineering, University of Ottawa, Canada; 2005.
51. Manickam S, Abidi SSR. Extracting clinical cases from XML-based electronic patient records for use in Web-based medical case-based reasoning systems. In: Patel V, Rogers R, Haux R, editors, *Medinfo*; September, London. Amsterdam: IOS Press; 2001 (CD-Rom). Available from: http://www.cs.dal.ca/~sraza/papers/MEDINFO01_CBR.pdf [31 October 2005].
52. Morris B. Case-based reasoning, West Virginia University. *AI/ES Update* 1995;5(1).
53. Craw S. *Case-based reasoning for tablet formulation.* Available from: http://www. comp.rgu.ac.uk/staff/smc/papers/bpc01.pdf [October 31 2005].
54. Frize M, Walker R. Clinical decision support systems for intensive care units using case-based reasoning. *Med Eng Phys* 2000;22:671–677.
55. Ennett CM. Imputation of missing values by integrating artificial neural networks and case-based reasoning. PhD thesis, Systems and Computer Engineering, Carleton University, Ottawa, Canada; 2003.
56. Meis PJ, Goldenberg RL, Mercer BM, Iams JD, Moawad AH, Miodovnik M, et al. The preterm prediction study: Risk factors for indicated preterm births. *American Journal of Obstetrics and Gynecology* 1998;178(3):562–567.
57. Papile LA, Burstein J, Burstein R, Koffler H. Incidence and evolution of subependymal and intraventricular hemorrhage: a study of infants with birth weights less than 1,500 gm. *J Pediatr* 1978;92(4):529–534.
58. Ewing G, Freer Y, Logie R, Hunter J, McIntosh N, Rudkin S, et al. Role and experience determine decision support interface requirements in a neonatal intensive care environment. *J Biomed Inform* 2003;36(4–5):240–249.
59. Frize M, Yang L, Walker RC, O'Connor A. Conceptual framework of knowledge management for ethical decision-making support in neonatal intensive care. Trans Inf Technol Biomed 2005;9(2):205–215.
60. Turner M, Zhu F, Kotsiopoulus I, Russell M, Bennett K, Brereton P, et al. Using Web service technologies to create an information broker: an experience report. In: *Proceedings of the 26th International Conference on Software Engineering*, 23–28 May 2004, Edinburgh, Scotland; pp. 552–561.
61. Hoffman D. Marketing + MIS = e-service. *Commun ACM.* 2003;46:29–34.

62. Lea D, Vinoski S. Middleware for Web services. *IEEE Internet Comput* 2003;7:28–29.
63. Berners-Lee T, Hendler J, Lasilla O. The semantic Web. *Sci Am.* 2001; 34–43. Available from: http://www.sciam.com/article.cfm?articleID=00048144-10D2-1C70-84A9809EC588EF21 [31 October 2005].
64. Lee Y, Patel C, Chun SA, Geller J. Compositional knowledge management for medical services on semantic Web. In: *Proceedings of the 13th International World Wide Web Conference*, May 2004, New York, NY; pp. 498–499.
65. Kwon OB. Meta Web service: building Web-based open decision support system based on Web services. *Expert Syst Appl* 2003;24:375–389.
66. Catley C, Frize M, Petriu DC. (2005) Semantic Web services for healthcare. *Handbook of Research on Informatics in Healthcare and Biomedicine*. Idea Group Reference: Lazakidou A, In press (June 2005).
67. Turner M, Budgen D, Brereton P. Turning software into a service. *IEEE Comput* 2003;36:38–44.
68. Catley C, Petriu DC, Frize M. A UML framework for Web services-based clinical decision support. In: *Proceedings of the 14th International Conference on Intelligent and Adaptive Systems*, 20-22 July 2005, Toronto, Canada. pp. 174–179.

Biographies

Syed Sibte Raza Abidi holds a BEngg degree in electronic engineering from NED University of Engineering & Technology, Karachi, Pakistan, and an MSc degree in computer engineering from University of Miami, Florida, USA, secured in 1986 and 1989 respectively. He received a PhD degree in computing sciences from University of Surrey, UK, in 1994. He is currently an Associate Professor and Director of Health Informatics at the Faculty of Computer Science in Dalhousie University, Canada. He leads the NICHE (kNowledge management and Information Customization for Healthcare Enterprises) research group. His research interests include knowledge management, health informatics, information personalization, and data mining. He is involved in both government and industry-funded research projects. He currently holds research grants from the National Science and Engineering Research Council, Canadian Foundation for Innovation, Nova Scotia Health Research Foundation, Agfa Inc. Prior to his current appointment he worked in England and Malaysia, and his research projects were funded by the European Strategic Program for Research in Information Technology (ESPRIT), WHO, UN, the Malaysian Government's program on Intensified Research in Priority Areas, and various industry-funded projects. He has served as an invited reviewer for a number of health informatics and computer science journals, conferences, and research grants proposals. He has published over 100 peer-reviewed papers in peer-reviewed journals and conferences and has supervised around 30 graduate students. He is the recipient of the VHK International Award for Innovation in Medical Informatics (Hannover, 2000) for his work on the intelligent personalization of healthcare information. He has twice received the Best Paper Award in the "IT for Healthcare" track at the IEEE Hawaii International Conference on System Sciences (HICSS-38 and HICSS-39) in 2005 and 2006.

Rajeev K. Bali. Dr. Bali is currently a Reader at Coventry University, UK. He is the leader of the Knowledge Management for Healthcare research subgroup which works under the Biomedical Computing and Engineering Technologies (BIOCORE) Applied Research Group. He is an invited reviewer for several journals, conferences, and organizations. His primary research interests are in healthcare knowledge management, clinical governance, e-health, change management, organizational behavior, and medical informatics. He has recently published a text on Clinical Knowledge Management. Dr. Bali has served as an invited reviewer and associate editor for several journals, including the Transactions on Information Technology in Biomedicine, and was the Publications Chair for the IEEE–EMBS Information Technology Applications in Biomedicine (ITAB) conference 2003, held in Birmingham, UK. He was the invited Guest Editor for a special issue on "Advances in Clinical and Healthcare Knowledge Management" for the IEEE Transactions on Information Technology in Biomedicine (TITB) in 2005 and is the Associate Editor of the International Journal of Networking and Virtual Organisations. He was a member of the UK's National Knowledge Service's Heart Failure Knowledge Mobilisation Project Advisory Board. Past and current KM projects include ICTs and KM for organizational decision-making in healthcare organizations, KM to increase uptake of the NHS Breast Screening Programme, using KM to improve paramedic assessment and management of suspected AMIs and a Malaysian telemedicine implementation framework.

Cameron Barr acquired his Bachelor of Mechanical Engineering in 1999, from Carleton University in Ottawa, Canada. He has spent several years as a contract consulting engineer in the areas of impact biomechanics, injury research, and product development. His principle work is in the study of mild traumatic brain injury and associated numerical indicators, but has contributed to the study of ballistic treats and pediatric crash victim trauma. He has been a speaker at several injury biomechanics conferences and has been providing remote research support to the Application Service Provider group at ISPJAE in Cuba since April, 2005.

Caroline De Brún (née Papi) holds a BA in Business Studies gained from Buckinghamshire College: a college of Brunel University, in 1993. She also holds a Diploma and MA in Library and Information Studies gained from the University of North London in 1997 and 1998 respectively. Caroline is a chartered member of the Chartered Institute of Library and Information Professionals (CILIP). She commenced her career by working in academic libraries before moving into medical librarianship. Caroline is currently the Information Scientist for the NHS National Library for Health Knowledge Management Specialist Library. She is a member of the teaching staff on the University of Oxford Postgraduate Certificate in Evidence-Based Health Care course, and is a guest lecturer for Loughborough University. She has also served as an invited reviewer for Health Information and Libraries Journal and for the Health Research Board in Ireland. Caroline's primary research interests are knowledge management in healthcare settings, clinical decision support systems, and primary care information skills training.

Frada Burstein is an Associate Professor in the School of IT at Monash University in Melbourne, Australia. She holds a Masters of Sci (Applied Math) from Tbilisi State University from Georgia (1978), USSR, and PhD in Technical Cybernetics and Information Theory from the Soviet Academy of Sciences (1984). She has researched and taught in the areas of knowledge management and decision-support systems at Monash University since 1992. At Monash University she has established and leads a Knowledge Management Research Program, including an industry-sponsored virtual laboratory for studying modern technologies for supporting knowledge creation, storage, communication, and application. Her current research interests include knowledge management technologies, intelligent decision support, cognitive aspects of information systems development and use, organizational knowledge and memory, and systems development research. Professor Burstein has been a Chief Investigator for a number of many research projects supported by grants and scholarships from the Australian Research Council and industry. Professor Burstein has published extensively in academic journals and collections of papers. She is an Area Editor for the *Decision Support Systems* journal, a member of the Editorial Board of the *Journal of Information and Knowledge Management*, and Associate Editor for the *Journal of Decision Systems*, Associate Editor for the *International Journal of Knowledge Management*. Professor Burstein has also been a member of the Scientific, Program and Organizing committee or chaired many international workshops and conferences on decision-support systems and knowledge management. Professor Burstein is a member of the Executive Committee Member for the Australian Council of Professors & Heads of Information Systems, Membership Chair for the Association of Information Systems Special Interest Group in DSS, and a secretary for the IFIP WG 8.3 (DSS).

Christina Catley was born in Ottawa, ON, Canada in 1976. She received the BEng degree and MASc degree in computer systems engineering from Carleton University, Ottawa, ON, Canada, earned in 2000 and 2002 respectively. She is currently working towards the PhD degree in electrical engineering (biomedical engineering focus) at Carleton University. Her PhD dissertation relates to developing a novel Web services-based approach for integrating perinatal databases and clinical decision-support tools for the clinical outcome prediction. She has published 14 papers in peer-refereed journals and conference proceedings. Ms Catley is registered as an Engineer in Training with the Professional Engineers of Ontario, and is a student member of IEEE (Institute of Electrical and Electronics Engineers) and ACM (Association for Computer Machinery). During the course of her PhD, she has received a Natural Sciences and Engineering Research Scholarship, two Ontario Graduate Scholarships, and the Canadian Engineering Memorial Foundation Graduate Engineering Scholarship.

Rajneesh Chowdhury holds a BA in Sociology from the University of Delhi and an MA in Sociology from the Jawaharlal Nehru University, India, qualifying in 2000 and 2002 respectively. Following this, he joined the University of Hull and qualified with an MSc in Management Systems with Distinction in 2003. Rajneesh has previously worked on challenging research projects funded by the National Health Service, and has also conducted extensive research on the Indian Prime Minister's office. He is presently an Associate in the Knowledge Transfer

Partnership program between the University of Hull and the West Hull Primary Care Trust. Appointed to lead one of a select 20 projects under the Department of Health, Rajneesh is presently working on the design and implementation of a cardiac informatics protocol in Hull. He is also studying for a PhD in the University of Hull. His area of research interest is critical systems thinking, health informatics, and healthcare knowledge management. Rajneesh has published widely in peer-reviewed journals and has presented research papers extensively in regional, national, and international conferences. He also heads a multi-lingual medical informatics project for the West Hull Primary Care Trust. In 2004, he was nominated to the Department of Trade and Industry for the award of Business Leader of Tomorrow, for making an outstanding contribution to the field of health informatics.

Gouenou Coatrieux holds an engineer degree in electronics and industrial informatics from the École Nationale Supérieure des Sciences Appliquées et de Technologie, Lannion, France, and an MSc degree in signal, telecommunications, image, and radar from Rennes I University, France, both gained in 1999. He also holds a PhD in signal processing and telecommunications from the University of Rennes I, France, obtained in 2002. Dr. Coatrieux, is currently an assistant professor in the Image and Information Processing department, at the GET École Nationale Supérieure des Télécommunications de Bretagne, and is a member of the LaTIM, INSERM U650 laboratory. He is an invited reviewer for several conferences and journals, including the *IEEE Transactions on Information Technology in Biomedicine*. His primary research interests concern medical information systems security, watermarking, electronic patient record, and healthcare knowledge management.

Annette Copper holds a BSc (Hons) in sociology and an MSc in social science research methods, both gained from the University of Leicester, in 1996 and 1998 respectively. She is currently completing an MSc in knowledge organization and management at the University of Central England. She first worked in the voluntary sector, then at the University of Wolverhampton as a research administrator. She came to work at the NHS Modernisation in Leicester, initially as an information professional specializing in using the Internet as a resource tool and then as a knowledge resources manager deploying information and knowledge management tools and techniques across the organization to improve organizational culture and output. Her primary interests are knowledge management and learning organizations, and bridging policy, research, and decision making in healthcare management.

Antonio Miguel Cruz was born in Marianao, Ciudad Havana, Cuba, in July 1971. He holds a Nuclear Engineering degree and an MSc. in Bioengineering, both gained from the University of Nuclear Sciences and "José Antonio Echeverría" (ISPJAE) Technical University, Havana, Cuba, in 1995 and 1997 respectively. He also holds a PhD in Bioengineering from (ISPJAE) Technical University, Havana, Cuba, gained in 2003. He is currently a Senior Lecturer and Course Tutor in Clinical Engineering, Object Oriented Programming, Medical Informatics, and Advanced Maintenance subjects. He is the leader of the Computing Development for Clinical Engineering research group which works at Bioengineering Department (CEBIO). He was reviewer of the 8th and 9th World Multi-Conference on Systemics, Cybernetics and Informatics WMSCI 2004 and 2005, Miami, Florida. His primary research interests are in healthcare knowledge management, data mining, fuzzy logic, intelligent computational methods for planning, and medical informatics. He has more than 25 technical paper published. He is Member of the Cuban Bioengineering Society and the Caribbean Medical Association. He was student finalist in the 2000 World Congress on Physical Medics and Bioengineering competition, Chicago, USA. He received the Cuban Bioengineering Society Award in 1997 and 2005.

Alex Czerwinski holds a BSc degree in Information Technology from Staffordshire University in the UK, awarded in 1992. He commenced his career working for International Computers Ltd. (ICL) in Staffordshire, UK, initially working on client-server systems within both the utilities and media sectors, before moving onto Project Management of e-Business solutions for a number of 'blue chip' companies. In 2003 he joined the North West Midlands Cancer Network as a Service Improvement Facilitator involved in re-engineering secondary core processes. Alex currently works for Shropshire and Staffordshire Strategic Health Authority as the Choose and Book Programme Manager, tasked with the implementation of the CfH Booking and Choice Programme.

Ernesto Rodríguez Denis is Professor of Electronics Instrumentation and Electronics Measurement at "José Antonio Echeverría" (ISPJAE) Technical University, Havana, Cuba. He obtained his PhD in Measurements from the University of Prague. He is Coordinator of Bioengineering Center (CEBIO), ISPJAE, and a Member of the Cuban Bioengineering Society and Caribbean Medical Association and Clinical Engineering Council.

Ashish N. Dwivedi holds a BA in Management and a MBA with Distinction gained in 1993 and 1995 respectively. He also holds a MSc in IT for management and a Ph.D in healthcare knowledge management, both from Coventry University, UK, gained in 2000 and 2004 respectively. He has worked for several organizations including Sundaram Finance Ltd (SFL) at New Delhi, India and University College, Northampton, UK. Dr. Dwivedi is currently a Lecturer at the Business School, University of Hull. At Hull, Dr. Dwivedi is also associated with the management of the high-tech Management Learning Laboratory and is the programme leader for a newly created Masters in Knowledge Management (MSc in KM). His primary research interests are in knowledge management, organisational behaviour, healthcare management and information and communication technologies. Dr. Dwivedi has published his work in a number of academic journals including the IEEE Transactions on Information Technology in Biomedicine, Journal on Information Technology in Healthcare, OR Insight, International Journal of Healthcare

Technology and Management and International Journal of Electronic Healthcare. Dr. Dwivedi is a member of the editorial board of the International Journal of Networking and Virtual Organisations. Recently, he has also served as the Special Issue editor of the IEEE Transactions on Information Technology in Biomedicine.

Dr. Alan Eardley has a PhD in strategic IT management gained from Southampton University in 2000, an MSc in Computing Science from Aston University awarded in 1990 and a BA degree in Business from Staffordshire University awarded in 1984. Alan worked for 15 years in production and IT in the engineering and manufacturing sectors before becoming an academic at Staffordshire University in 1984. He developed and led undergraduate programmes in Business and IT for twelve years and was Leader of the IT for Strategic Management group and the Head of Information Systems Division. Alan's teaching and research interests are currently focused on the strategic use of IT and Knowledge Management in a variety of business sectors. He is currently Head of Postgraduate Research Studies in the Faculty of Computing, Engineering and Technology and where he teaches research methods and supervises postgraduate students in the above areas.

Gabby Fennessy holds a BA (South Australian Institute of Technology), an MSc (University of Wales) in information management, and a PhD in knowledge management in health care from Monash University gained in 2002. Gabby has had broad work experience in health services research, evaluation, and project management. In recent years Gabby has been working in the field of women's health and the continuing professional development for healthcare professionals. Gabby's prime areas of research interest are knowledge management, clinical effectiveness, professional competencies, and health policy related to professional development and workforce.

Schubert Foo is Professor and Vice Dean of the School of Communication & Information at Nanyang Technological University (NTU), Singapore. He received his B.Sc., M.B.A. and Ph.D. from the University of Strathclyde, UK. He is a Chartered Engineer, Chartered IT Professional, Fellow of the Institution of Mechanical Engineers and Fellow of the British Computer Society. He is a Board Member of the National Archives of Singapore and the National Library Board. Dr. Foo has over 140 publications in the research areas of multimedia technology, Internet technology, multilingual information retrieval and digital libraries. He is also a member of the Editorial Advisory Board of the Journal of Information Science and Journal of Information and Knowledge Management, among others.

Monique Frize holds a BASc degree in electrical engineering from the University of Ottawa (Canada, 1966), an MPhil in engineering in medicine from Imperial College of Science and Technology (UK, 1970), an MBA from Université de Moncton (Canada, 1986), and a Doctorate from Erasmus Universiteit in Rotterdam (The Netherlands, 1989). She was a biomedical engineer at Notre-Dame Hospital (Montreal) for 8 years, and Director of Regional Clinical Engineering Services in

Moncton, NB, for 10 years. Then Dr. Frize was appointed Professor in electrical engineering and Chairholder, Northern Telecom/NSERC Chair for women in engineering, University of New Brunswick (Fredericton, NB, 1989). In 1997, she was appointed to the NSERC/Nortel Chair for women in science and engineering in Ontario for 5 years; since 1997 she has been Professor, Systems and Computer Engineering at Carleton University and Professor, School of Information Technology and Engineering at University of Ottawa. She is the Leader of the Medical Information technologies Research Group (MIRG), a Visiting Professor at Coventry University, 2002–2007, and Affiliated Scientists at the Ottawa Hospital Research Institute (OHRI). Dr. Frize is on the Editorial Board of *Biomedical Engineering Online* (IEEE), a member of the Engineering & Physical Sciences Research Council (UK), a Senior Member of IEEE, a Fellow of the Canadian Academy of Engineering, and registered member of Professional Engineers Ontario. She was inducted as Officer of the Order of Canada in 1993. Dr. Frize's research interests are in the area of clinical decision-support systems, thermal medical imaging, and clinical engineering. She has published over 135 papers in peer-referred journals and conference proceedings.

Oliver Harding graduated in medicine from the University of Glasgow in 1990. He trained as a general practitioner before going into public health medicine, in which field he has worked as a consultant within the National Health Service in Scotland for the past 4 years. He is currently seconded to the Information Services Division of National Services Scotland, where his work has focused largely on the development of the new Scottish Public Health Observatory. His remit also includes exploring risk factors, inequalities, and systems thinking in health and healthcare.

Chu Keong Lee is currently Lecturer at the Division of Information Studies, School of Communication and Information, Nanyang Technological University of Singapore. He is a chemical engineer by training, and holds a bachelor's degree from National University of Singapore and a master's degree from Nanyang Technological University. He is also the Managing Editor of the Journal of Information and Knowledge Management. His current teaching assignments include graduate courses in the areas of knowledge management, business information services, and information sources and searching. His research areas are knowledge management, scientometrics and bibliomentrics.

Laurent Lecornu was born in Rennes in 1967. He holds an MSc in signal processing and telecommunications from the Rennes I University, France, gained in 1990. He also holds a PhD in signal processing and telecommunications from the same university, gained in 1995. Since 2002, Dr. Lecornu has been assistant professor in the Image and Information Processing department at the GET École Nationale Supérieure des Télécommunications de Bretagne, and is a member of the LATIM, INSERM U650. His primary research interests are image processing, image indexing, and medical databases data mining. Dr. Lecornu is an IEEE member.

Dr. Jay Liebowitz is Full Professor in the Graduate Division of Business and Management at Johns Hopkins University. He is the Program Director of the Graduate Certificate in Competitive Intelligence at Johns Hopkins University. He is Founder and Editor-in-Chief of *Expert Systems With Applications: An International Journal*, published by Elsevier. Previously, Dr. Liebowitz was the first Knowledge Management Officer at NASA Goddard Space Flight Center, the Robert W. Deutsch Distinguished Professor of Information Systems at the University of Maryland-Baltimore County, Chair of Artificial Intelligence at the U.S. Army War College, and Professor of Management Science at George Washington University. He has published over 30 books and over 200 articles dealing with expert/intelligent systems, knowledge management, and information technology management. His newest books are *Strategic Intelligence: Business Intelligence, Competitive Intelligence, and Knowledge Management* (Auerbach Publishing/Taylor & Francis, April 2006), *What They Didn't Tell You About Knowledge Management* (Scarecrow Press/Rowman & Littlefield, May 2006), *Communicating as IT Professionals* (Prentice Hall, 2006), and *Addressing the Human Capital Crisis in the Federal Government: A Knowledge Management Perspective* (Butterworth-Heinemann/Elsevier, 2004). He is the Founder and Chair of The World Congress on Expert Systems. Dr. Liebowitz was a Fulbright Scholar, the IEEE-USA Federal Communications Commission Executive Fellow, and the Computer Educator of the Year by the International Association for Computer Information Systems. He has consulted and lectured worldwide for numerous organizations, and he can be reached at jliebow1@jhu.edu.

Simon de Lusignan qualified in medicine at Barts in London, MB BS; and he also completed an integrated BSc in biochemistry. He subsequently completed GP training and obtained MRCGP. Simon has remained active as a GP, albeit part time. Simon also became a GP trainer and undergraduate tutor for students from St George's in southwest London. Simon has always been interested in IT; he developed his practice's IT in the late 1990s. He subsequently established an informatics research group at St George's. He also completed a Health Informatics MSc at Surrey University and then an MD thesis on the barriers to using IT in clinical practice. Simon is research active in biomedical informatics; he also heads the primary care informatics working group of EFMI (European Federation for Medical Informatics). His research is in four theme areas: using routinely collected clinical data for quality improvement, health service planning and research; how to use IT most effectively in the clinical consultation; knowledge management, especially the use of digital libraries; and eHealth.

Raouf Naguib is Professor of Biomedical Computing and Head of the Biomedical Computing Research Group (BIOCORE) at Coventry University. He has published over 200 journal and conference papers and reports in biomedical image processing and the applications of artificial intelligence and evolutionary computation in cancer research. He has also published a book on digital filtering, and co-edited a second book on the applications of artificial neural networks in cancer diagnosis, prognosis, and patient management, which is his main area of research interest. He was awarded the Fulbright Cancer Fellowship in 1995–96, when he carried out research in the USA, at the University of Hawaii in Mãnoa, on the applications of artificial neural networks in breast cancer diagnosis and prognosis. Professor Naguib is a member of several national and international research committees and boards, and has recently served on the Administrative Committee of the IEEE Engineering in Medicine and Biology Society (EMBS). He has also recently been selected to join the UK EPSRC Peer Review College and is a reviewer for the EU Directorate-General Information Society, eHealth. Professor Naguib has recently been appointed as Adjunct Research Professor at the University of Carleton, Ottawa, Canada.

Martha R. Ortiz Posadas holds a BSc degree in biomedical engineering from the Universidad Autónoma Metropolitana-Iztapalapa, Mexico in 1984; she has an MSc in systems, planning, and informatics from the Universidad Iberoamericana, Mexico, in 1990 and a PhD in Sciences from the Universidad Autónoma Metropolitana-Iztapalapa in 1999. She commenced her career by working in several medical equipment companies and in public hospitals doing medical technology management; then she moved to academia. Dr. Ortiz Posadas is currently a full time professor at the Electrical Engineering Department at Universidad Autónoma Metropolitana-Iztapalapa. Her primary research interests are in mathematical modeling of medical problems using the logical-combinatorial approach of pattern recognition theory, and clinical engineering related with medical technology management. She is member of the Medical Informatics research subgroup which works under the Biomedical Images and Signals Processing research group. She is also the leader of the Clinical Engineering research group. Dr. Ortiz Posadas has served as an invited reviewer for several international and national conferences and organizations and as a researcher. She has been recognized as a member of the Sistema Nacional de Investigadores (SNI). This distinction is offered by the Mexican government to the best researchers in their areas of interest.

John Puentes holds an electronics engineering degree gained from Simón Bolívar University, Caracas, Venezuela, in 1991, and an MSc in image processing and artificial intelligence gained from the École Nationale Supérieure des Télécommunications de Bretagne, France, in 1992. He also holds a PhD in signal processing and telecommunications from the Rennes I University, France, gained in 1996. After varied engineering, consultancy, and project management experience in biomedical and telecommunications multinational companies, he moved to the Image and Information Processing department at the GET École Nationale Supérieure des Télécommunications de Bretagne, where he is currently assistant professor and associate researcher of the French Institute of Health and Medical Research (LaTIM, INSERM U650). He is an invited associate editor and reviewer for several international journals, conferences, and organizations. His primary research interests are medical decision-support systems, knowledge-based systems, image indexing, and the application of multimedia emerging technologies to medical information processing. Dr. Puentes is an IEEE member.

Judas Robinson was born in Dundee. He studied pre-clinical medicine and Physiological Sciences at St John's College, Oxford, matriculating in 1989 and obtaining an honors degree in 1993. Judas went on to live abroad, and studied for a short period at the Albert-Ludwigs University, Freiburg, Germany. Here, he gained his first experience of Internet programming, an interest which he has pursued in the intervening years. After returning to England, Judas worked on the Primary Care National Electronic Library for Health, then part of the National Electronic Library for Health, based at St George's, University of London. Judas is now studying full time for a PhD at St George's and his research topic is the evaluation of healthcare digital libraries.

María Caridad Sanchez is Professor of Computer Sciences at "José Antonio Echeverría" (ISPJAE) Technical University, Havana, Cuba. She graduated in 1975 in Computer Sciences from ISPJAE. She obtained a Computer Sciences Master's degree in 1997 from ISPJAE. She is a Member of the Cuban Bioengineering Society and Caribbean Medical Association.

Ann Wales has worked within library services in the NHS in England and Scotland for many years, and is currently the Programme Director for Knowledge Management for NHS Education for Scotland.

Robin C. Walker was educated in the UK at King's School, Macclesfield, before receiving the degree MB, ChB in medicine in 1971 from the University of Manchester. His postgraduate work in pediatrics and neonatal–perinatal medicine was at Dalhousie University, Halifax, NS, and he received his FRCPC (Fellow of the Royal College of Physicians and Surgeons of Canada) in pediatrics in 1977, as well as subsequently the designation FAAP (Fellow of the American Academy of Pediatrics). Dr. Walker was Director of Perinatal Pediatrics at The Moncton Hospital, Moncton, NB, and Chief of Neonatology at Queen's University in Kingston, ON, before moving to Ottawa, where he is a Full Professor of Paediatrics at the University of Ottawa and Medical Director of Critical Care at the Children's Hospital of Eastern Ontario. His research as Co-Principal Investigator of the Medical Information Technology Research Group and as a member of the Steering Committee of the Canadian Neonatal Network is in decision-support systems using artificial intelligence tools in neonatal medicine, as well as evidence-based approaches to improving practice in neonatal intensive care. Dr. Walker has published over 160 peer-reviewed papers and conference abstracts, as well as having given over 140 invited presentations at regional, national, and international events. He is the immediate Past President of the Canadian Paediatric Society and Chair of the Committee on Pediatric Education of the American Academy of Pediatrics. He was awarded the Commemorative Medal for the Queen's Golden

Jubilee in recognition of ("his commitment to the right of all children to a healthy start in life"). The International Pediatric Association asked him to serve as a North American representative in its launch of a "Global Movement of Pediatricians for Newborn Health."

Nilmini Wickramasinghe (PhD, MBA, GradDipMgtSt, BSc. Amus.A (piano) Amus.A (violin)). Currently, Dr. Wickramasinghe researches and teaches in several areas within Information Systems, including knowledge management, e-commerce and m-commerce, and organizational impacts of technology. In addition, Dr. Wickramasinghe focuses on the impacts of technologies on the healthcare industry. She is well published in all these areas and regularly presents her work throughout North America, as well as in Europe and Australasia. Dr. Wickramasinghe is the US representative of the Health Care Technology Management Association (HCTM), an international organization that focuses on critical healthcare issues and the role of technology within the domain of healthcare. She is the associate director of the Center Management Medical Technologies (CMMT), a unique research think tank that focuses on groundbreaking issues in the healthcare domain and holds an associate professor position at the Stuart Graduate School of Business, IIT.

Zhichang Zhu's normal education stopped when he was sixteen, due to China's "Cultural Revolution." Without a first degree, he obtained an MSc in Information Management (1990) and a PhD in Management Systems and Sciences (1995) from the University of Hull, sponsored by British scholarships. Zhichang has been a Maoist Red Guard, farm laborer, shop assistant, lorry driver, corporate manager, assistant to the dean of a business school, software engineer, systems analyst, IS/IT and business consultant, in China, Singapore, Sri Lanka, and England. Zhichang is currently teaching corporate strategy for MBA programs at the University of Hull Business School (UK). He has also held visiting positions as research professor in Knowledge Management at the Japan Advanced Institute of Science and Technology (Ishikawa, Japan), research professor in International Business Management at the International East–West University (Honolulu and Los Angles, USA), research professor in Systems Management at the South China Normal University (Guangzhou, China), lecturing professor in Innovation and Entrepreneurship at the Friedrich Schiller University (Jena, Germany), external examiner for PhD theses for the Cape Town University (South Africa). Zhichang has delivered invited keynote speeches and guest lectures at international conferences, universities, and research institutes in China, Germany, Hong Kong, Indonesia, Ireland, Japan, the Gulf, and the US. Zhichang is an editor of the international journal *Systems Research and Behavioural Science*, an organizer of the comparative institutional research project sponsored by the Ford Foundation, the international Systems East & West project sponsored by the International Federation for Systems Research, the China–Japan–UK research project in systems methodologies sponsored by institutions of the three countries. Zhichang provides business consultancy for several

Chinese corporations in car-making, leather goods, and animal food industries, including for a Forbes 500 company. Zhichang has been researching and publishing in comparative management/systems studies, strategy/decision theory, information systems, and knowledge management, all from an institutional perspective, with over 60 articles published in refereed academic journals, edited books, and international conference proceedings.

Index

Accenture/NHS local IT service, 48, 49, 50, 51
access control list (ACL), 168
accreditation manual for hospitals
  environment of, 146
acute physiology and chronic health evaluation
  (APACHE), 235
Alberta Healthcare System, 124–127
  reformation in, 124
  regional health authorities in, 125
American Association of Otolaryngology, 123.
  See also cochlear implants
  and the National Health Service in Scotland,
  189
Application Service Provider (ASP), 142–145,
  149, 156
  design and development of, 149
    system description functions, 150
  features of, 149
    Web-based interface, 149
  for clinical engineering, 144–145
    stages in the development of, 145
    storage service provider model, 144
  installation and modules implementation of,
    156–158
  maintenance management, 143, 147, 152
    inspection and preventive, 152
  operational needs in, 145, 147, 149
  technology of, 143
    and healthcare environment, 143
arthroplasty, 99, 100
artificial intelligence, 7, 232, 234
artificial neural networks (ANN), 234, 240, 241
  and analyzing medical data, 241
  ANN system, 239, 248, 253
  estimation model, 241
  improving performance of, 241
  logarithmic-sensitivity index in, 241
  MATLAB software, 241

ASP information management goals, 145–147.
  See also Application Service Provider
ASP model, 147, 149–150, 155
  capital acquisition management feature of, 155
  inventory module in, 150
    inspection and preventive maintenance
      procedure, 152, 154
    institution directors, 157
    nurses and medical staff, 157
    user types of, 157
    universal medical device nomenclature
      system, 151

biomedical knowledge, 4, 8, 20
business intelligence, 90, 92, 98
  business-like healthcare, 125, 126
  infrastructure, 90, 92, 98
  knowledge-gathering/analyzing tools, 92

Canadian Council on Health Services
  Accreditation (CCHSA), 146
Canadian Neonatal Network (CNN) database,
  236, 254
capital acquisition management, 155, 157
Care Pathways Database, 186, 210. *See also*
  England
case-based image retrieval (CBIR), 172
case-based reasoning (CBR) system, 172, 242
  and CBR R4 Cycle, 242
  CBR–ANN system, 248
cerebral palsy (CP), 248
Clark–Nucleus, 122, 123
clinical care
  and knowledge management, 232, 233
  clinical data, access to, 234
  clinical decision support (CDS) system
    development, 251
  differential diagnosis in, 232

Health Informatics Series
(formerly Computers in Health Care)

(continued from page ii)

Printed in the United States
104772LV00003B/25-48/A

9 780387 335407